Orthotic Design and Fabrication for the Upper Extremity

A PRACTICAL GUIDE

Orthotic Design and Fabrication for the Upper Extremity
A PRACTICAL GUIDE

Katherine Schofield, DHS, OTR/L, CHT
Assistant Program Director and Associate Professor
Department of Occupational Therapy
Midwestern University
Glendale, Arizona

Deborah Schwartz, OTD, OTR/L, CHT
Product and Educational Specialist
Physical Rehabilitation
Orfit Industries
Antwerp, Belgium
Adjunct Professor
Department of Occupational Therapy
Touro University
New York, New York

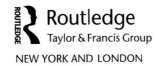

Routledge
Taylor & Francis Group

NEW YORK AND LONDON

Cover Artist: Katherine Christie

First published in 2019 by SLACK Incorporated

Published 2024 by Routledge
605 Third Avenue, New York, NY 10158

and by Routledge
4 Park Square, Milton Park, Abingdon, Oxon OX14 4RN

Routledge is an imprint of the Taylor & Francis Group, an informa business

© 2019 Taylor & Francis Group

Dr. Katherine Schofield has no financial or proprietary interest in the materials presented herein.
Dr. Deborah Schwartz is a full-time employee of Orfit Industries America, a manufacturer of thermoplastic materials.

Library of Congress Cataloging-in-Publication Data

Names: Schofield, Katherine (Katherine A.), author. | Schwartz, Deborah
   (Deborah A.), author.
Title: Orthotic design and fabrication for the upper extremity : a practical
   guide / Katherine Schofield, Deborah Schwartz.
Description: Thorofare, NJ : Slack Incorporated, 2019. | Includes
   bibliographical references and index.
Identifiers: LCCN 2019007687 (print) | ISBN 9781630915902 (hardcover : alk. paper)
Subjects: | MESH: Orthotic Devices | Upper Extremity | Equipment Design
Classification: LCC RD557 (print) | NLM WE 26 | DDC 617.5/7--dc23
LC record available at https://lccn.loc.gov/2019007687

ISBN: 9781630915902 (pbk)
ISBN: 9781003525509 (ebk)

DOI: 10.4324/9781003525509

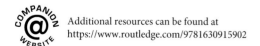

Additional resources can be found at
https://www.routledge.com/9781630915902

Dedication

I dedicate this book to those in my life who encouraged me along the way. This includes my husband, Dale; my sons, Austin and Andrew; my mom, Gretchen; and my sister, Lisa. Thank you for having faith in me.
—*Katherine Schofield*

I inherited my love of writing from my father, Bernard Shuman. My brother, Ellis, shares this passion as does my husband, Barry. I dedicate this book to Barry, who encourages and inspires me everyday, and to my children, Nadav, Talia, and Noam, who have offered me multiple opportunities to practice orthotic fabrication.
—*Deborah Schwartz*

Contents

Acknowledgments

I am so grateful that Deb agreed to work with me on this endeavor. I found a knowledgeable, passionate individual who loves teaching and making orthoses as much as I do! Thank you, Deb, for all of your support, perseverance, tenacity, friendship, encouragement, constructive feedback, and hard work. This would not have been possible without you!

Thank you Brien Cummings and the wonderful staff at SLACK Incorporated for supporting us through to the end of this long journey.

Thank you to my colleagues and mentors at Midwestern University in Glendale, Arizona, for their unending encouragement. I am blessed to have the opportunity to teach and inspire my occupational therapy students on a regular basis, and I am eternally grateful for their ongoing support and excitement about this project as it progressed. A special thank you to Jack Mullins and Jason Tinsley for their expertise and patience with video production; Dr. Chris Merchant for her support and encouragement; and Dr. Tana Brown for her suggestion that I needed a "project" to work on.

I also wish to express my gratitude and appreciation for my occupational therapy students: Allie Cammarata for her hard work and tireless attitude drawing all of our custom illustrations; Callie Surridge for having her camera ready for our photos; Carson Lund for his suggestions and help during our video shoot; and Brianne Van Buren and Cassie Durfee for their time and willingness to assist with our videos and photos.

—*Katherine Schofield*

Thank you to my wonderful writing partner and colleague, Katherine, for inviting me to join you on this creative journey.

Thank you to SLACK Incorporated and Brien Cummings for picking up the ball with this project.

Thank you to Orfit Industries for donating thermoplastic materials for our orthotic fabrication videos and for use of photos.

—*Deborah Schwartz*

About the Authors

Katherine Schofield, DHS, OTR/L, CHT is an Associate Professor and Assistant Program Director for Midwestern University's Occupational Therapy Program in Glendale, Arizona. She received her Bachelor of Science degree in Occupational Therapy in 1988 at the University of Alberta in Canada, her certification in hand therapy in 1993, as well as a Masters in Health Science degree in 2009 and a Doctorate in Health Science degree in 2012, both from the University of Indianapolis. Since beginning her career in 1988, Dr. Schofield has worked in physical rehabilitation, acute care, and outpatient upper extremity orthopedics. Dr. Schofield has more than 30 years of experience as a practicing clinician. She has presented at numerous local, state, national, and international conferences and postgraduate educational venues on various topics pertaining to upper extremity rehabilitation. She has publications in peer-reviewed journals on anatomy content and teaching pedagogy for occupational therapy students and orthotic instructional strategies. Dr. Schofield began her career at Midwestern University in 2000 as an adjunct professor while concurrently managing an outpatient hand therapy clinic. She has been a full-time professor since 2007. She is currently a member of the American Society of Hand Therapists, the American Occupational Therapy Association, the Arizona Occupational Therapy Association, and a past member of the American Association of Hand Surgeons.

Deborah Schwartz, OTD, OTR/L, CHT is a hand therapist with over 34 years of experience as a practicing clinician. She works with Orfit Industries America to promote product awareness and splinting education. Debby is an active member of American Society of Hand Therapists and has participated in International Federation of Societies for Hand Therapy meetings as well. She has presented on a variety of hand therapy topics both at national and international conferences and has written a number of articles for hand therapy publications, including the *British Journal of Hand Therapy, ADVANCE for OT*, www.exploringhandtherapy.com, and several research studies for the *Journal of Hand Therapy*. Debby regularly conducts splinting workshops for beginner, intermediate, and advanced splinting as well as introductory classes for occupational therapy students in university programs. Debby completed her doctoral studies in Occupational Therapy at Rocky Mountain University of Health Professions in Provo, Utah. She is currently writing several book chapters for hand therapy references.

Preface

Orthotic design and fabrication is a specialized skill that is often referred to as both an art and a science. It is regarded as a highly specialized and complex task that involves application of specific psychomotor skills, along with critical thinking and clinical reasoning abilities. The occupational therapist, occupational therapy assistant, physical therapist, or orthotist must apply knowledge of anatomy, biomechanics, and physiology and synthesize all of these topics with an understanding of the characteristics of low-temperature thermoplastic materials in order to create a suitable and therapeutic orthosis. The ability to form a moldable piece of thermoplastic material around the pertinent body part demands background knowledge, a sense of artistry, and a client-centered focus. The rehabilitation practitioner must also be able to articulate the purpose and intent of the orthosis to the client because the outcome of orthotic intervention requires the client to accept and be able to use the finished product as prescribed. Collectively, this is quite an undertaking for a student or entry-level therapist to tackle!

Orthotic Design and Fabrication for the Upper Extremity: A Practical Guide is designed for occupational and physical therapy students, entry-level practitioners, and practitioners who wish to acquire core knowledge of orthotic utilization in practice and/or improve their orthotic fabrication skills. Its emphasis is on providing students and therapists with the necessary knowledge to design common immobilization orthoses used in current practice, along with detailed step-by-step instructions on design and fabrication in a digital video format.

This textbook, with the accompanying digital instructional videos, allows students and new practitioners to actively engage with the materials in the classroom, clinic, or hospital environment. The digital videos outline the steps of making a particular orthosis and can be viewed multiple times on a tablet, laptop computer, smart phone, or watch. The written component provides a foundation for understanding the pertinent anatomical and biomechanical principles of common orthoses in practice.

These 11 chapters complete a comprehensive orthotics course, or they can be incorporated into other courses (along with rehabilitation, biomechanical, physical dysfunction, and/or orthopedic content). The first three chapters cover foundational knowledge critical to orthotic design and fabrication: anatomy, biomechanical principles, orthotic concepts, and low-temperature thermoplastic material characteristics. Each of the following eight chapters highlights common upper extremity orthoses. Students can easily access a particular orthosis and gather all of the necessary information about it. Educators can assign specific orthoses by chapter as time permits.

SPECIAL FEATURES

This textbook includes special features designed to provide students with methods to enhance their understanding of the content and apply this to practice. *Orthotic Design and Fabrication for the Upper Extremity: A Practical Guide* offers the following:

- **Key Terms:** An alphabetical list of key terms appears at the beginning of each chapter. These terms are in bold-faced print the first time they appear in the text. A full definition is located in the Glossary at the back of the book.
- **Helpful Hints:** This feature provides students with practical information that they can apply when learning about a particular orthosis.
- **Multiple-Choice Questions:** Review questions located at the end of Chapters 3 through 11 allow students to test their knowledge of a particular orthosis. Answers are found at the end of each respective chapter.
- **Evidence:** Key articles from the current evidence are highlighted to support the use of the orthosis in clinical practice.
- **Case Studies:** Two case studies located at the end of Chapters 4 through 11 allow students to apply and clinically reason through orthotic concepts and apply these to clinical practice.
- **Orthosis Assignments/Learning Activities:** A variety of activities/assignments located at the end of Chapters 4 through 11 allow students the opportunity to experience wearing an orthosis for a period of time, assess effectiveness, and evaluate fit and appearance of their completed orthoses.
- **Instructional Videos:** Links to detailed instructional videos are included in each chapter (except Chapter 2), outlining the specific steps necessary to fabricate the highlighted orthoses. Many chapters offer multiple variations of each orthosis. The videos are broken down so that students can master each segment and watch multiple times as needed.

Current and future occupational therapy, occupational therapy assistant, and physical therapy students must be competent in their ability to design and fabricate common orthoses used in clinical practice. It is our hope that this textbook and the accompanying instructional videos will provide readers with a user-friendly, fun, and clear resource that will help in the development of orthotic design and fabrication skills.

Part One

FOUNDATIONS OF ORTHOTIC DESIGN

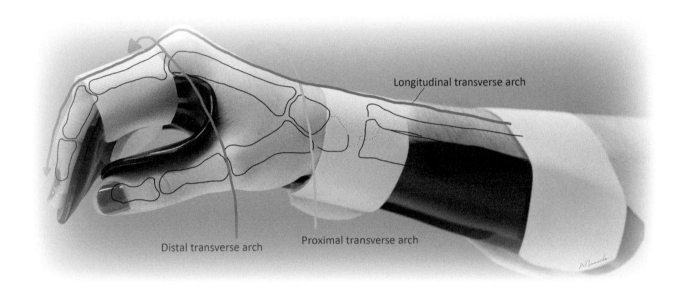

Longitudinal transverse arch

Distal transverse arch

Proximal transverse arch

CHAPTER 1

Orthotic Fabrication
Principles and Practice

Key Terms

Dorsal	Mobilization orthosis	Serial static
Dynamic orthoses	Orthosis	Static
Health Care Common Procedural Coding System codes (HCPCS codes)	Orthoses	Static progressive
	Orthotic fabrication	Ulnar
Immobilization orthosis	Orthotic intervention	Volar
L-codes	Radial	

Learning Outcomes

Upon completion of this chapter, you will be able to:

1. Define the terms *orthosis*, *orthoses*, and *orthotic*.

2. Identify the common purposes of orthotic intervention for the upper extremity.

3. Describe the different orthotic designs: static/immobilization, serial static, dynamic (mobilization), and static progressive (mobilization).

4. Explain the key elements of effective documentation and reimbursement associated with orthotic intervention.

5. Explain evidence-based practice and orthotic intervention.

6. List the common precautions and contraindications associated with orthotic intervention.

7. Describe the key elements associated with determining orthotic wearing schedules and client education.

Introduction

An **orthosis** is an external rigid or semi-rigid device that is used to support, align, prevent or correct deformity, improve function, or restrict movement of a part of the body following injury, disease, or surgical intervention. **Orthoses** is the correct term for more than one orthosis. The term *orthotic* is used as an adjective to describe the process of orthoses in rehabilitation: **orthotic intervention** refers to use of an orthosis as an intervention strategy; **orthotic fabrication** refers to the process, or science, of creating an orthosis. A practitioner would consider an orthotic intervention for a client to serve one or more of many possible purposes (Box 1-1).

Schofield, K., & Schwartz, D. *Orthotic Design and Fabrication for the Upper Extremity: A Practical Guide* (pp 3-14). © 2019 Taylor & Francis Group.

Box 1-1. Purposes of Orthotic Intervention

PREVENT

- Maintain tissue length to prevent contractures
- Prevent joint positions that cause compression of nerves, skin, and other soft tissues

PROTECT

- Protect a healing fracture
- Protect a repaired tendon, ligament, or other structure to promote optimal healing

IMPROVE FUNCTION

- Assist and support weak muscles
- Block or transfer power to enhance exercise and joint/soft tissue motion
- Improve joint alignment and stability
- Provide symptom relief (pain/swelling) after an injury or surgery
- Substitute for weak or paralyzed muscles

CORRECT

- Improve joint alignment
- Reduce joint stiffness and/or soft tissue tightness
- Remodel scar tissue

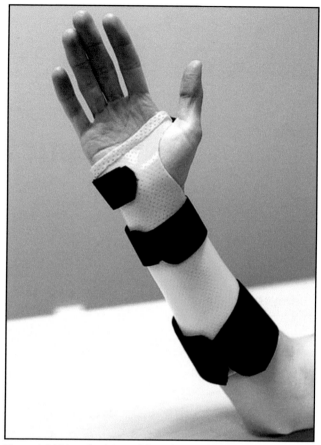

Figure 1-1. This orthosis immobilizes the wrist but allows for full finger and thumb movement.

A variety of allied health care professionals are qualified to fabricate and provide custom orthoses. Orthotic design and fabrication are integral components of an occupational therapist's and occupational therapy assistant's scope of practice. Physical therapists specializing in upper extremity (UE) rehabilitation often provide orthotic services, as well as certified orthotists whose education and training specializes in the fabrication and fit of orthoses.

Orthotic fabrication is often referred to as both an art and a science. The *science* of orthotic design and fabrication requires knowledge of the principles of anatomy, biomechanics, and wound healing; of disease, injury, and treatment protocols following surgical intervention; and of the psychosocial aspects of injury and disease. The practitioner must have the ability to address the individual client's biological/physical goals and needs of an orthosis to optimize the function of musculoskeletal and/or neuromuscular structures and make every effort to make the orthosis align with his or her goals and lifestyle needs. The *artistry* of orthotic design and fabrication involves creating the pattern for a particular orthosis and then synthesizing this with an understanding of the characteristics of low-temperature thermoplastic materials to create a suitable orthosis. The practitioner must use knowledge of proper strapping techniques, possess appropriate hands-on fabrication skills, and consider the overall aesthetic appearance of the finished product. Forming a moldable piece of material around the pertinent body part demands artistry and a client-centered focus because the outcome of orthotic intervention requires the client to accept and be able to use the finished product as prescribed. In summary, skillful orthotic design and fabrication by the practitioner yields an end product that (1) meets the clinical and functional needs of the client, (2) is professional in appearance and design, (3) is of value to the client in the treatment of the condition, (4) is aesthetically pleasing to the client, and (5) is cost effective.

Orthotic Designs

The overall purpose of a given orthosis will determine its design. In general, orthoses used in occupational therapy or physical therapy practice can be grouped into two categories: orthoses that *immobilize* body structures, and orthoses that *mobilize* a joint, muscle, or soft tissue. **Immobilization orthoses**, also known as *static orthoses*, have no moveable parts and are used to immobilize a

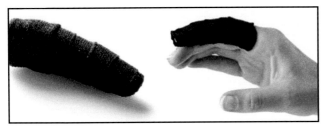

Figure 1-2. This serial static proximal interphalangeal extension orthosis positions the proximal interphalangeal joint in maximum extension and is remolded on a regular basis as joint motion improves. (Reprinted with permission from Orfit Industries.)

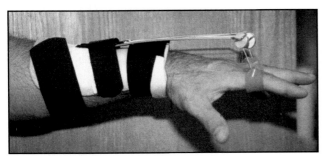

Figure 1-3. Muscles innervated by the radial nerve may become paralyzed or weak following injury to the radial nerve. This dynamic metacarpophalangeal extension mobilization orthosis helps to support these muscles and facilitates grasp and release hand function.

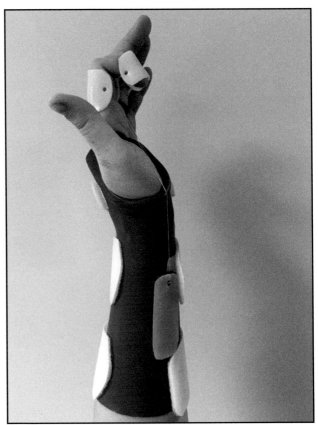

Figure 1-4. This static progressive composite digit flexion mobilization orthosis applies mobilization force to the metacarpophalangeal, proximal interphalangeal, and distal interphalangeal joints to improve digit flexion.

body part, prevent movement, encourage rest of injured structures, and provide support (Figure 1-1). **Mobilization orthoses** typically have additional adjustable parts called *outriggers*, such as turnbuckles, hinges, or others, and are designed to apply low load stress to contracted, stiff tissues to improve joint and tissue movement or to facilitate UE function by substituting for weak or paralyzed muscles (Figures 1-2 through 1-4). These are further categorized by the specific type: **static**, **serial static**, **dynamic**, and **static progressive** (Table 1-1).

Orthotic Intervention Terminology

The practitioner must consider descriptive terminology that is used to help accurately describe an orthosis provided to a client. This helps to clarify the orthosis being requested by the referral source, optimize understanding of the purpose and intent of the orthosis, assist with billing and reimbursement, and ensure accurate and complete documentation. The descriptive terms contained in Boxes 1-2 and 1-3 are commonly used by hand surgeons and practitioners and are based on the anatomical location and body segment included in the orthosis. The authors use this terminology consistently throughout this textbook to describe the type of orthoses.

Reimbursement and Documentation

In addition to the descriptive terms associated with orthotic provision, it is imperative for the practitioner to be aware of other factors that influence billing and reimbursement for orthoses provided to clients, specifically terms used to code and bill for the type of orthosis provided. In the United States, these include **HCPCS codes** and **L-codes** (see description following), as well as knowledge of the insurance contracts associated with the practice setting where service is provided (which L-codes are covered and at what rate). In addition, accurate and complete documentation of orthotic intervention(s) provided is essential to optimize reimbursement for services.

HCPCS CODES AND L-CODES

An HCPCS code, part of the Level II **Health Care Common Procedural Coding System**, is a five-character alphanumeric code. The first character is a letter that describes the type of service billed, and the other four numeric characters describe the specific type of service

Table 1-1

CATEGORIES OF ORTHOSES

IMMOBILIZATION ORTHOSES	MOBILIZATION ORTHOSES
Static: An orthosis without an outrigger or moveable components (see Figure 1-1).	Serial Static: Orthosis that holds a body part in its end range position to regain passive joint motion. It is periodically remolded to accommodate changes in joint position. This serial static orthosis is designed to improve PIP joint extension range of motion (see Figure 1-2).
	Dynamic: Orthosis that incorporates outriggers with variable tension such as springs, coils, or elastic components to assist in function or place force on stiff joints or soft tissue. This dynamic orthosis is designed to support the wrist and MCP joints in a functional position to improve hand function following injury to the radial nerve and paralysis of the wrist and digit extensor muscles (extensor carpi radialis longus, extensor carpi radialis brevis, extensor carpi ulnaris, and extensor digitorum; see Figure 1-3).
	Static Progressive: Orthosis that incorporates an outrigger with constant tension designed to progressively reposition a stiff joint in its maximum tolerable end range position. This static progressive orthosis is designed to apply a low load, constant force to the digit to improve flexion of the MCP, PIP, and DIP joints (see Figure 1-4).

Abbreviations: DIP, distal interphalangeal; MCP, metacarpophalangeal; PIP, proximal interphalangeal.

Box 1-2. Anatomical Location Terminology

Volar, anterior, or palmar	The front part of the body segment in anatomical position
Dorsal or posterior	The back part of the body segment in anatomical position
Radial	The same side as the thumb and radius
Ulnar	The same side as the fifth digit and ulna
Circumferential	Covers both the front and back of the body segment
Arm	The area between the shoulder and elbow
Forearm	The area between the elbow and wrist
Wrist	The area that includes the carpal bones, distal radius, and ulna
Hand	The area from the wrist to the fingertips
Fingers or digits	The area from the metacarpophalangeal joints to the tips of the fingers
Digits I to V	I = thumb, II = index finger, III = long or middle finger, IV = ring finger, V = small finger

provided (Box 1-4). L-codes are part of the HCPCS and are used to report and bill for fabrication and fitting of specific orthoses for the UE. Introduced by the U.S. Centers for Medicare & Medicaid Services, and revised in 2006 in conjunction with the American Society of Hand Therapists, these codes accurately describe common UE orthoses provided by occupational therapists and physical therapists. These codes collectively represent the evaluation, cost of materials, fabrication time, fitting, and adjustments required when making and fitting an orthosis for a client. Many private insurance carriers also follow these guidelines, but not all codes are accepted by all payers, including Medicare. When billing for an orthosis, the practitioner must select the most appropriate L-code and anatomical

Box 1-3. Orthoses Descriptors

Digit based	Orthosis includes one or more joints distal to the metacarpophalangeal joints (Figure 1-5).
Hand based	Orthosis includes one or more joints distal to the wrist (Figure 1-6).
Forearm based	Orthosis includes one or more joints distal to the elbow (Figure 1-7).
Arm based	Orthosis includes one or more joints distal to the shoulder (Figure 1-8).
Thumb based	Orthosis includes one or more joints of the thumb; may or may not include the wrist (Figure 1-9).
Dorsal based	Orthosis is located on the dorsal or posterior aspect of the body segment (Figure 1-10).
Volar based	Orthosis is located on the volar or anterior aspect of the body segment (Figure 1-11).
Ulnar gutter	Orthosis is on the ulnar aspect of the body segment (same side as ulna; Figure 1-12).
Radial gutter	Orthosis is on the radial aspect of the body segment (same side as radius; Figure 1-13).

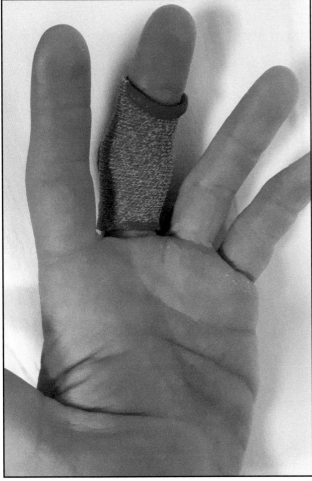

Figure 1-5. Digit-based orthosis. (Reprinted with permission from Anna Ovsyannikova.)

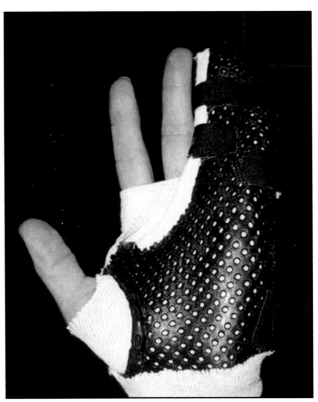

Figure 1-6. Hand-based orthosis.

heading that accurately describes the orthosis provided: S = shoulder, E = elbow, W = wrist, H = hand, F = finger, O = orthosis. Refer to Box 1-4 for L-codes and anatomical headings for common UE immobilization orthoses and anatomical headings.

DOCUMENTATION

Thorough documentation of orthotic services provided to a client is essential. It serves as a communication tool between the practitioner and third-party payers to optimize reimbursement, and it reinforces the medical necessity and efficacy of orthotic intervention. It is a means to communicate with other health care providers involved in a particular client's care. It is also a means to communicate directly with the client to optimize understanding of the purpose, care, and use of the orthosis provided. The practitioner must include a description of the orthosis and its purpose,

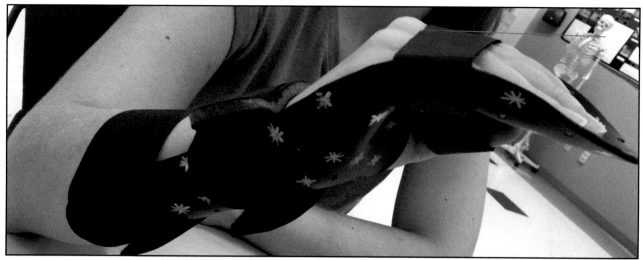

Figure 1-7. Forearm-based orthosis.

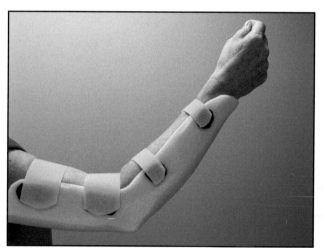

Figure 1-8. Arm-based orthosis.

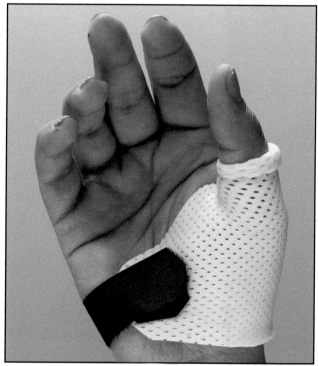

Figure 1-9. Thumb-based orthosis.

an outline of the recommended wearing schedule, and client instructions regarding care and use of the orthosis. A photograph of the completed orthosis on the client is also important to include in the record, along with a statement indicating that the client understands the orthosis purpose and how to don and doff the orthosis correctly. See the Appendix at the end of the chapter for an example of a handout to provide a client that includes these components.

Evidence-Based Practice and Orthotic Intervention

Evidence-based practice (EBP) is a critical element of effective health care delivery, including orthotic intervention, and helps the practitioner in his or her decision making when selecting the suitable orthosis for a client's situation.

EBP is a thoughtful, systematic approach that considers the practitioner's clinical experience, best available research evidence, and client goals and values when making clinical decisions about a client's care (Brown, 2017).

Integral to the process of using EBP is the practitioner's ability to critically appraise the quality of current available evidence based on study design. There are five levels of evidence that are commonly used to appraise current research, based on the Oxford Center for Evidence-Based Medicine (Box 1-5).

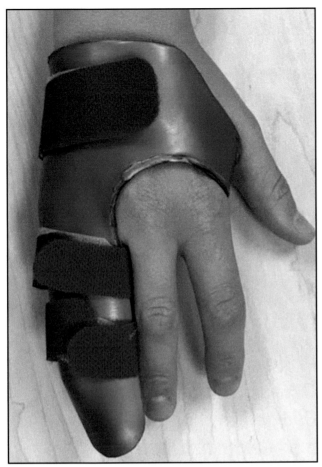

Figure 1-10. Dorsal-based orthosis.

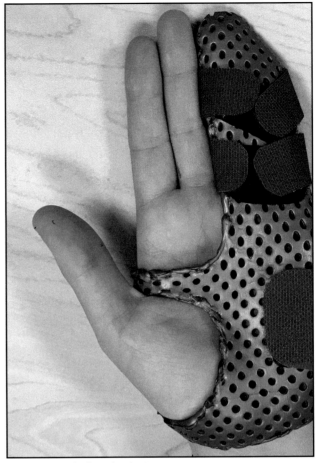

Figure 1-11. Volar-based orthosis.

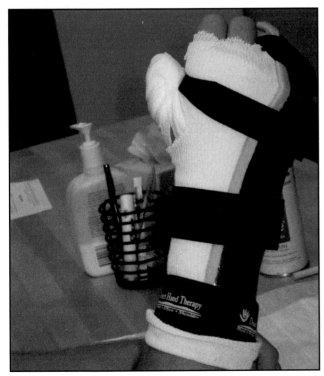

Figure 1-12. Ulnar gutter orthosis.

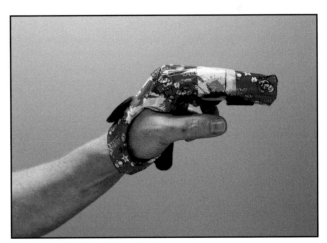

Figure 1-13. Radial gutter orthosis

Box 1-4. Codes and Anatomical Headings for Common UE Immobilization Orthoses

L3702 EO	Elbow Orthosis, custom fabricated without joints
L3763 EWHO	Elbow Wrist Hand Orthosis, custom fabricated without joints
L3808 WHFO	Wrist Hand Finger Orthosis, custom fabricated without joints
L3906 WHO	Wrist Hand Orthosis, custom fabricated without joints
L3913 HFO	Hand Finger Orthosis, custom fabricated without joints
L3933 FO	Finger Orthosis, custom fabricated without joints

This information was current at the time of publication. It is the practitioner's responsibility to work directly with his or her local insurance carriers to determine which L-codes are covered and keep abreast of changes in coverage and guidelines set forth by the U.S. Centers for Medicare & Medicaid Services.

Box 1-5. Levels of Evidence

Level I	Systematic review of randomized trials
Level II	Randomized trial
Level III	Nonrandomized controlled cohort/ follow-up study
Level IV	Case series, case-control study, or historically controlled study
Level V	Mechanism-based reasoning

It is the practitioner's responsibility to stay informed of the most current and high-level evidence in the literature to support the use of orthoses when choosing this as an intervention strategy. The decision to use an orthosis for a client must take into account this evidence, the practitioner's level of experience, and the needs and values of the client. Moreover, when designing an orthosis, the practitioner must consider the client's daily activities, roles, and routines as carefully as possible. Even the best designed orthosis that is supported with high levels of evidence will collect dust in a drawer or end up in the trash if it is deemed uncomfortable or unsuitable by the client or if he or she does not understand its value, benefit, or purpose. Students and practitioners should access and review current literature often to stay abreast of the evidence available. Some useful databases to access research include PubMed, Medline (OVID), Cumulative Index of Nursing and Allied Health Literature (CINAHL), OT Search, Cochrane Database of Systematic Reviews, OTSeeker, Google Scholar, Pedro (Physiotherapy Evidence Database), and EBSCOhost.

Disclaimer: All of the evidence presented in this textbook is current as of the date of writing. The authors have done their best to review and research the most up-to-date databases in an effort to present the best research and literature to support the therapeutic interventions for each population. They likewise advise each reader to do independent literature searches for the most up-to-date research as it relates to orthotic interventions.

Principles of Effective Orthotic Intervention: Education, Precautions, and Orthotic Design

It is very important for the practitioner to consider the client's needs and goals when choosing an orthosis as an intervention strategy. Educating the client on the purpose of his or her orthosis, the prescribed wearing schedule, how to care for it, donning and doffing, and specific instructions on what to do if he or she experiences problems is critical to optimize outcomes and compliance. The practitioner must also be aware of any preexisting conditions, or comorbidities, that the client may present with that would affect use of an orthosis. Finally, being client centered, or matching the orthosis to the client's needs and personal preferences, is an important consideration to optimize the effectiveness of an orthosis.

CLIENT EDUCATION

Educating the client is a vital component of orthotic intervention. A client who does not understand the purpose and care of his or her orthosis will, at best, not derive any benefit from it. Alternatively, a client who lacks full understanding of the need to use his or her orthosis as prescribed may cause undo harm. No practitioner wants to receive a phone call from a referring physician informing him or her that the client's condition has been adversely affected by incorrect use of the orthosis.

Components of client education include the following:

- Name or description of the orthosis
- Education on the client's condition
- Education on reasons of orthosis intervention
- Detailed wearing schedule (all night, day and night, removal for hygiene only)
- List of precautions for the client to be aware of: skin redness, pressure areas, discomfort in the orthosis, increased swelling, color changes in the extremity
- Contact information for the practitioner (name of the practitioner, phone number, email of clinic)
- Photograph of the orthosis on the client highlighting proper positioning (this is easy to do now because most clients have a smart phone)
- Orthosis cleaning and care, including keeping the orthosis away from excessive heat
- Compensatory techniques if needed (e.g., if the dominant hand is restricted)

If the client is unable to understand the instructions, a family member or caregiver should be provided with these instructions to ensure that the orthosis is worn and used as prescribed. All of this information should be given verbally and in writing to the client or caregiver, and a copy kept in the client's record. See the Appendix at the end of the chapter for a sample client education handout.

It is important to take the time to evaluate a client following orthotic fabrication and immediately address any problems that arise. Ideally, have the client wear the orthosis in the clinic for 10 to 15 minutes to ensure that all problem areas are addressed before he or she leaves. Additional factors to consider after issuing the orthosis for a given client are shown in Table 1-2.

Clients should be instructed to contact the practitioner immediately if any problems arise. This is particularly important if the client will not be returning for any follow-up care.

PRECAUTIONS PERTINENT TO ORTHOTIC FABRICATION

The practitioner must thoroughly evaluate the client before orthotic provision to ensure that the orthosis is a safe and effective intervention strategy. If the client presents with any comorbidities that may affect use of the orthosis, the practitioner should seek clarification from the referring physician before orthotic provision. The following are precautions that warrant further consideration:

- Compromised cognitive state regarding wear and care of the orthosis

- Allergic reaction to the material used (the client may develop a rash following provision of the orthosis)
- Diminished or absent sensation in the extremity
- Unclear diagnosis or unclear prescription request
- Compromised circulation in the area where the orthosis is applied (history of peripheral vascular disease, recent arterial repair, or noted color changes in the skin)

EFFECTIVE ORTHOTIC DESIGN

Taking the time to consider the impact that an orthosis will have on a client's daily occupations will go a long way to optimize compliance and the outcomes that the orthosis is intended to achieve. Making the orthosis look professional and polished and keeping the design simple and straightforward can be accomplished with relative ease (Table 1-3).

Summary

- The goals of an orthosis will vary depending on the client's needs and the diagnosis.
- There are two main categories of UE orthoses: immobilization and mobilization orthoses.
- EBP plays a very important role in orthotic intervention.
- Knowledge of the key anatomical structures and biomechanical principles will help the practitioner understand how an orthosis will influence these structures and assist in determining the most appropriate orthotic design and wearing schedule.
- A practitioner must use appropriate L-codes and terminology when documenting orthotic services and for billing and reimbursement (for those practicing in the United States).
- It is important for a practitioner to design a client-centered orthosis and to evaluate the fit and comfort to optimize compliance.

Test Your Knowledge

1. Explain the difference between the terms *orthotic* and *orthosis*.
2. Describe how orthotic design and fabrication is both an art and a science.
3. Compare the difference between an immobilization and mobilization orthosis.

Table 1-2

ORTHOSIS PROBLEMS AND SOLUTIONS

PROBLEM	POTENTIAL SOLUTION
Color changes (skin turns red, purple, or pale/white since wearing the orthosis) or temperature changes (skin feels warmer or cooler to the touch since wearing the orthosis)	These may indicate compression or constriction of the sensory nerves or blood vessels due to tight strapping or a tight-fitting orthosis. Loosen the straps, flare away the orthosis edges, and recheck the fit.
Skin integrity: breakdown of skin or highly fragile skin	Use perforated and/or lightweight materials and issue a stockinette sleeve for wearing under the thermoplastic orthosis. Consider a dorsal approach if the volar skin is highly sensitive or vice versa. Make sure the straps hold the limb securely in place and that the limb does not rotate inside the orthosis.
Edema	If edema in the limb is significant, use an elastic wrap initially to hold the orthosis in place on the extremity. The wrap should be applied in a distal to proximal direction to help the flow of fluids into the venous system for drainage. Once the edema subsides, hook-and-loop straps may be applied. Additionally, the orthosis may need to be remolded to accommodate for the reduction in edema.
	A circumferential or dorsal orthotic design may be most appropriate when edema is present in the hand to avoid uneven pressure distribution and collection of edema between the straps. Alternately, lightweight cotton bias wrap or Coban (lightweight elasticized, self-adherent tape) may be used to secure the orthosis on the extremity. In addition, extra padding may be necessary for orthoses designs that cover the dorsal aspect of the hand to protect the thin anatomical structures.
Improper positioning of joints	Check to see that the orthosis maintains the correct positioning of all joints. In particular, pay attention to radial or ulnar deviation at the wrist, too much wrist flexion, and thumb positioning. Unless otherwise specified, the client should be able to oppose the thumb to the index finger easily.
Red markings on the skin along the border of the orthosis and/or on bony prominences	Take care to flare away edges and pad where needed so that the orthosis does not cause red marks on the skin. Carefully heat and flare out areas that directly cover bony prominences. Do not place pads on the underside of the orthosis without first flaring out the area because the padding will create unwanted compressive and shear forces.

Table 1-3

EFFECTIVE ORTHOTIC DESIGN

KEEP IT SIMPLE	Make sure the orthosis is simple in design to do the required job. Avoid unnecessary components and stick to basic design principles.
EASY ON, EASY OFF	The orthosis should be easy to put on and take off. The straps should not interfere with function.
NO UNNECESSARY JOINTS INCLUDED	Do not include uninvolved joints in a simple orthosis unless this is necessary to increase the leverage or mechanical advantage.
AESTHETICS	Do your best to make the orthosis look professional: • Cut with smooth scissor strokes to avoid uneven edges. • Do not leave markings on the orthosis. • Make all edges smooth and round all corners.
DURABLE	Choose a material that will last for the expected duration of orthosis wear.

4. Describe an orthosis using descriptive terminology that:
   - Immobilizes the wrist only
   - Immobilizes the wrist and metacarpophalangeal joints
   - Immobilizes the elbow, forearm, and wrist
   - Immobilizes the thumb carpometacarpal and metacarpophalangeal joints

5. Describe the five levels of evidence commonly associated with EBP.

6. What is an L-code?

7. Describe how a therapist can make an orthosis as client centered as possible.

8. List the important factors to include when educating a client on the wear and care of his or her orthosis.

Reference

Brown, C. (2017). *The evidence-based practitioner: Applying research to meet client needs.* Philadelphia, PA: F.A. Davis Company.

Suggested Reading

American Occupational Therapy Association. (n.d.). *Evidence-based practice and research.* Retrieved from https://www.aota.org/Practice/Researchers.aspx

American Society of Hand Therapists. (n.d.). *Coding.* Retrieved from https://www.asht.org/practice/durable-medical-equipment-dme/orthotics/coding

Holm, M. B. (2000). Our mandate for the new millennium: Evidence-based practice. *American Journal of Occupational Therapy, 54*(6), 575-585.

McKee, P. R., & Rivard, A. (2011). Biopsychosocial approach to orthotic intervention. *Journal of Hand Therapy, 24*(2), 155-163.

Oxford Centre for Evidence-Based Medicine. (2016). *OCEBM levels of evidence.* Retrieved from http://www.cebm.net/index.aspx?o=5653

Rosner, A. L. (2012). Evidence-based medicine: revisiting the pyramid of priorities. *Journal of Bodywork & Movement Therapies, 16,* 42-49. doi:10.1016/j.jbmt.2011.05.003

Sackett, D. L., Rosenberg, W. M., Gray, J. A., Haynes, R. B., & Richardson, W. S. (1996). Evidence based medicine: What it is and what it isn't. *British Medical Journal, 312*(7023), 71-72.

Appendix

CLIENT EDUCATION HANDOUT: WEAR AND CARE OF YOUR ORTHOSIS

Client Name: _____ Date: _____

Your custom orthosis was made by: _____

Name of your orthosis: _____

The purpose of your orthosis is: _____

Your orthosis should be worn: _____

Notify your therapist as soon as possible if you notice any of the following:

- Skin redness
- Pain while wearing your orthosis
- Increased swelling
- Color changes in your fingertips
- Tingling or numbness in your hand
- Skin rashes, itchy areas, or other areas of irritation

If you can take your orthosis off during your recovery, please note:

- Do not place your orthosis near a heat source such as a hot car, in the dishwasher or microwave, or near a hot radiator. The heat may melt your orthosis.
- Do not adjust or change your orthosis in any way, unless your therapist tells you to.
- You can clean your orthosis with an antibacterial wipe or cool water and soap. The straps and socks can be hand washed and left to air dry.

IT IS VERY IMPORTANT THAT YOU WEAR YOUR ORTHOSIS AS PRESCRIBED BY YOUR DOCTOR AND THERAPIST. IF YOU HAVE ANY QUESTIONS, PLEASE CONTACT YOUR THERAPIST OR CLINIC IMMEDIATELY.

Client Signature: _____

Therapist Name: _____ Phone: _____

Email: _____

CHAPTER 2

Anatomical and Biomechanical Principles of Orthotic Intervention

Key Terms

Annular pulleys	Effort force	Opposition
Axis	Equilibrium	Palmar aponeurosis
Biomechanics	Extensor mechanism	Prehension
Bony prominences	Extrinsic muscles	Resistance force
Bowstringing	First-class lever	Second-class lever
Brachial plexus	Flexor and extensor retinaculum	Shear force
Camper's chiasm	Fulcrum	Skin creases
Central slip	Intrinsic muscles	Synovial joint
Circumduction	Lateral bands	Tensile force
Compressive force	Lever systems	Third-class lever
Cruciate pulleys	No man's land	Valgus
Cubital fossa	Oblique retinacular ligament	Varus
Cubital tunnel		

Learning Outcomes

Upon completion of this chapter, you will be able to:

1. Review the anatomy of the upper extremity as a basis for understanding clinical conditions that affect function.

2. Identify the key anatomical structures (bones, joints, muscles, nerves, and soft tissues) that are influenced by an orthosis for the upper extremity.

3. Describe the biomechanical principles associated with orthotic intervention for the upper extremity.

4. Explain how each stage of wound healing is affected by orthotic intervention.

5. List the common precautions and contraindications associated with orthotic intervention.

6. Describe the key elements associated with determining orthotic wearing schedules and client education.

Schofield, K., & Schwartz, D. *Orthotic Design and Fabrication for the Upper Extremity: A Practical Guide* (pp 15-39).
© 2019 Taylor & Francis Group.

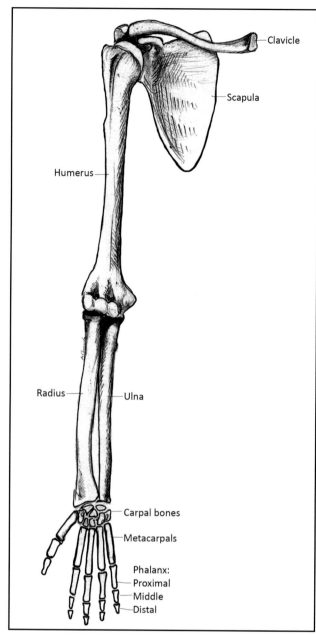

Figure 2-1. Bones of the UE.

Introduction

In order to design an effective and well-fitting orthosis, the practitioner must have a thorough foundation of upper extremity (UE) anatomy, wound healing, and biomechanical principles. More importantly, this requires the ability of the practitioner to apply this knowledge to meet the client's particular needs. This chapter presents an overview of UE anatomy and wound healing concepts. The anatomical structures specific to each orthosis in this textbook are highlighted in the instructional videos. Readers are encouraged to refresh their knowledge of specific UE anatomical structures, including bones, muscles (including nerve innervations), joints, ligaments, surface landmarks, and digital anatomy, and of the healing time frames of each of these structures.

It is also critical for a practitioner to consider the biomechanical principles surrounding orthotic design when using orthoses to treat a client's condition. This knowledge will help the practitioner understand how the orthosis will influence anatomical structures involved and assist them in determining appropriate orthosis designs and wearing schedules. Thorough knowledge of biomechanical concepts related to orthotic fabrication will assist the practitioner in designing a comfortable, effective, and cosmetically pleasing orthosis.

Overview of Upper Extremity Anatomy

The anatomical structures of the UE are influenced by wearing any type of orthosis. It is critical for the practitioner to understand what these structures are, where they are located, and how an orthosis affects them.

BONES AND JOINTS

Depending on its purpose, UE orthoses acts on the bones, joints, and soft tissue structures of the elbow, forearm, wrist, hand, thumb, and digits (Figures 2-1 and 2-2). The majority of joints in the UE are **synovial joints**. This type of joint is the most common in the body and is designed for movement. These joints permit free motion between the bones they join together. There are eight elements found in all synovial joints (Figure 2-3).

The concavity, or curvature, of the metacarpal and carpal bones on the volar aspect of the hand make up the three hand arches: proximal transverse, distal transverse, and longitudinal. The proximal transverse arch forms a rigid arch at the carpometacarpal (CMC) joints of digits II through V, whereas the distal transverse arch and longitudinal arches are more mobile and contribute to mobility and functional posture of the palm and digits (Figure 2-4A). When an orthosis includes the wrist and hand, it is critical for the practitioner to accommodate these arches to allow for optimal support and alignment (Figure 2-4B). The distal transverse arch must not be obstructed in orthoses that do not include the digits to allow for full, unrestricted movement of the fingers (Figure 2-4C). Note the oblique orientation of the distal transverse arch with the hand in a fist, as compared with a more horizontal orientation with the fingers in extension (Figure 2-4D).

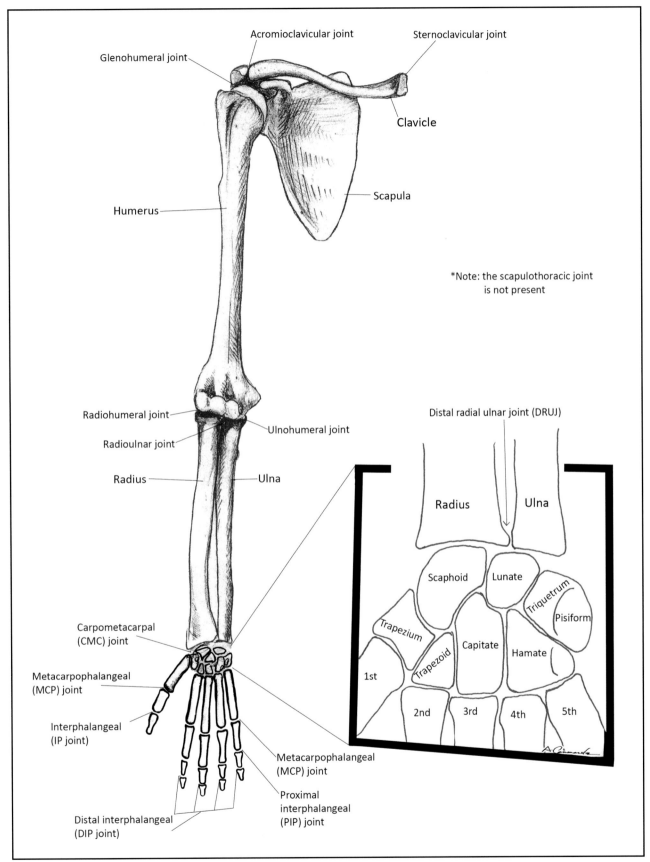

Figure 2-2. Joints of the UE.

Figure 2-3. Components of a synovial joint.

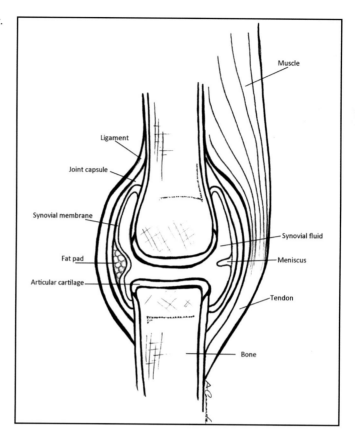

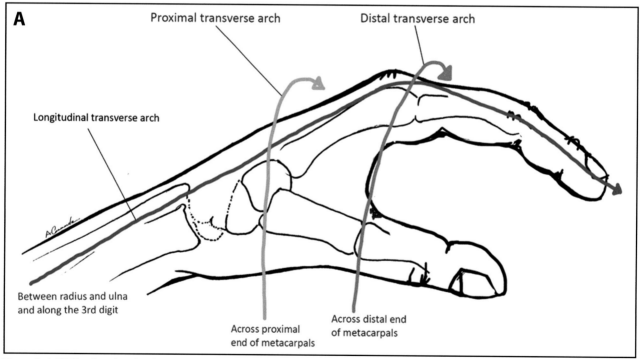

Figure 2-4. (A) The three hand arches are outlined here. *(continued)*

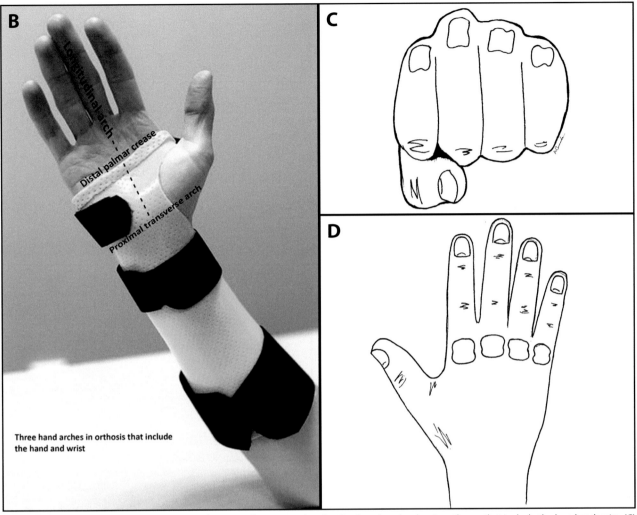

Figure 2-4 (continued). (B) It is important to observe and accommodate for the three hand arches in orthoses that include the hand and wrist. (C) Note the oblique orientation of the metacarpal heads when the digits are flexed: higher on the radial side, lower on the ulnar side. (D) Note the horizontal orientation of the metacarpal heads when the digits are in extension.

BONY PROMINENCES

Defined, **bony prominences** are areas where a bone lies immediately below the surface of the skin (Box 2-1 and Figure 2-5). It is critical for the practitioner to locate all of the prominences that will be covered or affected in some way by a UE orthosis. If not addressed properly, the thermoplastic material and straps of the orthosis can apply excessive **compressive** and **shear forces** over the prominences and create pressure areas and discomfort for the client. Left unchecked, these excessive forces can lead to tissue breakdown and pain. The practitioner should take care to use highly conforming thermoplastic materials so it conforms well to the bony anatomy, flare the thermoplastic material away from the bony prominence, and consider use of padding on the inside of the orthosis *after* the area is flared to avoid unwanted pressure.

NERVE INNERVATIONS

An orthosis for the UE can influence virtually all the nerve pathways in the arm, forearm, and hand. Nerve innervation to all UE muscles arises from the **brachial plexus** (Figure 2-6A through D). The three terminal branches of the brachial plexus form the peripheral nerves that innervate the majority of the muscles of the arm and all muscles of the forearm and hand.

FOREARM AND HAND CONNECTIVE TISSUES

By virtue of design, an orthosis for the UE affects connective tissues in the forearm, wrist, and hand. It is important for the practitioner to understand these structures and how an orthosis influences them.

Box 2-1. Upper Extremity Bony Prominences

Medial epicondyle

Lateral epicondyle

Olecranon

Ulnar head

Ulnar styloid

Metacarpal heads

Pisiform

Scaphoid tubercle

Radial styloid

Dorsal proximal and distal interphalangeal joints

Thumb CMC joint/base of first metacarpal

Thumb metacarpophalangeal and interphalangeal joints (dorsal aspects)

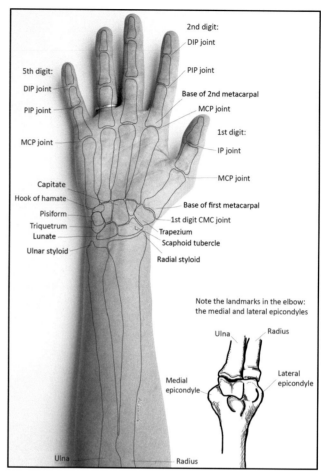

Figure 2-5. UE bony prominences are important to observe when fabricating an orthosis.

The skin on the volar surface of the hand is distinctly different from the skin on the hand's dorsal surface. The palmar/volar skin is thick and immobile and serves to stabilize and protect the underlying structures. The palmar skin attaches to the underlying **palmar aponeurosis**, a thin, strong layer of fascia attached to the palmaris longus tendon that helps to form the palmar **skin creases** and assists with grasp (Figure 2-7).

The skin on the dorsal aspect of the hand, conversely, is thin and mobile and allows the underlying tendons of the extensor digitorum to glide freely across the metacarpals and the fingers to flex and extend freely (Figure 2-8).

Due to the relative laxity of the dorsal skin, edema tends to accumulate on the dorsal aspect of the hand following injury. The practitioner must take care to accommodate for this edema when fabricating an orthosis that includes the hand and wrist (Figure 2-9).

Upper Extremity Anatomy by Region

ELBOW AND FOREARM

The elbow contributes significantly to UE function and is the key to positioning the hand and wrist in space.

Elbow Joint

The elbow joint is a complex structure that consists of three separate joints—the radiohumeral, ulnohumeral, and proximal radioulnar—contained in a single joint capsule. The radiohumeral joint is formed by the articulation between the capitulum of the distal humerus and the proximal end of the radius, the radial head. The ulnohumeral

joint is formed by the trochlea of the distal humerus and the proximal end of the ulna, the trochlear notch (Figure 2-10).

Both the radiohumeral and ulnohumeral joints are highly congruent and act together to form a modified hinge joint where elbow flexion and extension occur. Normal range of motion (ROM) in the elbow is 0 to 150 degrees, and the majority of this movement occurs at the ulnohumeral joint.

Forearm Joints

The proximal radioulnar joint, also located within the elbow capsule, is the articulation between the radial head of the radius and the radial notch of the ulna. This joint is linked directly to the radiohumeral and radioulnar joints by the elbow capsule, but the movement produced differs. This articulation, along with the distal radioulnar joint at the wrist, allows for forearm pronation and supination and does not contribute to elbow motion. Acting together, all three joints allow the hand to be placed in a wide variety of positions and contribute to the stability of the UE during weightbearing activities such as using a walker or cane, shifting one's weight in a chair, or pushing and pulling activities.

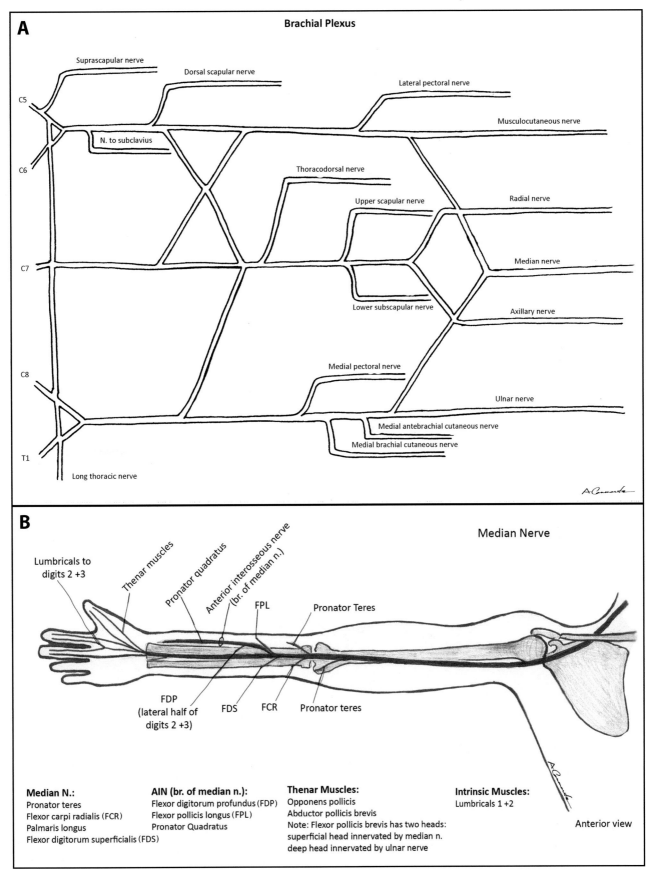

Figure 2-6. (A) Outline of the brachial plexus and terminal branches. (B) Median nerve, (C) radial nerve, and (D) ulnar nerve. The musculocutaneous nerve is not shown. *(continued)*

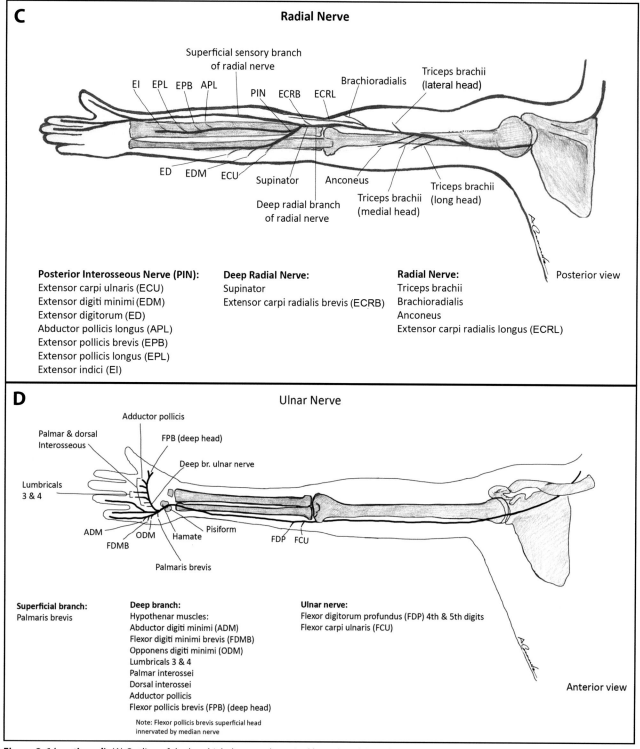

C   Radial Nerve

Superficial sensory branch of radial nerve

EI   EPL   EPB   APL   PIN   ECRB   ECRL   Brachioradialis   Triceps brachii (lateral head)

ED   EDM   ECU   Supinator   Anconeus   Triceps brachii (medial head)   Triceps brachii (long head)

Deep radial branch of radial nerve

Posterior view

Posterior Interosseous Nerve (PIN):
Extensor carpi ulnaris (ECU)
Extensor digiti minimi (EDM)
Extensor digitorum (ED)
Abductor pollicis longus (APL)
Extensor pollicis brevis (EPB)
Extensor pollicis longus (EPL)
Extensor indici (EI)

Deep Radial Nerve:
Supinator
Extensor carpi radialis brevis (ECRB)

Radial Nerve:
Triceps brachii
Brachioradialis
Anconeus
Extensor carpi radialis longus (ECRL)

D   Ulnar Nerve

Adductor pollicis

Palmar & dorsal Interosseous   FPB (deep head)

Deep br. ulnar nerve

Lumbricals 3 & 4

ADM   ODM   Hamate   Pisiform   FDP   FCU

FDMB

Palmaris brevis

Superficial branch:
Palmaris brevis

Deep branch:
Hypothenar muscles:
Abductor digiti minimi (ADM)
Flexor digiti minimi brevis (FDMB)
Opponens digiti minimi (ODM)
Lumbricals 3 & 4
Palmar interossei
Dorsal interossei
Adductor pollicis
Flexor pollicis brevis (FPB) (deep head)

Note: Flexor pollicis brevis superficial head innervated by median nerve

Ulnar nerve:
Flexor digitorum profundus (FDP) 4th & 5th digits
Flexor carpi ulnaris (FCU)

Anterior view

Figure 2-6 (continued). (A) Outline of the brachial plexus and terminal branches. (B) Median nerve, (C) radial nerve, and (D) ulnar nerve. The musculocutaneous nerve is not shown.

Due to the high degree of conformability between each of the three joints and the single joint capsule configuration, injury to these joints and other associated soft tissues can lead to significant loss of joint movement in elbow flexion/extension and/or forearm pronation and supination.

With the UE in anatomical position (humeral adduction, elbow extension, forearm supination), the forearm tends to deviate laterally in relationship to the humerus. This lateral deviation is termed the *carrying angle* or **valgus** of the elbow, and it is normally between 10 and 15 degrees from the longitudinal **axis** of the distal humerus

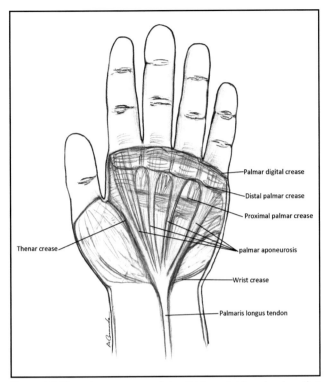

Figure 2-7. The palmar aponeurosis is a thick, unyielding structure that helps to form the skin creases in the palm and assists with grasp.

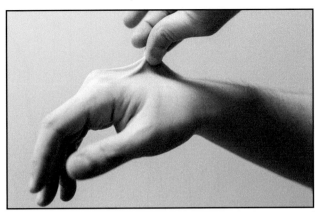

Figure 2-8. The thin, mobile skin on the dorsal aspect of the hand allows the extensor tendons to move and glide freely during digit movement.

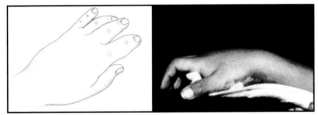

Figure 2-9. Edema tends to accumulate on the dorsal aspect of the hand due to the laxity of the skin. It is important to accommodate for this when fabricating an orthosis.

Figure 2-10. The radiohumeral and ulnohumeral joints of the elbow are contained in the elbow joint capsule.

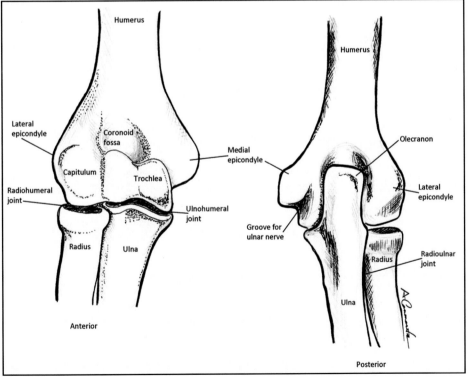

and the mid-forearm between the radius and ulna. This angle is attributed to the medial and distal orientation of the trochlea of the humerus in relation to the capitulum (Figure 2-11).

It is very important to accommodate the carrying angle when fabricating elbow extension orthoses to ensure that the joints and soft tissues are positioned correctly. A less common deviation is cubitus **varus**, or gunstock deformity,

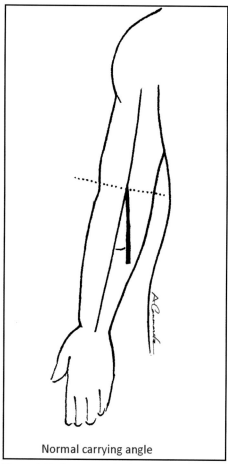

Figure 2-11. Carrying angle: the oblique orientation of the humerus in relation to the radius and ulna with the UE in anatomical position.

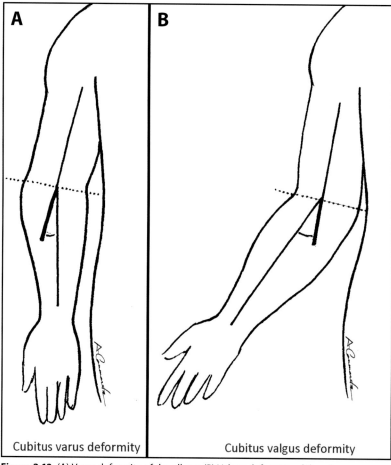

Figure 2-12. (A) Varus deformity of the elbow. (B) Valgus deformity of the elbow.

Normal carrying angle

Cubitus varus deformity

Cubitus valgus deformity

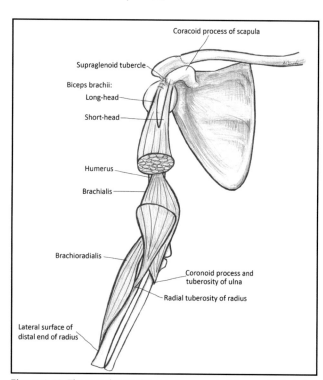

Figure 2-13. The muscles on the anterior aspect of the arm include the brachialis, biceps brachii, and brachioradialis.

Coracoid process of scapula

Supraglenoid tubercle

Biceps brachii:

Long-head

Short-head

Humerus

Brachialis

Brachioradialis

Coronoid process and tuberosity of ulna

Radial tuberosity of radius

Lateral surface of distal end of radius

where the forearm deviates medially in relation to the distal humerus. Collectively, the terms *valgus* and *varus* are derived from the Latin *turned outward* and *turned inward*, respectively (Figure 2-12).

The elbow has very strong ligamentous support on the medial and lateral aspects of the joint. The medial collateral ligament complex contributes to stability of the joint and helps limit valgus stresses, whereas the lateral collateral ligament complex helps to limit varus stresses. Injury to these structures can therefore significantly affect stability and movement of the elbow.

Soft Tissue Structures

Muscles in the upper arm are divided into two compartments: anterior and posterior. The anterior compartment, shown in Figure 2-13, comprises muscles that flex the elbow (biceps brachii, brachialis, and brachioradialis) and help flex and adduct the glenohumeral joint (coracobrachialis). The musculocutaneous (biceps brachii and brachialis) and radial (brachioradialis) nerves innervate this compartment. The three heads of the triceps brachii (long, lateral, and medial), innervated by the radial nerve, make up the posterior compartment of the arm.

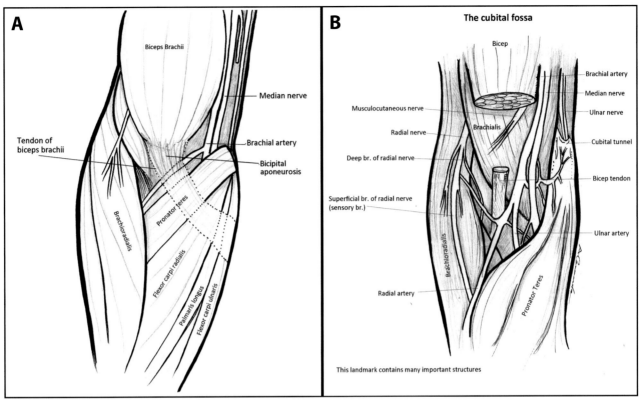

Figure 2-14. The cubital fossa contains many important anatomical structures.

The volar aspect of the elbow contains a number of important soft tissue structures and is termed the **cubital fossa**. This fossa, or hollow, is bordered by the brachioradialis muscle laterally, pronator teres muscle medially, biceps brachii superiorly, and biceps tendon inferiorly (Figure 2-14A and B). Contents of the cubital fossa include the median nerve, brachial artery, and distal biceps tendon.

The posterior aspect of the elbow, in contrast, is bony in nature and consists of the olecranon process in the center, the lateral epicondyle laterally, and the medial epicondyle medially. When the elbow is flexed at 90 degrees, these three structures form a triangle. In extension, they form a straight line (Figure 2-15).

The area between the medial epicondyle and the olecranon is referred to as the **cubital tunnel**, and the ulnar nerve travels through this area on its course from the arm into the forearm (Figure 2-16). Collectively, the bony structures and the ulnar nerve can be subject to irritation and pressure from an elbow and forearm immobilization orthosis and must be protected during fabrication.

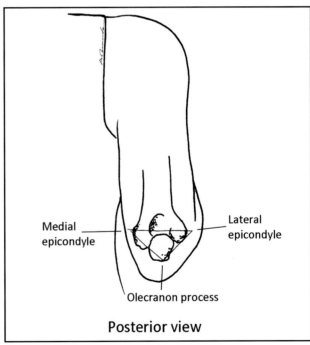

Figure 2-15. Note the triangle formed by the olecranon, medial and lateral epicondyles with the elbow flexed at 90 degrees and the straight line formed with the elbow extended.

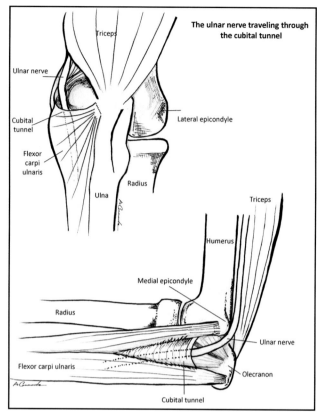

Figure 2-16. The ulnar nerve travels in a space between the medial epicondyle and the olecranon. These structures must be protected in orthoses that include the elbow.

WRIST

The wrist joint is made up of several distinct joints: distal radioulnar, radiocarpal, midcarpal, and CMC joints of digits II to V (Figure 2-17).

Soft Tissue Structures

Muscles

Muscles in the forearm and hand can be divided into extrinsic and intrinsic groups. **Extrinsic muscles** originate proximally in the forearm and insert on or distal to the wrist. Muscles on the dorsal or posterior aspect of the forearm are commonly referred to as the *extrinsic extensors* (Figure 2-18); muscles on the volar or anterior aspect are *extrinsic flexors* (Figure 2-19). **Intrinsic muscles** originate and insert distal to the wrist (Figure 2-20).

Refer to Table 2-1 for a complete list of forearm and wrist muscles and their nerve innervations.

Muscles in the intrinsic group work in a synergistic manner to provide stability for effective coordination, dexterity, and power (Table 2-2).

Flexor and Extensor Retinaculum

The retinacula collectively are strong fibrous bands that serve to hold the tendons that cross the wrist close to the

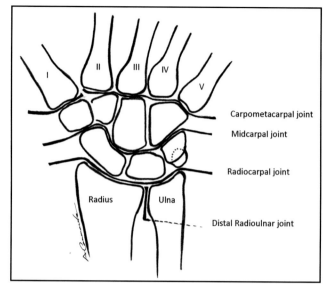

Figure 2-17. Note the joints that make up the wrist: distal radioulnar, radiocarpal, midcarpal, and CMC joints of digits II through V.

wrist joint axis during movement. This helps to optimize the forces that the muscles are able to generate during flexion and extension of the wrist and fingers. The **flexor retinaculum** courses across the volar aspect of the wrist and is continuous with the transverse carpal ligament. The eight flexor digitorum superficialis (FDS) and profundus tendons (each muscle has four tendons), the flexor pollicis longus tendon, and the median nerve run beneath the flexor retinaculum. Wrist and hand orthoses are commonly prescribed for conditions that affect these structures, such as tendonitis, carpal tunnel syndrome, and hand trauma (Figure 2-21).

The **extensor retinaculum**, located on the dorsal aspect of the wrist, lies on top of the extensor tendons of the wrist and fingers (Figure 2-22). Six distinct compartments under the extensor retinaculum serve to group the tendons together according to their function (Box 2-2). Hand and wrist immobilization orthoses may be prescribed for treatment of inflammation of the tendons in these compartments.

THUMB

The human thumb is critical to hand function and contributes significantly to grip, pinch, and fine motor movements. The CMC joint, or basal joint, formed by the base of the first metacarpal and trapezium, is considered to be the most important joint of the thumb and hand. This joint possesses a wide arc of motion, largely due to the saddle shape of the joint surfaces. Combined with strong ligamentous support and intrinsic musculature, this relationship permits movements unique to this joint, **circumduction** and **opposition**, along with stability during pinching and gripping tasks.

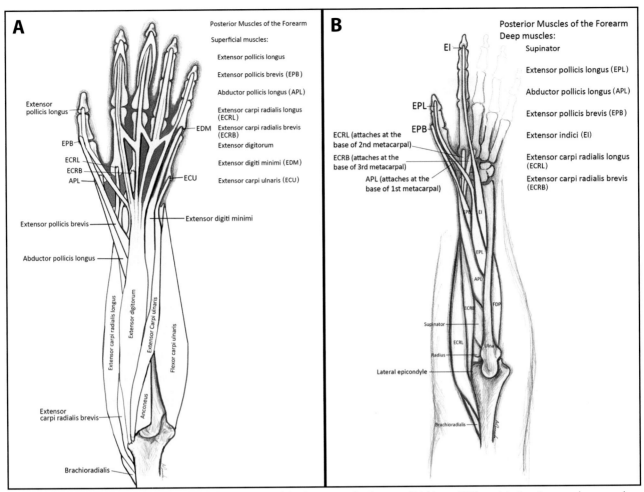

Figure 2-18. (A) The extrinsic extensors on the dorsal aspect of the forearm and wrist: superficial layer. (B) The extrinsic extensors: deep muscles.

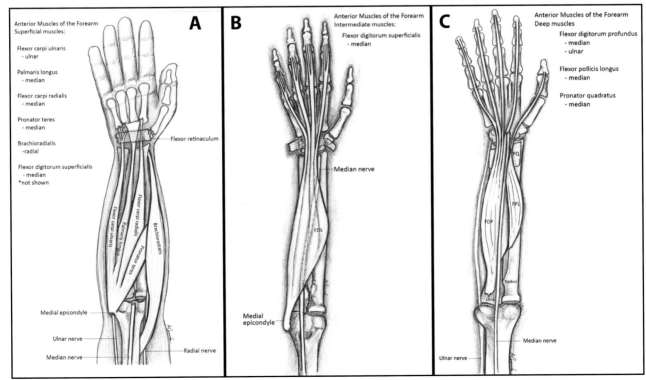

Figure 2-19. (A) The extrinsic flexors on the volar aspect of the forearm and wrist: superficial layer. (B) The extrinsic flexors: intermediate layer. (C) The extrinsic flexors: deep layer. FDP, flexor digitorum profundus; FDS, flexor digitorum superficialis; FPL, flexor pollicis longus; PQ, pronator quadratus.

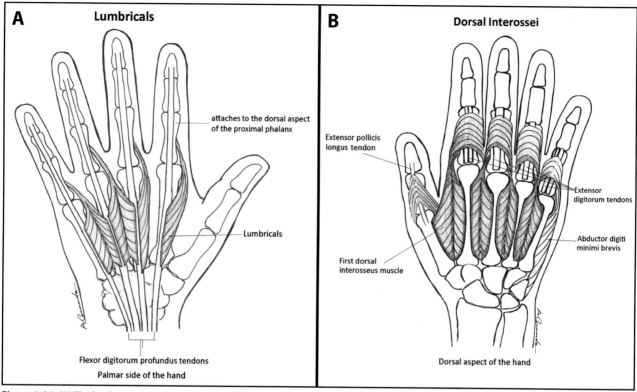

Figure 2-20. (A) The lumbrical and volar interossei muscles lie in the palm. (B) The dorsal interossei muscles are located between the metacarpals.

Table 2-1

MUSCLES OF THE ARM AND EXTRINSIC MUSCLES OF THE FOREARM AND HAND

VOLAR ARM		DORSAL ARM	
The brachialis and biceps brachii both work together to flex the elbow; the biceps also supinates the forearm when the elbow is flexed.		The triceps is the only muscle that extends the elbow.	
Muscle	*Nerve Supply*	*Muscle*	*Nerve Supply*
Biceps brachii	Musculocutaneous	Triceps brachii (long, lateral, and medial heads)	Radial
Brachialis	Musculocutaneous		
Brachioradialis	Radial		
VOLAR FOREARM EXTRINSIC FLEXOR MUSCLES		**DORSAL FOREARM EXTRINSIC EXTENSOR MUSCLES**	
This group of muscles collectively flex the wrist, digits, and thumb.		This group of muscles collectively extend the wrist, thumb, and fingers.	
Muscle	*Nerve Supply*	*Muscle*	*Nerve Supply*
Flexor carpi radialis	Median	Extensor carpi radialis longus	Radial
Flexor carpi ulnaris	Ulnar	Extensor carpi radialis brevis	Deep radial
Palmaris longus	Median	Extensor carpi ulnaris	Posterior interosseous (radial)

(continued)

Table 2-1 (continued)

MUSCLES OF THE ARM AND EXTRINSIC MUSCLES OF THE FOREARM AND HAND

Muscle	Nerve Supply	Muscle	Nerve Supply
Flexor digitorum superficialis	Median	Extensor digitorum	Posterior interosseous
Flexor digitorum profundus	Index/long: Anterior interosseous Ring/small: Ulnar	Extensor indicis	Posterior interosseous
Flexor pollicis longus	Anterior interosseous	Extensor digiti minimi	Posterior interosseous
		Extensor pollicis longus	Posterior interosseous
		Extensor pollicis brevis	Posterior interosseous
		Abductor pollicis longus	Posterior interosseous

Table 2-2

INTRINSIC HAND MUSCLES

MUSCLE	NERVE SUPPLY
Lumbricals	Median (index/long), ulnar (ring/small)
Palmar interossei	Deep ulnar
Dorsal interossei	Deep ulnar
Thenar muscles: abductor pollicis brevis, flexor pollicis brevis, opponens pollicis	Recurrent median
Adductor pollicis	Deep ulnar
Hypothenar muscles: abductor digiti minimi, flexor digiti minimi, opponens digiti minimi	Deep ulnar

The thumb axis is based at the CMC joint, and the first metacarpal is pronated and flexed approximately 80 degrees with respect to the other hand metacarpals. This unique positioning of the first metacarpal in relation to the other four metacarpals allows for circumduction, or movement of the thumb CMC joint in a circular fashion. Opposition refers to the combined movements of thumb abduction, metacarpophalangeal (MCP) joint flexion, internal rotation, and radial deviation of the proximal phalanx over the MCP joint, collectively allowing the thumb pad to come into contact with the pads of each finger. **Prehension** refers to the ability to reach, grasp, and manipulate objects with the thumb and the fingers together. The thumb is an essential component in the ability to use the hands for this function. Any disease or trauma involving the thumb can result in considerable loss of function due to instability, pain, or weakness.

The thumb bones include the trapezium, first metacarpal, and proximal and distal phalanges (Figure 2-23). The

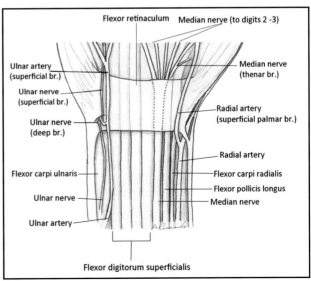

Figure 2-21. The flexor retinaculum helps to hold the flexor tendons of the wrist and digits close to the wrist joint axis during movement.

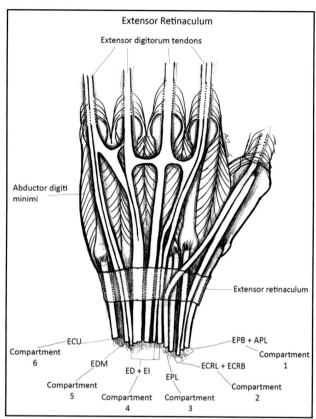

Figure 2-22. The extensor retinaculum helps to hold the extensor tendons of the wrist and digits close to the wrist joint axis during movement. There are six distinct compartments.

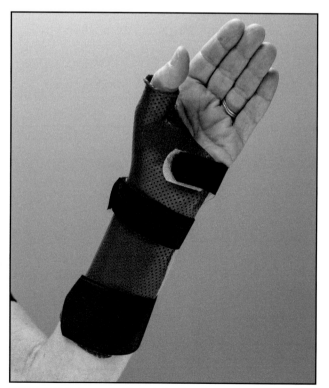

Figure 2-24. Orthoses that include the thumb must also accommodate the hand arches.

Box 2-2. Extensor Tendon Dorsal Compartments

1: Abductor pollicis longus (APL) and extensor pollicis brevis (EPB)

2: Extensor carpi radialis longus (ECRL) and brevis (ECRB)

3: Extensor pollicis longus (EPL)

4: Extensor digitorum (ED) and extensor indicis (EI)

5: Extensor digiti minimi (EDM)

6: Extensor carpi ulnaris (ECU)

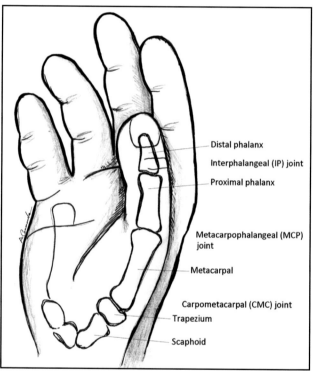

Figure 2-23. The bones and joints of the thumb: first CMC, MCP, and IP joints.

joints involved are the first CMC and MCP joints; the interphalangeal (IP) joint may also be affected if it is included in the orthosis.

An orthosis that supports the thumb must also support the proximal and distal transverse arches fully and reflect the oblique orientation of the metacarpal heads with the fingers fully flexed. The thermoplastic material should conform intimately to the palm to support these concave arches (Figure 2-24).

The bony prominences affected by a thumb orthosis include the base of the first metacarpal, radial styloid, second metacarpal base, pisiform, scaphoid tubercle, and ulnar head if the orthosis includes the wrist (Figure 2-25).

The muscles influenced directly by a thumb immobilization orthosis include the abductor pollicis brevis, flexor

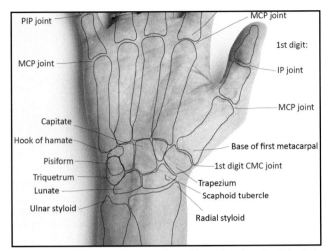

Figure 2-25. Bony prominences affected by a thumb orthosis include the base of the first and second metacarpals, radial styloid, and scaphoid tubercle.

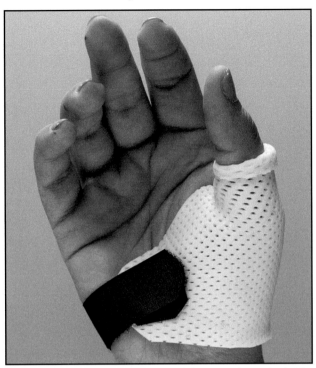

Figure 2-26. The thumb CMC joint should be covered completely. The area around the pisiform can be trimmed to optimize comfort.

Table 2-3

MOTOR AND SENSORY FUNCTION OF THE THUMB

	MOTOR	SENSORY
MEDIAN NERVE	Thumb abduction (abductor pollicis brevis), MCP flexion (superficial head of flexor pollicis brevis), IP flexion (flexor pollicis longus), opposition (opponens pollicis)	Volar aspect of thumb, entire volar aspect of index and long fingers, radial half of ring finger
ULNAR NERVE	Thumb adduction (adductor pollicis), MCP flexion (deep head of flexor pollicis brevis), index finger abduction (first dorsal interosseous)	Ulnar, volar aspect of ring finger, entire small finger
RADIAL NERVE	Thumb CMC extension (EPL, EPB, APL), MCP extension (EPB, EPL), IP extension (EPL), abduction (APL)	Dorsal radial aspect of thumb, dorsal aspect of web space

All three peripheral nerves—median, ulnar, and radial—contribute to motor and sensory function of the thumb (Table 2-3).

Injury to one or more of these nerves, particularly the median and/or ulnar nerves, can have debilitating effects on prehensile function.

All thumb immobilization orthoses should cover the thumb CMC joint in order to provide adequate support; the orthosis can be trimmed more on the ulnar side of the hand near the pisiform (Figure 2-26). The distal palmar crease should be completely cleared to allow for full finger ROM in the orthosis. The MCP joint and/or IP joint crease should be fully visible if these joints are not included in the orthosis to allow for full, unrestricted movement (Figure 2-27A and B).

DIGITS

The digital anatomy is quite complex. In order to properly design and fabricate an orthosis that includes the digits, the practitioner must have knowledge of this anatomy. This section will focus on the following:

- Proximal interphalangeal (PIP) and distal interphalangeal (DIP) joint anatomy

- Flexor and extensor zones of injury

- Muscles that move the digits

- Key soft tissue structures: **annular** and **cruciate pulleys**, **extensor mechanism**, **lateral bands**, **central slip**, **oblique retinacular ligament**

pollicis brevis, adductor pollicis, opponens pollicis, flexor pollicis longus, EPL and EPB, and APL. Also affected are the flexor carpi radialis, flexor carpi ulnaris, ECRL and ECRB, and ECU if the orthosis includes the wrist. A wrist and thumb orthosis also immobilizes the wrist joint, which includes the distal radioulnar, radiocarpal, midcarpal, and second through fifth CMC joints.

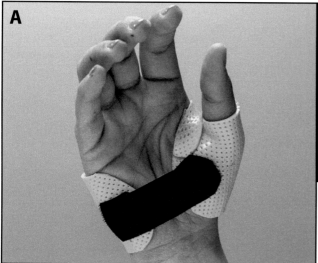

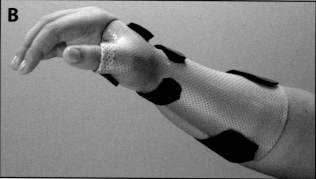

Figure 2-27. (A) A thumb immobilization orthosis directly influences the thenar muscles. (B) A thumb immobilization orthosis that includes the wrist also influences the flexor and extensor muscles of the thumb and wrist.

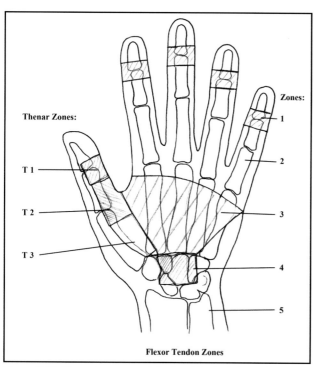

Figure 2-28. The volar aspect of the hand is divided into five zones to help identify the anatomical structures, specifically flexor tendons, intrinsic muscles, and pulleys. (Illustration by Allie Cammarata.)

Proximal Interphalangeal and Distal Interphalangeal Joints

The PIP joints are hinge joints that allow only flexion and extension. The radial and ulnar collateral ligaments provide joint stability by resisting radial (lateral) and ulnar (medial) forces. The volar plate is a unique structure on the volar surface of the PIP joint that prevents hyperextension and assists with joint stability. It has been described as accordion-like because it folds in and on itself during flexion. On the dorsal aspect of the joint, the common extensor tendon contributes to the PIP joint capsule fibers and the central slip. The lateral bands are extensions of the intrinsic muscles; they converge onto the dorsal aspect of the middle phalanx, forming the terminal portion of the extensor digitorum, which inserts onto the distal phalanx. These and the transverse retinacular ligament form the extensor mechanism of the PIP joint. The DIP joints are also hinge joints, which means that only flexion and extension occur at this joint. They also have collateral ligaments, but no volar plate.

Volar Hand: Flexor Zones

The volar, or palmar, surface of the hand, including the digits, is divided into five zones for easy identification of anatomical structures involved in injury (Figure 2-28). Zone 1 is distal to the FDS insertion. Zone 2 spans from the insertion of the FDS just distal to the PIP joint to the distal palmar crease near the metacarpal head. It is sometimes referred to as **no man's land** due to the challenge of repairing an injured flexor tendon and the other assorted structures in this zone. In Zone 2, the FDP and FDS travel in the same tendon sheath and are typically injured together. Zone 3 is within the palm itself and is often associated with neurovascular injury. Zone 4 is the carpal tunnel itself. Finally, Zone 5 is the area proximal to the wrist.

Dorsal Hand: Extensor Zones

The extensor tendons are also divided into zones (Figure 2-29). The eight zones are over the digits and hand, making for easy identification of anatomical structures involved. Odd-numbered zones (Zones 1, 3, 5, 7) correspond to the DIP, PIP, MCP, and wrist joints, and even-numbered zones (Zones 2, 4, 6, 8) correspond to the shafts of the bones (middle and proximal phalanges, metacarpals, radius, and ulna).

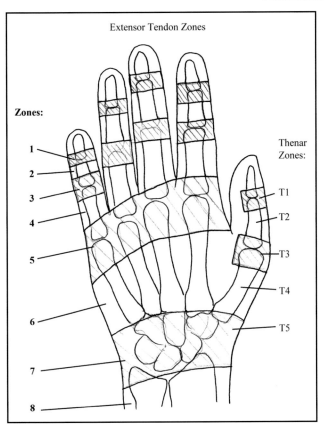

Figure 2-29. The dorsal aspect of the hand is similarly divided into eight zones to identify the extensor tendon(s) and other anatomical structures. (Illustration by Allie Cammarata.)

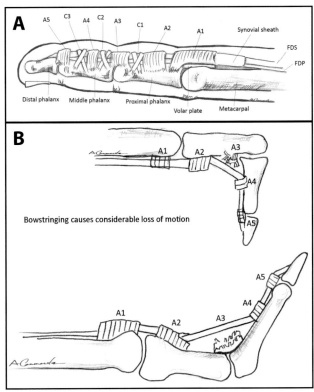

Figure 2-30. (A) The annular and cruciate pulleys of the digits help to hold the flexor tendons close to the joint axes of the MCP, PIP, and DIP joints during active movement. (B) Injury to one or more pulleys can cause bowstringing of the associated tendon(s) and considerable loss of joint movement.

Movement of the Digits

Flexion

The PIP joints flex by contraction of the FDS, and the DIP joints flex with contraction of the flexor digitorum profundus (FDP). The FDS and FDP tendons run together inside a tendon sheath into the fibro-osseous canal of each digit. The tendon sheath provides both lubrication and an important source of nutrition to the largely avascular tendons. The fibro-osseous canal is formed by the metacarpals and phalanges and by the unique pulley system and tendon sheath. The pulley system consists of five annular (circular) pulleys and three cruciate (cross-shaped) pulleys and functions to keep the flexor tendons close to the bone and joint axes during movement (Figure 2-30A). Their significance is in preventing **bowstringing** during active digit flexion. Bowstringing refers to loss of the critical pulley function causing movement of the flexor tendon away from the PIP joint's normal axis of motion during digit flexion. This can cause considerable loss of joint movement (Figure 2-30B).

The FDS tendon lies superficial to the FDP profundus until it reaches the first annular pulley in the vicinity of the metacarpal head. At that point, the profundus emerges through a split in the superficialis known as **Camper's chiasm**; this split allows the profundus to continue to its attachment on the volar surface of the distal phalanx, where it flexes the DIP joint. It also assists with PIP joint flexion. The two tendon slips of the superficialis attach onto the base of the middle phalanx, and thus flex the PIP joint.

Extension

The extensor mechanism of each finger is complex and made up of extensor tendons and multiple fibers and ligaments that are interwoven together and difficult to separate. Other nomenclature used to describe this structure include the extensor expansion, extensor or dorsal aponeurosis, and dorsal apparatus. The tendon components of this structure include the extensor digitorum communis on the dorsal aspect of each digit and the extensor indicis proprius and EDM for the second and fifth digits, respectively. The extensor digitorum communis attaches by a tendinous slip to the proximal phalanx, extending the MCP joint. The central slip, a continuation of the extensor tendon, attaches to the base of the middle phalanx and contributes to PIP extension. The lateral bands, coming from either side of the midline, contribute to extension of the PIP and DIP joints through their attachment to the extensor mechanism and the terminal tendon. The oblique retinacular ligament is a unique dorsal structure that attaches to the sides of the proximal phalanx on the volar surface and connects distally

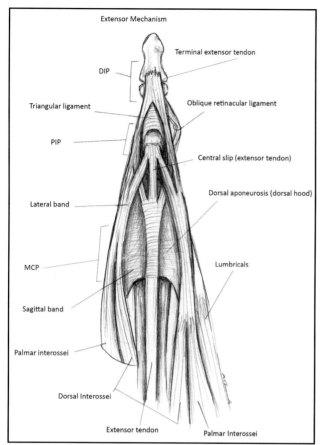

Figure 2-31. The extensor mechanism is complex and made up of the extensor tendon, ligaments, and multiple fibers intricately connected to provide balanced muscle forces across the MCP, PIP, and DIP joints.

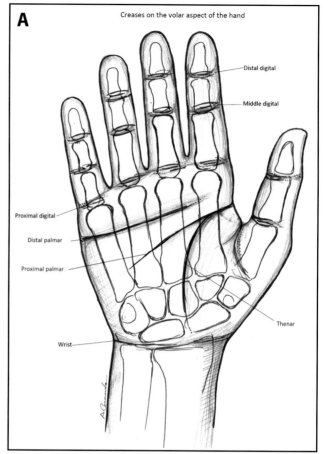

Figure 2-32. (A) Note the creases in the palm and volar aspect of the digits, and their relationship to the underlying joints. *(continued)*

to the lateral bands. It lies volar to the PIP joint's lateral axis and dorsal to the DIP joint's lateral axis. As a result of this unique configuration, it contributes to PIP flexion and DIP extension, connecting the two movements.

The intrinsic muscles (the lumbrical muscles and volar and dorsal interossei) contribute to extension of the PIP and DIP joints through their attachment onto the lateral bands and extensor mechanism. The lumbrical muscles are unique in that they originate from the FDP tendons in the palm and insert into the extensor expansion of each adjacent finger. Due to their origin from tendon and insertion into soft tissue, they act as a dynamic stabilizer between the digital flexors and extensors (Figure 2-31).

Abduction and Adduction

The movements of abduction and adduction of the digits is provided by the attachments of the volar and dorsal interossei. The dorsal interossei originate proximally between adjacent metacarpals and insert distally to the proximal phalanx or to the extensor mechanism. They produce MCP abduction and contribute to PIP and DIP extension. The palmar or volar interossei originate from a metacarpal

bone and insert distally to the proximal phalanx or to the extensor mechanism. They produce MCP adduction and contribute to PIP and DIP extension through the extensor mechanism.

Anatomical Landmarks

The practitioner should be able to identify and accommodate the pertinent anatomical landmarks when fabricating an orthosis for a client. The visible skin creases correspond to where the joints of the elbow, wrist, and hand move. These creases should be covered completely if the goal of the orthosis is to immobilize and stabilize a given joint. Conversely, creases that correspond to joint movement should be left uncovered to allow for full, unrestricted movement of joints not included in the orthosis, such as the thenar and distal palmar creases. Specifically, the thermoplastic material should be flared away from the thenar crease to allow the thenar muscles to contract; the distal palmar crease should be cleared completely to allow for full MCP joint flexion and fisting (Figure 2-32).

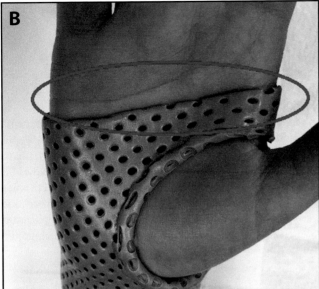

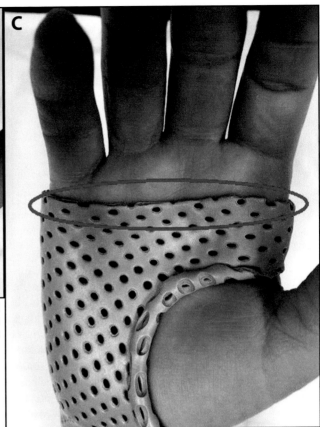

Figure 2-32 (continued). (B) Skin creases must be observed and cleared completely to allow for joints not included in the orthosis to move freely. (C) Skin creases that are covered by an orthosis will limit joint movement.

Wound Healing Principles and Tissue Response to Stress

Following injury, orthoses are often used as an intervention strategy and consequently influence healing of affected structures. It is important for the practitioner to have thorough knowledge of wound healing principles and how the healing structures respond to stresses placed upon them from an orthosis.

The correct choice of orthosis depends significantly on the stage of healing the client's tissue presents in at the time. Wounds of the body typically heal in a set pattern, known as the three main stages of healing (Box 2-3).

In stage 1, the *inflammatory phase*, initially all wounds and injuries cause an inflammatory reaction where edema and white blood cells invade the wound. This initial stage of healing can last less than 1 week but may take longer to resolve depending on the client's general health and the presence of complicating factors such as infections, number of tissues involved, and mechanism of injury. The first phase of healing requires protection and proper positioning for best healing of the injured part. The correct and most appropriate orthotic approach is typically immobilization to allow for rest and resolution of the edema.

Box 2-3. Stages of Healing

INFLAMMATORY PHASE

- Increased blood flow to area of injury; signs of inflammation, including erythema, heat, edema, and pain
- Use of orthoses to protect, support, position, and reduce pain and edema

PROLIFERATION OR FIBROPLASIA PHASE

- Formation of new granulation tissue with collagen and network of blood vessels; wound closure
- Active exercises and possibly light functional activities to help decrease edema and regain mobility

MATURATION OR REMODELING PHASE

- Final phase of wound healing when wound has closed; involves remodeling of collagen fibers to allow motion and gliding of tissues
- May need increased stretching and orthotic intervention to regain full ROM when limited by scar and shortening of soft tissue

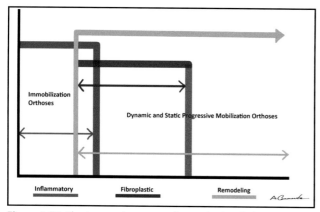

Figure 2-33. The type and purpose of an orthosis will depend on the stage of wound healing.

During the stage 2, the *fibroplasia phase*, the predominate cell type is the fibroblast, the cell that contributes to the collagen production for wound healing. The wound is full of new vascular growth and granulation tissue. This is laying the groundwork for the synthesis of new collagen tissue. The collagen tissue begins to synthesize and becomes stronger and more abundant. This phase of healing usually lasts about 4 to 6 weeks with a reduction in edema and pain and the beginning of restoration of movement and function in the involved extremity. Orthoses that apply a low load of force or stress on involved joints to improve PROM may be applied during this phase.

Stage 3, the last phase of healing, termed the *scar maturation phase* or *remodeling phase*, is where the scar collagen fibers increase, mature, and reorganize. It is in this phase that mobilization orthoses are most effective. However, care must be taken to avoid application of too much force; orthoses that apply excessive force can lead right back to a renewal of the inflammatory process. The connective tissue of the body responds most favorably to low loads of prolonged stress or force application. Practitioners can help to influence and promote the reorganization of this tissue to accommodate this stress and allow for patterns of joint motion critical to function.

It should be noted that the timing of each healing stage may vary according to the client's specific situation, general health and well-being, and individual reaction to the injury or trauma. The purpose of a given orthosis will determine its influence on the wound healing process. In general, immobilization orthoses are typically used during the first two stages of wound healing to rest and protect healing structures. Mobilization orthoses are typically applied in the late fibroplastic or remodeling phases to improve joint motion and lengthen soft tissue (Figure 2-33). However, there are instances where mobilization orthoses are used immediately following an injury or surgery. These include following flexor or extensor tendon repairs, joint arthroplasties (joint replacement), and muscle paralysis or weakness following injury to a peripheral nerve. These orthoses are discussed in more detail in Chapter 10.

Biomechanical Principles

Biomechanics is the study of mechanics, or forces, on the musculoskeletal system. Orthotic design and fabrication involve application of external forces on body structures with orthotic materials, so it is important for the practitioner to fully understand how these forces influence these structures. Doing so will optimize orthosis fit, comfort, durability, and effectiveness. Conversely, improper application of these principles can cause undue harm to the underlying subcutaneous tissues, resulting in pain and discomfort for the client, frustration for the practitioner and client, and potential loss of function. Effective orthotic design and fabrication requires knowledge and application of certain core biomechanical principles. These include the following:

- **Lever systems**
- Mechanical advantage
- Force type and distribution
- State of **equilibrium**

LEVER SYSTEMS

Most orthoses commonly used in UE rehabilitation represent lever systems that affect joint movement. A lever is a rigid structure or object that can rotate or move around a fixed axis when force is applied to it. There are three different types or classes of lever systems: **first**, **second**, and **third class**. Each lever system has the following three components:

1. The axis, or **fulcrum**
2. The **effort force**
3. The **resistance force**

Most orthoses used in UE clinical practice are first-class lever systems, and comprise three components, explained next.

Fulcrum

The specific joint that the orthosis immobilizes, or acts on, can be considered the fulcrum. For example, in a wrist immobilization orthosis, the wrist is the fulcrum. This is located between the effort force and resistance force, with the force of application opposite to the forces on either side.

Effort Force

This is the segment of the orthosis that provides the effort, or force, needed to support the fulcrum. It is typically the body segment proximal to the fulcrum. In the wrist orthosis example, the part of the orthosis proximal to the wrist that rests on the forearm is the effort force. For an orthosis that supports the elbow, the proximal portion on the arm is the effort force.

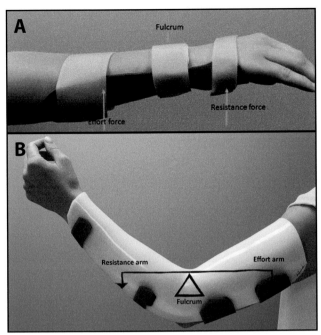

Figure 2-34. (A) A wrist immobilization orthosis represents a first-class lever system. (B) An elbow and wrist immobilization orthosis also represents a first-class lever system.

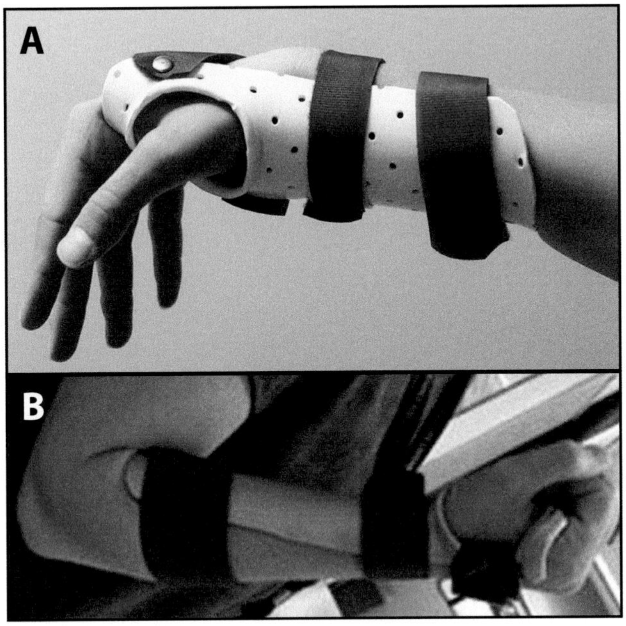

Figure 2-35. (A) Note the short effort arm on this wrist immobilization orthosis and how the wrist is not supported adequately. (B) Note the excessively long effort arm and how this can potentially impede full elbow movement.

Resistance Force

This is the segment of the orthosis that resists the effort force. It is typically the body segment distal to the fulcrum. Using the wrist orthosis as an example, the hand represents the resistance force. For the elbow orthosis example, the portion of the orthosis on the forearm and wrist is the resistance force (Figure 2-34).

All of the forces applied to body structures must be balanced in order for the orthosis to be effective and comfortable. More specifically, the effort force must equalize the resistance force in order to support the fulcrum effectively; a long and wide effort arm is needed to counteract and balance a shorter resistance arm. In the wrist orthosis example, the forearm component must be long and wide enough to support the hand and wrist effectively (see Figure 2-34A). If it is too short, the wrist will move in the orthosis when the client uses his or her hand. Unwanted forces will be created on the proximal and distal ends of the orthosis, making it uncomfortable for the client (Figure 2-35A). If the effort force is too long, it will potentially impede uninvolved joint motion (Figure 2-35B).

FORCE TYPES AND DISTRIBUTION

A well-designed orthosis should distribute forces evenly. This optimizes the comfort and effectiveness of the orthosis. Ill-fitting orthoses can create potentially damaging shear and compressive forces on tissues. Shear forces are created when two external forces are applied parallel to a

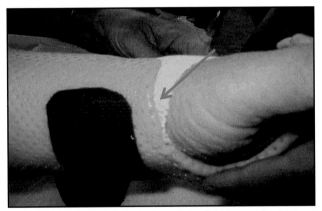

Figure 2-36. Pressure area over the radial styloid formed from a hand and wrist immobilization orthosis.

structure. Examples are development of a blister after wearing a new pair of shoes or on the ulnar styloid from unwanted movement of the orthosis on the wrist (Figure 2-36). Compressive forces are created when two forces are applied perpendicular to a structure, causing the two parts to come together. Examples of this type of force are development of skin redness from a wristwatch that is too tight or skin redness from ill-fitting straps (Figure 2-37). Finally, **tensile forces** are created when two forces are applied perpendicular to a structure, causing parts of a structure to pull apart. Examples of this type of force are forces created at the elbow when hanging from a monkey bar, or on application of tensile force to a fractured bone to facilitate healing (Figure 2-38).

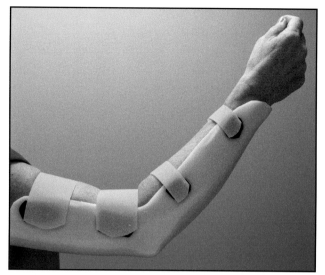

Figure 2-37. Pressure created by straps applied too tightly.

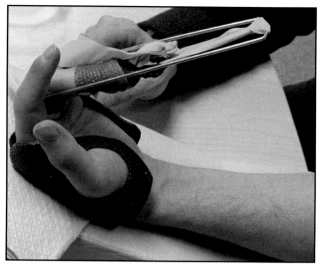

Figure 2-38. Tensile forces are created at the PIP joint with this specialized orthosis used to treat a complex finger fracture.

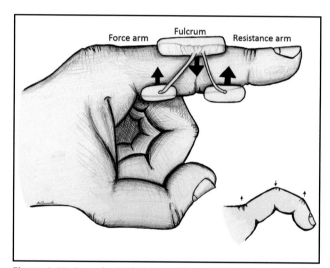

Figure 2-39. An orthosis that immobilizes a joint must provide balanced forces on either side of the joint to properly support the joint and optimize comfort and stability of the orthosis.

Principles of force distribution pertaining to orthotic design and fabrication include the following:

- Balanced effort and resistance arms = balanced lever system (Figure 2-39)
- Flared and smooth edges, especially on proximal and distal ends of orthosis
- For forearm-based orthoses, an effort arm that spans half the width and two-thirds the length of the forearm to distribute forces over a large surface area (Figure 2-40)
- Use of thermoplastic material that conforms well and evenly over body structures, particularly bony prominences, across hand arches, and over muscle tissues

- Use of wide, soft straps to distribute the forces over a large area
- Proper strap placement for optimal support and security

STATE OF EQUILIBRIUM

When an object is at rest and does not move, it is in a state of equilibrium. To effectively support a joint or other body structure, an orthosis must place that structure in equilibrium. Doing so optimizes comfort, effectiveness, and client compliance. Principles of equilibrium pertaining to orthotic design and fabrication are included in Box 2-4.

Summary

- Knowledge of the specific regional anatomy of the UE guides the practitioner to understand each clinical condition and how the orthotic intervention will contribute to the healing process.
- Knowledge of the stages of healing will allow the practitioner to determine which orthosis might be appropriate for the specific client's condition.
- Understanding the biomechanical principles of orthotic fabrication will help the practitioner to match the design and construction of the orthosis to adequately support the intended anatomical structures.
- This chapter offers a general review of the UE anatomy; the reader is encouraged to seek out more explicit details to match individual needs.

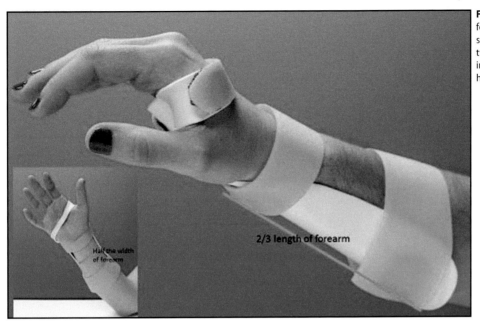

Figure 2-40. The effort arm of most forearm-based immobilization orthoses should span half the width and two-thirds the length of the forearm in order to support the wrist (and/or hand) adequately.

Box 2-4. Principles of Equilibrium for Orthotic Design

LEVER SYSTEM COMPONENT	EFFECT/CONSEQUENCE
• Effort arm too short	• Allows fulcrum to move
• Effort arm too long	• Impedes uninvolved joint motion
• Resistance arm too short	• Does not support the fulcrum effectively
• Resistance arm too long	• Immobilizes joints unnecessarily
• Straps too narrow	• May create excessive pressure on underlying tissue
• Straps too wide	• May not match and conform to anatomy
• Use circumferential straps when appropriate	• Provide optimal security of orthosis to anatomy

Test Your Knowledge

1. Explain how the anatomy of the UE might influence the orthotic design.

2. Explain why it is important to contour an orthosis to match the arches of the hand.

3. Identify the three components of a lever system and explain how this contributes to well-constructed orthoses.

4. Describe the three phases of wound healing.

5. Draw an example of an orthosis that represents a first-class lever system.

6. Describe how the mechanical advantage might be affected by orthotic design.

Suggested Reading

Coppard, B. M., & Lohman, H. (2014). *Introduction to orthotics: A clinical reasoning and problem-solving approach* (4th ed.). St. Louis, MO: Elsevier Mosby.

Drake, R. L., Vogl, A. W., & Mitchell, A. W. M. (2005). *Gray's anatomy for students*. St. Louis, MO: Elsevier Health Sciences.

Fess, E., Gettle, K., Philips, C., & Janson, J. R. (2005). Mechanical principles. In *Hand and upper extremity splinting: Principles and methods* (3rd ed., pp. 161-184). St. Louis, MO: Elsevier Mosby.

Jacobs, M. A., & Austin, N. M. (2014). *Orthotic intervention for the hand and upper extremity* (2nd ed.). Baltimore, MD: Lippincott Williams & Wilkins.

Jenkins, D. B. (2002). *Hollingshead's functional anatomy of the limbs and back* (8th ed.). Philadelphia, PA: Saunders.

Lippert, L. S. (2011). *Clinical kinesiology and anatomy* (5th ed.). Philadelphia, PA: F.A. Davis Company.

Schultz-Johnson, K. (1996). Splinting the wrist: Mobilization and protection. *Journal of Hand Therapy, 9*(2), 165-177.

The Basics

Key Terms

Activation time	Memory	Thermoplastic
Conformability/drapability	Resistance to stretch	Velcro hook
Low-temperature thermoplastic material (LTTM)	Rigidity	Velcro loop
	Surface impressionability	Working time

Learning Outcomes

Upon completion of this chapter, you will be able to:

1. List and describe different characteristics of thermoplastic materials used for orthotic fabrication.

2. Describe methods for testing each of the thermoplastic material characteristics.

3. Outline the equipment needed to design and fabricate an orthosis.

4. Describe three safety precautions to consider when fabricating an orthosis.

5. Describe three ergonomic considerations for the orthotic fabrication process.

6. Outline the steps involved when designing an orthosis.

7. Outline the steps of pattern making.

8. List the steps involved in evaluating a completed orthosis.

Introduction

Today, practitioners take advantage of the multitude of products and materials available on the market for orthotic fabrication. **Low-temperature thermoplastic material (LTTM)** is the most commonly used material for orthotic fabrication by occupational therapists, occupational therapy assistants, and physical therapists. By definition, **thermoplastic** means materials that are activated by heat. They become softened and can be molded and formed around body parts. As they cool, they harden in whatever shape they have been formed. Temperatures for heating LTTM range between 140° to 160°F (60° to 65°C) and are tolerated well on the skin. LTTM is available in a wide variety of thicknesses, colors, and styles. Orthoses can also be formed from neoprene and other fabric-like materials or from a combination of thermoplastic and fabric-like materials. Practitioners should continually educate themselves on what new materials are available. Newer products typically offer some advantage over older materials. For example, new products might have longer **working times** (the material stays soft longer to allow the practitioner more time to

Schofield, K., & Schwartz, D. *Orthotic Design and Fabrication for the Upper Extremity: A Practical Guide* (pp 41-53).

mold the orthosis), quicker **activation times** (the time it takes for the thermoplastic material to soften), more color choices, and even lighter-weight versions than older materials. Moreover, practitioners should become familiar with the different characteristics of materials, the advantages and disadvantages of each characteristic, and the clinical utility and applicability of each. Sales representatives and product specialists from each company that sell orthotic materials and supplies are good sources of information about the products they carry.

Characteristics of Low-Temperature Thermoplastic Material

LTTM typically comes in 18 x 24-inch sheets. It is available for purchase in single sheets, double sheets, or cases of four sheets. Extra-large sheets are also available in 24 x 36-inch sizes. Samples can also be ordered in 6 x 9-inch or 9 x 12-inch sizes when a single orthosis is to be fabricated or for testing an unfamiliar product.

It is critical to be familiar with the various characteristics of the different materials. Each type of material offers the practitioner different benefits for making an orthosis that is appropriate for a particular client and his or her specific condition. Learning how to work with different materials takes time and is as important as understanding the specifics of a client's condition and the most appropriate treatment protocol that applies to a particular client. Selecting the proper LTTM for a specific orthosis will make the fabrication process easier. The client will also likely be more comfortable wearing the orthosis and more inclined to adhere to the prescribed wearing schedule. Refer to Table 3-1 for a summary of LTTM.

The following terms are the key characteristics of LTTM:

- **Memory**: Memory refers to the ability of the material to return to its original size and shape once it has been stretched out and then reactivated/reheated (Figure 3-1). Orthoses that require frequent remolding should be made from materials with high memory because the material will revert back to the original pattern size. This is a good feature for the new practitioner as well because the orthosis can be remolded if necessary without needing to use additional material.

- **Rigidity**: This refers to how strong and supportive the material is on its own (Figure 3-2). Materials with high rigidity are best suited for larger orthoses, larger clients, and those clients who present with strong deforming forces such as high muscle tone. Less rigid materials are better suited for smaller clients and smaller body parts.

- **Resistance to stretch**: This refers to how easy or difficult it is to stretch the material around the body part

(Figure 3-3). Material with high resistance to stretch will require a firm handling of the material in order to work with it, whereas material with low resistance to stretch requires a gentle handling approach because the material is likely to stretch beyond the needed size. Low-resistance materials tend to have more drapability and conform well to intricate anatomical features. Care is required with handling not to overstretch these materials during orthotic fabrication because they rarely have memory and cannot be remolded easily.

- **Conformability/drapability**: These two terms refer to the ability of the material to conform or drape and mold around contours of the individual's anatomy (see Figure 3-3). Material with high conformability will mold easily around joints and bony prominences without much effort, letting gravity assist. Material with limited conformability and drape should not be selected for intimate fitting orthoses. These low-conforming materials may be better suited for larger orthoses where a high degree of conformability is not required.

- **Surface impressionability**: This refers to the surface of the material and whether it easily marks up with fingerprints and etching or has a dense and strong surface that is not easily marked (Figure 3-4). Softer materials may easily be left with indentations and marks from the practitioner's fingerprints as the material is handled. This can create pressure on the inside of the orthosis and adversely affect the appearance of the completed orthosis. Materials with a matte or glossy finish are collectively easier to handle but tend to be more rigid and less conformable.

Other important variations in LTTM are reflected in the thickness, the presence or absence of a nonstick coating, and the presence or absence of perforations:

- Thickness: LTTM is typically available in several thicknesses: 1/8 inch, 3/32 inch, 1/12 inch, and 1/16 inch (Figure 3-5). The thickness of the material will have a direct effect on the rigidity of the finished orthosis. In general terms, the practitioner should select a thicker material to support a larger body part or make a large multiple joint orthosis and a thin material to support a smaller client or a smaller body part. Forearm- and hand-based orthoses may be fabricated from medium-weight materials, but thick and thin materials may also be used. Use thinner materials for small pediatric orthoses, finger orthoses, circumferential orthoses, and for clients who need light support as appropriate.

- Solid or perforated: LTTM comes in a large assortment of solid or perforated patterns and designs. Perforated materials allow ventilation of the skin and may be more comfortable for clients in warmer climates or for those who perspire a great deal, have open wounds, or have very sensitive skin. Each manufacturing company calls the perforation patterns by different terminology

Table 3-1

TYPES OF LOW-TEMPERATURE THERMOPLASTIC MATERIAL AND THEIR APPLICATIONS

MATERIAL FEATURES	HANDLING	APPLICATIONS
Elastic materials with full memory and elasticity	Typically, latex-free products turn translucent or shiny when heated. They offer a moderate resistance to stretch. Available in 1/8-, 1/12-, and 1/16-inch thicknesses. Can be coated (not sticky) or noncoated (sticky). Resistant to finger printing. Require no reinforcing and are self-bonding.	Orthoses that will require remolding on subsequent visits (for positioning changes, edema management, and similar indications). Appropriate for all small finger orthoses, thumb orthoses, resting hand orthoses, wrist and wrist/thumb orthoses, and circumferential designs and large orthoses (elbow, knee, long arm, ankle/foot), as well as for AFOs and fracture bracing depending on material thickness.
Plastic materials with high drape and conformability	These have excellent conformability and drape but minimal memory and low rigidity. May have low to moderate resistance to fingerprinting. Use gravity to assist in orthotic fabrication. Available in 1/8-, 1/12-, and 1/16-inch thicknesses.	Appropriate for the fabrication of large to very small orthoses, depending on the thickness of the material, but require care in handling large pieces. Good choice for wrist orthoses, wrist/thumb orthoses, hand-based orthoses, and all orthoses where excellent conformity and intimate fit are required.
Rubber-based materials	Can be worked aggressively without fingerprinting. These products offer excellent rigidity without reinforcement. Some can be softened in a hot-air oven as well as in hot water. Heat in oven at 175°F (80°C) for 2 to 3 minutes.	Ideal for medium to large orthoses such as antispasticity orthoses and contracture management, functional position orthoses, resting mitt orthoses, back supports, body jackets, and shoe orthotics.
Materials with moderate to high resistance to stretch and excellent rigidity	Excellent resistance to markings and fingerprints. Materials can withstand firm handling during fabrication. Maintain positioning even against high tone and spasticity. Maximum resistance to stretch. Some have memory and some do not. Need to test for this.	Appropriate for most types of orthoses, especially large and rigid orthoses and orthoses for spasticity, including long arm orthoses, elbow orthoses, forearm orthoses, wrist orthoses, and wrist/thumb orthoses. Might also be a good choice of material for back bracing and ankle supports.
Lightweight materials	Lightweight products that might weigh 15% to 30% less than other materials.	Finger, toe, and thumb orthoses, hand- and wrist-based orthoses. Lightweight wrist orthoses are especially suited for pediatric clients.
Silicone products and inserts	Latex-free products that can be combined with LTTM.	Indications for use are burns and hypertrophic scars.
LTTM in rolls of different widths	These products offer great moldability, conformability, and rigidity. No need to make a pattern; just cut and wrap around the limb. Rigidity is increased by the addition of multiple layers.	All types of finger orthoses and hand-based orthoses and some types of wrist and forearm supports, built up handles for utensils and functional aids for ADL.

Abbreviations: ADL, activities of daily living; AFO, ankle-foot orthosis.

Figure 3-1. Example of LTTM with memory.

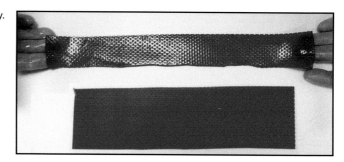

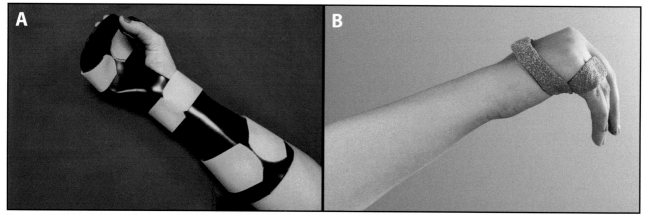

Figure 3-2. (A) Rigid LTTM provides needed support to counteract large opposing forces (such as a heavy, large hand or clients who have spasticity). (B) Less rigid materials are more suited for smaller orthoses or those that require an intimate fit.

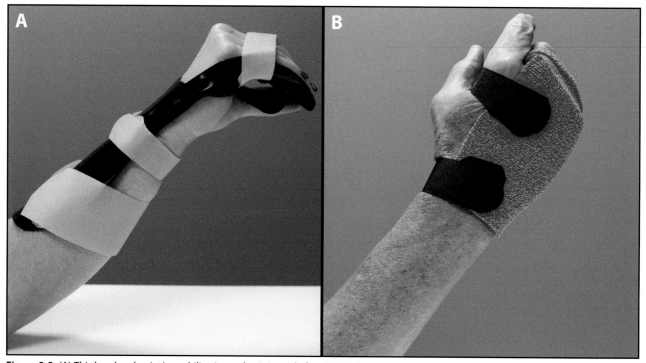

Figure 3-3. (A) This hand and wrist immobilization orthosis is made from LTTM that is resistant to stretch. The material does not conform as well around bony prominences and other anatomical landmarks but provides the necessary support for immobilizing large hands or multiple joints. (B) This hand-based fourth- and fifth-digit immobilization orthosis (also known as an *ulnar gutter*) is made from LTTM that is less rigid and conforms well over the metacarpophalangeal joints and the arches of the hand.

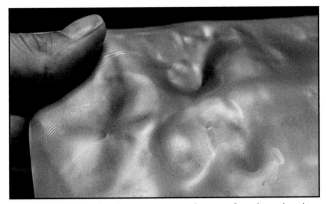

Figure 3-4. Note that fingerprints can be transferred to the thermoplastic material. Always handle the material using broad, smooth strokes to avoid this.

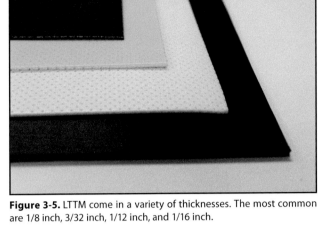

Figure 3-5. LTTM come in a variety of thicknesses. The most common are 1/8 inch, 3/32 inch, 1/12 inch, and 1/16 inch.

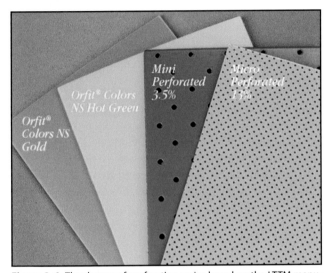

Figure 3-6. The degree of perforation varies based on the LTTM manufacturer. Note the descriptors used: microperforated and mini perforated.

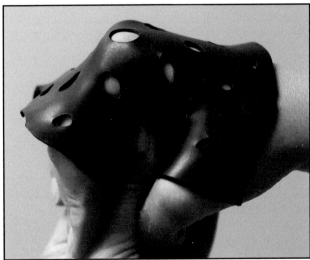

Figure 3-7. A localized area of weakness may be created when perforated material is stretched. A solid material may be more suitable.

and names. Materials may also vary in the amount of perforations present (Figure 3-6). Make sure to check the supplier's catalog or website to verify the desired perforation style. Solid materials have no perforations, offer more rigidity, and may be more suited for orthoses where the material requires significant stretching to conform to the body part. Stretching perforated materials may cause a localized area of weakness in the material (Figure 3-7).

- Nonstick coating: Most materials today are coated to allow greater ease in handling. The coating can be removed when desired by scraping, sanding, filing, or with using a special solvent. Removing the coating before bonding straps, adhering two pieces of LTTM together, or attaching outriggers is important. Material that is not coated may be very sticky and tacky on the skin, but it bonds more easily to outriggers and

attachments. Newer coatings claim to be antibacterial and may be more resistant to smells and dirt.

- Working and activation time: Each material has a specific activation time prior to molding and an optimum working time after activation in hot water (150° to 160°F [60° to 65°C]). Typically, this allows the practitioner ample time to mold the material into the proper position before the material begins to harden. The practitioner should check the information provided by the manufacturer for specific information for each product.

  ∘ Thicker material (3.2 mm or 1/8 inch) will take longer to activate and remain soft and malleable for longer than thinner material (1.6 mm or 1/16 inch).

  ∘ Thicker material should be slightly warmed or softened prior to cutting out patterns, then reheated fully prior to molding.

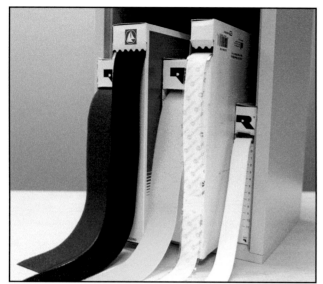

Figure 3-8. Velcro strapping come in a variety of colors, sizes, and material choices.

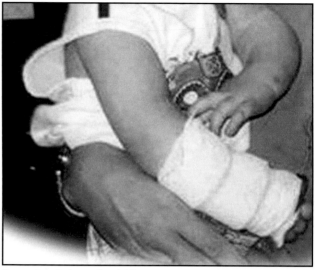

Figure 3-9. Orthoses for children may need to be designed to discourage them from removing the orthosis, such as using Coban wrap (3M) or an Ace bandage (3M) or covering the orthosis with stockinette.

TESTING OF LOW-TEMPERATURE THERMOPLASTIC MATERIAL

If a practitioner is unsure of the characteristics of any LTTM, it is relatively easy to perform several quick tests to learn its specific properties. Refer to the Appendix at the end of the chapter for step-by-step instructions on how to test the different properties of LTTM.

MATERIAL MANUFACTURERS AND DISTRIBUTORS

LTTM is manufactured and distributed by a variety of different companies. Each company's website is a valuable source of information. The reader is encouraged to check these for new product information, techniques for working with materials, and instructions. In addition to LTTM, these companies carry most of the additional materials and products necessary for orthotic fabrication.

Strapping Materials

Strapping materials should hold the orthosis securely onto the relevant body part so that the orthosis does not move on the client's extremity. Strapping must be sized according to the size of the body part. Strapping generally comes in 1- and 2-inch widths but can be cut to lesser widths as needed. Strapping is typically cut from **Velcro loop** (Velcro BVBA), and adhesive **Velcro hook** is placed on the orthosis to anchor the Velcro loop straps. There is a wide choice of colors, sizes, and materials that can be used as strapping (Figure 3-8).

Special attention to strapping is indicated for certain conditions. Curious children may take their orthoses off when they should be left on. In this case, modifications can be made to the straps so young children cannot remove their orthoses (Figure 3-9). Clients with arthritis may have difficulty pulling on the strapping to don and doff their orthoses, and adaptations to the strapping methods to make them easier to handle may be required (Figure 3-10).

- Velcro loop: Loop is available in different widths (1/2 inch, 1 inch, or 2 inches) and a variety of colors. Straps can be cut easily to customize width and accommodate for particular client needs. This material is very durable and strong but often needs to be replaced as straps get lost or become dirty.

- Velcro hook: Hook, as with loop, is also available in different widths and colors. It is most commonly sold with an adhesive back so it adheres easily to the orthosis itself.

- Velfoam (Alimed), neoprene, and other soft materials: These types of materials are useful for clients with sensitive or enlarged bony prominences, sensitive skin, or open or fragile wounds, and for young children.

Work Space Requirements and Ergonomic Considerations

Prior to orthotic fabrication, the practitioner will need to have a proper work space and all of the necessary equipment and materials available to him or her. Preparation and design of this work space will depend on the following:

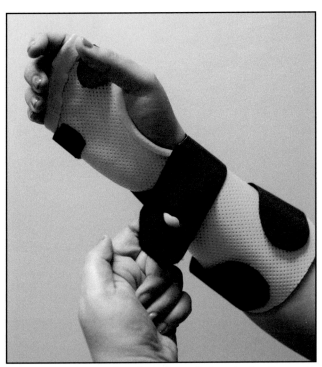

Figure 3-10. Straps can be adapted to make it easier for clients with arthritis to apply and remove their orthoses.

Box 3-1. Ergonomic Considerations

- Have all materials and equipment within reach.
- Have your client seated comfortably near the splint pan.
- Position the client's extremity in the correct position prior to removing the material from the splint pan.
- Position yourself close enough to the client's extremity so that you are not compromising your back or neck as you fabricate the orthosis.

- The department budget (for capital equipment and ongoing supply costs)
- The approximate number of orthoses made each month
- Types of orthoses made. Materials used for pediatric clients will differ from those used for adults, as will materials used for clients with neurological impairments compared with orthopedic conditions. Choice of material color, thickness, weight, memory, and rigidity, as well as different strapping materials, will allow the practitioner to customize the orthosis to his or her client's particular needs. Conversely, precut orthotic patterns save time, are more suitable for practitioners with less experience, and are useful in settings where only one or two types of orthoses are made (such as resting hand and wrist orthoses). Keep in mind that specialty materials typically cost more; selecting materials that meet the needs of the majority of clients will keep costs down and standing inventory fluid.
- Practitioner experience. Prefabricated orthoses and precut materials will be easier for those with little or no experience with orthotic fabrication. Practitioners need to consider the cost and whether these products will meet their clients' needs when making decisions about which type of orthoses to provide.

If necessary, a rolling cart with all necessary equipment is useful in acute care settings because it allows practitioners to fabricate an orthosis in a client's room. A separate space allocated specifically to orthotic fabrication is more suitable in an outpatient clinic where orthoses are provided on a regular basis and clients are positioned easily near the equipment. Outpatient settings where orthoses are provided on a less frequent basis may find portable equipment more useful so available space can be used judiciously.

Ergonomic considerations apply not only to the client receiving an orthosis, but also to the practitioner who is making the orthosis (Box 3-1).

Equipment Essentials

Proper equipment and supplies are essential when considering orthotic design and fabrication (Box 3-2).

Safety Considerations

It is important for the practitioner to be careful around sources of heat. Splint pans and heat guns are electrical appliances that are potential causes of injury if not attended to correctly. Cover the splint pan with a lid when it is not in use to minimize water evaporation and prevent steam from heating up the work space. Turn the heat gun to the cool setting when finished. Fellow colleagues and clients can be injured if the practitioner is not attentive to these details. Be careful around sharp objects! You will be working with scissors, knives, and other assorted cutting tools. Never leave them unattended on the table or counter. Clients, especially children, can harm themselves when picking up these instruments. Sharp tools should always be supervised. Check the water temperature and the material before placing activated LTTM directly on the client. The client's skin may be more sensitive due to the effect of the injury, the disease process, or his or her emotional state.

It is important to maintain all equipment in proper working order. Make sure to clean the splint pan regularly, turn off appliances when they are not in use, and keep the work area clean and uncluttered. Always clean and put away any tools when finished. Throw scraps of material away so

Box 3-2. Equipment Essentials

SPLINT PANS OR HEAT PANS

Choices include specialty splint pans from distributors or a small, commercially available electric skillet or frying pan. A hydrocollator is also a suitable option. This works well for most orthoses. Specialized mesh material can be used to place over the hot packs so the material does not stick or fall through the metal slots while heating (Figure 3-11). Keep in mind that the water can be too hot for some thermoplastic materials and is often dirty.

HEAT GUN

Essential for spot heating material and finishing edges (Figure 3-12).

SCISSORS

Most important piece of equipment for a practitioner to have! It is important to invest in a few good pairs of scissors specifically for orthotic fabrication. They need to be sharp, easy to clean, and durable. Allocate one pair for the LTTM and straps and another for cutting adhesive Velcro. The adhesive sticks to the scissor blades and makes it difficult to cut the LTTM smoothly. Consider having a smaller pair on hand, along with bandage scissors for cutting plaster of Paris material and smaller orthoses (Figure 3-13).

TOWELS

Necessary for drying the material when it comes out of the hot water. Some practitioners place a pillowcase on top of towels to avoid having the towel fibers adhere to or leave imprints on the LTTM. Others prefer to lay the material directly on the counter and blot dry with a towel.

MESH OR LINER FOR PANS

Prevents the LTTM from sticking to the heating source (see Figure 3-11).

SPATULA

Useful for removing the material from the splint pan.

PATTERN-MARKING PENS

Wax pencils are helpful for drawing patterns on material. An awl also works well and does not mark the material as much. Avoid using permanent markers, pens, and lead pencils because the marks cannot be removed once the orthosis is made.

OTHER

Hammer, needle-nose pliers, awl, hole puncher, X-ACTO knife (Elmer's Products), sewing machine for custom-made straps.

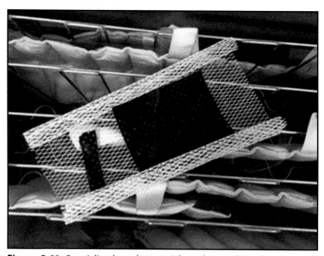

Figure 3-11. Specialized mesh material can be used to place over the hot packs so the material does not stick or fall through the metal slots while heating. (Reprinted with permission from Chris Reynolds, PT, CHT.)

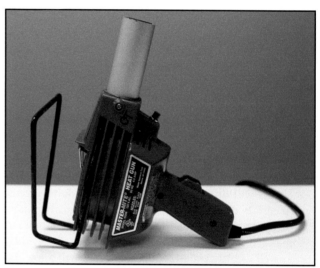

Figure 3-12. A heat gun.

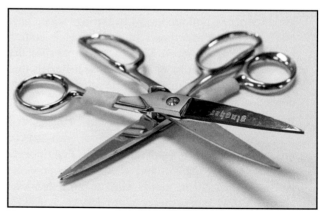

Figure 3-13. Scissors for cutting LTTM and small scissors.

they do not interfere with the process. Keep the work space neat and clean for fellow colleagues and clients.

Orthotic Fabrication Methods

The instructional videos that accompany this textbook will highlight the specific anatomical landmarks, pattern making, and step-by-step fabrication instructions. The general process is described next.

Orthotic Fabrication Steps

1. Pattern making
2. Material selection
3. Client positioning
4. Molding techniques
5. Finishing steps
6. Orthosis evaluation and check-out

Orthotic fabrication begins after the practitioner has determined which design is most suited to the client's condition, specific needs, and physician referral specifications. The process starts with designing the pattern, followed by selecting the LTTM, positioning the client, activating and molding the LTTM to the client, fitting and adjusting the orthosis, applying straps, and ending with an evaluation of the orthosis for fit and comfort. The final step in this process is educating the client on the purpose, wearing schedule, and care of the orthosis.

PATTERN MAKING

Pattern making is essential for designing an effective orthosis. This process allows the practitioner to visualize the completed orthosis, use the appropriate amount of material, and custom fit the orthosis to the individual client. In this way, mistakes, improper sizing, and wasting of materials are avoided. The client places his or her involved hand on a paper towel. If he or she is unable to do this due to pain or discomfort, the opposite hand may be used. In some instances, the practitioner's hand can be used if necessary, and the resultant pattern checked and adjusted accordingly on the client's hand. Sizing corrections are then made to the pattern before tracing the pattern onto the LTTM.

General pattern-making steps for forearm-based orthoses include the following:

- Draw an outline of the entire hand, digits, and thumb and mark the relevant anatomical landmarks on the paper pertaining to the orthotic design.

- Beginners should mark both sides of the wrist (ulnar head and radial styloid), 2 inches distal to the anterior elbow crease (this corresponds to approximately

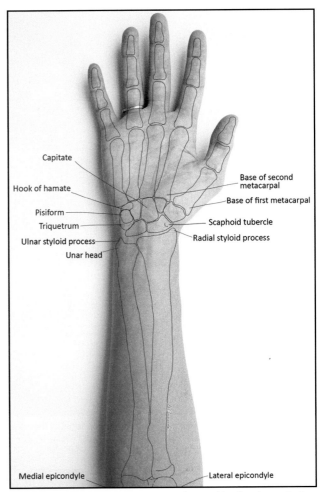

Figure 3-14. An example of common anatomical landmarks used when making forearm-based orthoses.

two-thirds the length of the forearm), the metacarpophalangeal (MCP) joints of the second and fifth digits, and the first web space. Other anatomical landmarks include the carpometacarpal joint of the thumb and the web space between the second and third digits; these are used for the wrist and hand immobilization orthosis pattern. Mark these landmarks regularly on all patterns until you become more familiar with what specific points you need for each orthosis (Figure 3-14). (The relevant anatomical landmarks will be clearly marked for each orthotic design in the instructional videos.)

- When drawing the forearm, it is helpful to place the marking pen at a 45-degree angle to the paper to mark extra width along the forearm lines. This will ensure that enough material is available to cover at least half the circumference of the forearm's width. Alternatively, you can use the tip of your small finger as a guide to measure the wrist and forearm width: two finger widths on both sides the wrist, and three on both sides of the proximal forearm (Figure 3-15).

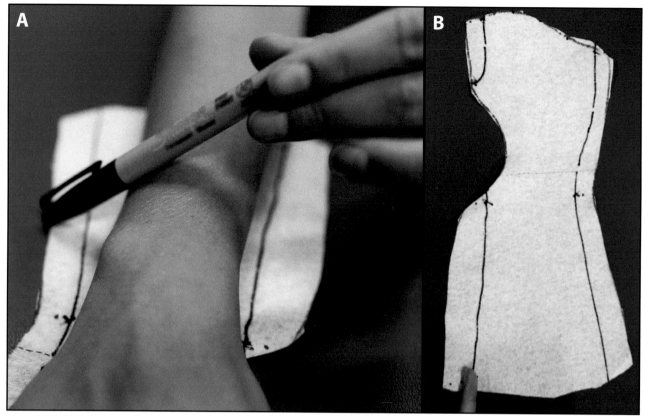

Figure 3-15. (A) Hold the marking pen at a 45-degree angle to the wrist and forearm to ensure that the orthosis is at least half the width of the wrist and forearm. (B) Use the small fingertip to approximate the width of the forearm, wrist, and hand.

MATERIAL SELECTION

A variety of factors are important to consider when selecting an appropriate LTTM. These include the material thickness, degree of conformability and stretch, presence of memory, and material color.

- Thickness
  - ◦ 1/8 inch, 3.2 mm solid or perforated. This is preferable for clients who require rigidity and support.
  - ◦ 3/32 inch, 2.4 mm, or 1/12 inch. This is preferable for smaller clients or for conditions needing less rigid support, and for circumferential designs (the additional material on both the volar and dorsal surfaces provides adequate support for the wrist).
  - ◦ 1/16 inch, 1.6 mm. This is for pediatric clients or for conditions needing light support, and for circumferential designs (the additional material on both the volar and dorsal surfaces provides adequate support for the wrist).
- Good conformability and drape
- Moderate degree of stretch
- Memory for conditions requiring frequent adjustments

- Colored material for client preference to optimize client compliance and adherence to wearing schedule of orthosis

CLIENT POSITIONING

- The client should be seated with the elbow resting comfortably on table, preferably near the splint pan.
- The practitioner should have easy access to the client's extremity. Often, the corner of the table allows for the best access. The client's forearm should be in supination to allow gravity to assist with molding the wrist and forearm.
- The client's wrist should be positioned in neutral to slight extension (unless his or her condition requires a different position).
- The client's digits should be relaxed to allow the material to conform to the hand arches. This also allows the wrist to fall comfortably into extension. Try to avoid having the client extend the digits during molding; this tends to flatten the hand arches (Figure 3-16).

See the demonstration video for more information.

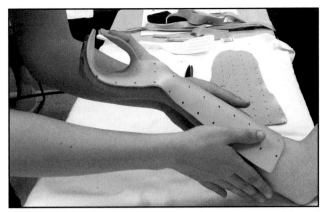

Figure 3-16. Place the client's forearm in supination when possible, and allow the client to relax the fingers during the molding process. This will allow the material to conform well to the contours of the wrist and forearm with gravity and conform to the hand arches, which allows the wrist to rest in slight extension.

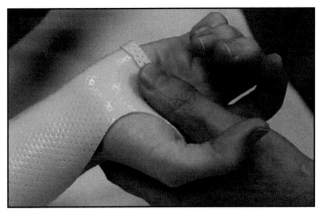

Figure 3-17. Placing your hand through the client's web space and your thumb lightly in the middle of the palm just proximal to the distal palmar crease will help maintain the wrist position and facilitate proper molding of the LTTM in the palm.

MOLDING TECHNIQUES

General instructions for molding are as follows:

1. Check the water temperature in the splint pan and make sure it is 150° to 160°F. Water that is too hot will overheat the LTTM, which can cause the material to overstretch and imprint more easily. Water that is not hot enough will not activate the LTTM adequately. Place the material in the water. Typical activation time is 45 to 60 seconds; thicker material takes longer, and thinner material takes less time.

2. Remove the LTTM from the hot water by lifting one corner out with a spatula, and then carefully lift the material out using both hands. Transfer it to a flat working surface nearby. It is helpful to have a pillowcase or towel on this surface to help absorb the excess water. A pillowcase is preferable because warm LTTM can pick up the imprint of the towel. Avoid holding the material vertically when removing it from the splint pan because it will stretch too much. Additionally, do not transfer the material from the pan to the working surface with the spatula. This will leave imprints.

3. Dry briefly on a towel or pillowcase. If a sticky LTTM is being used, transfer material directly to a nonporous surface and pat dry. Be careful not to press down firmly on the towel because the material will stick to it and may pick up unwanted lint from the towel. As mentioned, a pillowcase can be placed over the towel surface to avoid these problems.

4. Check the temperature of the LTTM prior to placing it on the client. This can be done by testing it on your own forearm or placing it lightly on the client's skin.

5. Accommodate for bony prominences (e.g., the ulnar head or radial styloid) by padding these areas with TheraPutty (Fabrication Enterprises, Inc.) or other padding material prior to molding. Alternatively, these areas can be addressed by flaring the areas prior to removing the orthosis or spot heating with a heat gun and bumping the material outward while maintaining the position until the material cools.

6. Place the LTTM on the client's hand. Take care to align the material in the center of the palm and/or wrist and forearm and mold carefully in the palm to accommodate for the hand arches. Take care not to stretch the material too much proximally or distally.

7. Use broad, smooth strokes with your hands to avoid fingerprints and indentations. Positioning the forearm in supination allows the LTTM to conform to the forearm and hand with the help of gravity and allows the wrist and digits rest in a functional position (wrist extension, relaxed digit flexion). This helps to preserve the hand arches during molding. It is helpful to place your hand through the client's first web space and hold your thumb lightly in the middle of the client's palm just proximal to the distal palmar crease. This will help control the wrist position and accommodate for the hand arches (Figure 3-17).

FINISHING TECHNIQUES: EDGES AND STRAPPING

Strapping must always be matched to the size of the client. For most adults, straps should be 1.5 inches wide at the wrist and proximal forearm to optimize security of the orthosis and assist in force distribution. Proximal strapping should be angled to accommodate the muscles of the forearm. Straps placed circumferentially at the wrist optimize wrist support and security. For straps across the metacarpals of the hand, care should be taken to position this strap just proximal to the metacarpal heads and align it

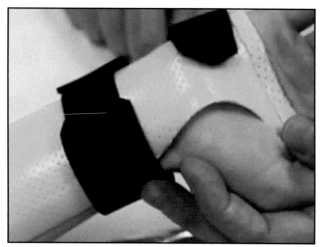

Figure 3-18. Be sure to cover the Velcro hook completely with the strapping material to enhance security of the strap on the orthosis. Exposed hook Velcro can also snag on clothing or blankets, and this should be avoided.

correctly (higher on the radial side, lower on the ulnar side of the hand). The adhesive hook Velcro should be covered completely with the strapping material. This will avoid the Velcro from snagging on clothing or blankets and will make the straps more secure. Be sure to round strap corners (Figure 3-18).

ORTHOSIS EVALUATION AND CHECK-OUT

It is critical for the practitioner to evaluate the finished orthosis to ensure that it meets the needs of the client. The following points should be considered upon completion of an orthosis:

- Is the orthosis comfortable?
- Does the orthosis cause any discomfort? Are there any red areas on the client's skin upon removal of the orthosis?
- Does the orthosis allow for full mobility of joints not included in the orthosis?
- Does the client understand the purpose and wearing schedule of the orthosis?
- Does the client understand how to care for the orthosis?
- Does the client know whom to contact if he or she has questions about the orthosis?

Summary

- Knowledge of the important characteristics of LTTM will help the practitioner choose the most appropriate material for each client and treatment protocol.

- A clinic must ensure adequate working space and appropriate equipment to enable the fabrication of orthoses for clients.
- Safety precautions for clients and practitioners are important when working with heated equipment and sharp instruments.
- Ergonomic considerations are important to protect both client and practitioner from unnecessary strain and discomfort during the fabrication process.
- Pattern making should be practiced often until the practitioner is familiar with all of the important anatomical landmarks.

Test Your Knowledge

SHORT ANSWER

1. Identify three to four safety precautions that pertain to orthotic fabrication.
2. Explain three to four ergonomic considerations that pertain to orthotic fabrication.
3. List the equipment needed to design and fabricate a custom orthosis.
4. Suggest a scenario in which a practitioner might offer a client soft strapping.
5. List the pattern-making process in four to five steps.

MULTIPLE CHOICE

6. When discussing LTTM, the term *drapability* refers to the material's ability to:
   a. Shrink to a smaller size
   b. Be remolded again and again
   c. Return to its former size after stretching
   d. Conform to the anatomy

7. When discussing LTTM, the term *surface impression-ability* refers to:
   a. The coating of the material.
   b. Whether there are fingerprints in the material.
   c. The color of the material.
   d. The ability of the material to become activated.

8. When discussing LTTM, the term *resistance to stretch* refers to:
   a. The coating of the material.
   b. How easy or difficult it is to pull the material.
   c. How easy or difficult it is to drape the material.
   d. The ability of the material to become activated.

9. A client with a very edematous wrist may require an orthosis made from a material that has _____ so that the orthosis can be remolded often.

   a. A nonstick coating.

   b. High memory.

   c. High drape.

   d. High resistance to stretch.

Appendix

STUDENT ASSIGNMENTS

1. Define all of the key terms used in this chapter.

2. Perform the testing of material characteristics on a sample piece.

3. Practice making a pattern from a fellow student's hand.

4. Practice identifying the different properties of a sample of LTTM by following steps 1 through 9:

Testing Low-Temperature Thermoplastic Material
Begin by placing a small sample piece (4 x 5 inches) of the material in hot water (140° to 160°F) and watch the following:
1. Does the sample turn transparent? If yes, the product has memory. If no, the product may still have memory, but you will need to stretch it when it is soft, wait until it hardens out of the water, and then place it back in the hot water to see if the material shrinks back to the original size.
2. Is the sample coated? When softened, fold the material in half and press together. Wait until it is cooled before trying to peel it apart. If it comes apart easily when cool, it has a non-stick coating. If it does not come apart but remains bonded, it has no coating.
3. Is the material rigid? Thicker materials are typically more rigid than thinner versions of the same material. For example, a 1/8-inch material will be more rigid than a 1/16-inch material. You can test the rigidity of the sample piece either before you heat it up or after it has hardened. Is it easy to bend in half, or does it stay very strong?
4. How long does it take for the product to soften and become fully activated? This is the activation time.
5. How much working time did you have with the sample piece? The working time is calculated as the amount of time you can still mold the material around the anatomy after it is activated.
6. How well does the sample conform? Test the material's conformability by molding the activated sample over your flexed MCP joints. Can you see the individual knuckles and bony outlines? If yes, the material has high conformability.
7. Test the resistance to stretch with the same exercise as step 6. How easy was it to handle the material as you molded it over the flexed MCP joints? Did you need a firm grasp of the material or only a gentle touch? The latter would imply low resistance to stretch.
8. Do your finger marks show on the material surface? This is a test of surface impressionability. Knowing this characteristic in advance will be helpful and make you more careful with overall handling and cutting.
9. Put the sample back into the hot water and recheck the memory. Does it return to its original shape? Even if it did not turn transparent but still shrinks back to the original size and shape, it does have memory.
Think about what types of orthoses could be fabricated from this sample.

Multiple Choice Answer Key

6. d

7. b

8. b

9. b

Part Two

ORTHOSES AS INTERVENTIONS

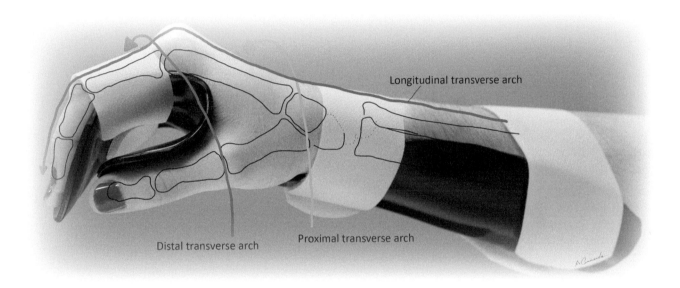

Longitudinal transverse arch

Distal transverse arch

Proximal transverse arch

CHAPTER 4

Wrist Immobilization Orthoses

Key Terms

Dorsal design	Osteoarthritis (OA)	Sprain
Flaccidity	Peripheral nerves	Tendinitis
Fracture	Rheumatoid arthritis (RA)	Volar design
Hypertonicity	Rigidity	Wrist cock-up
Hypotonicity		

Learning Outcomes

Upon completion of this chapter, you will be able to:

1. Describe the clinical conditions and goals for fabrication of a wrist immobilization orthosis.

2. Identify pertinent anatomical structures and biomechanical principles involved in a wrist immobilization orthosis and apply these concepts to orthotic design and fabrication.

3. Identify the four most commonly selected orthoses designs and describe the rationale for choosing one design over another.

4. Design suitable patterns for the four common types of wrist immobilization orthoses and identify the pertinent anatomical landmarks.

5. After reviewing the instructional videos:

   a. Outline the steps involved in the fabrication of a wrist immobilization orthosis.

   b. Complete the molding and finishing of a wrist immobilization orthosis.

   c. Evaluate the fit and function of a completed wrist immobilization orthosis and identify and address all areas needing adjustment.

6. Identify elements of a client education program following fabrication of a wrist immobilization orthosis.

7. Describe special considerations of wrist orthotic design and fabrication for special populations.

Schofield, K., & Schwartz, D. *Orthotic Design and Fabrication
for the Upper Extremity: A Practical Guide* (pp 57-80).
© 2019 Taylor & Francis Group.

Box 4-1. Common Goals of Wrist Immobilization Orthoses

PROTECTION

- Support and protect the wrist following surgical repair of structures.
- Support and protect the wrist after a fracture or ligament injury.
- Offer relief and joint protection from a painful tendinitis or arthritis.

POSITIONING

- Position the wrist to prevent prolonged wrist flexion posturing that can compress the median nerve.
- Position the wrist to prevent shortening of muscles and tendon(s) due to changes in muscle tone.

IMPROVE FUNCTION

- Support and position the wrist in slight extension to improve grasp and release hand function due to muscle paralysis or weakness.
- Use the orthosis as a base for outrigger attachments to create mobilization orthoses and/or adaptive equipment.

Introduction

The wrist is the cornerstone of the hand. It serves to balance muscle forces, promote anatomical alignment of the hand skeleton, and facilitate optimal grip and prehensile function. Proper wrist positioning and stability is critical for optimal hand function. Ten to 40 degrees of wrist extension allows the fingers and thumb to move freely and provides balance to the forearm extrinsic flexor and extensor muscles. Wrist immobilization orthoses offer support for injured bones, tendons, nerves, joints, ligaments, and other soft tissues crossing the wrist. These orthoses are used as a therapeutic intervention for a wide variety of upper extremity conditions and are common orthoses that practitioners provide for their clients.

When properly fabricated and fitted, wrist immobilization orthoses stabilize the wrist joint and allow full movement of the fingers and thumb, thereby enabling clients to perform light functional tasks without difficulty. There are several different wrist design options. The design chosen will depend on multiple factors, including the client's clinical condition, his or her functional needs, and specifications set by the referring physician.

Goals for Use of a Wrist Immobilization Orthosis

When fabricating a wrist immobilization orthosis, the practitioner must do the following:

- Be knowledgeable regarding the specific clinical condition or diagnosis
- Be knowledgeable about the expected clinical outcome following orthotic use
- Be aware of the goal(s) of the orthosis
- Use sound clinical reasoning to select the most appropriate design

The goals of a wrist immobilization orthosis will vary depending on the individual client's needs and clinical condition (Box 4-1).

Clinical Conditions and Wearing Schedules

The following section describes several clinical conditions commonly seen by practitioners where a wrist immobilization orthosis may be prescribed. Readers are encouraged to review the anatomy and biomechanical principles presented in Chapter 2 and the suggested reading provided for additional details regarding each clinical condition. Current evidence supporting wrist orthoses as an intervention strategy for each clinical condition is provided when available.

CARPAL TUNNEL SYNDROME

Carpal tunnel syndrome is the most common form of **peripheral nerve** compression in the upper extremity. In this condition, the median nerve becomes compressed within a narrow tunnel in the proximal palm that is formed by the carpal bones and covered by the transverse carpal ligament (Figure 4-1). In addition to the median nerve, nine tendons are enclosed in this tunnel (four slips of the flexor digitorum superficialis, four slips of the flexor digitorum profundus, and the flexor pollicis longus).

A number of factors can account for compression of the median nerve in this small tunnel, including the following:

- Swelling of the synovial tissues surrounding any of the nine tendons inside the carpal tunnel, a disease process such as **rheumatoid arthritis (RA)**, and/or diabetes
- Prolonged positioning of the wrist in flexion, which decreases the available space for the contents of the carpal tunnel to move freely
- Altered wrist anatomy from an injury such as a carpal bone or distal radius **fracture**

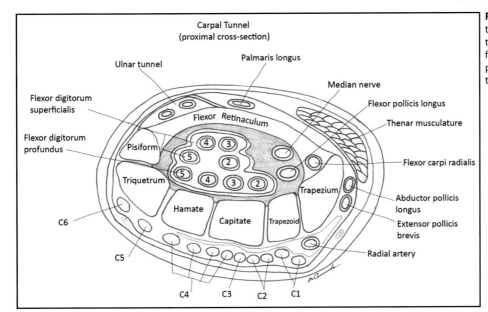

Figure 4-1. Contents of the carpal tunnel include the four tendons of the flexor digitorum superficialis, the four tendons of the flexor digitorum profundus, the flexor pollicis longus tendon, and the median nerve.

- Lumbrical muscles entering the carpal tunnel during full finger flexion

- Constant repetitive wrist motion causing friction between the flexor tendons and the flexor tendon sheaths causing inflammation within the carpal tunnel

All of these factors, plus additional health risk factors, may contribute to increased pressure on the median nerve and cause complaints of numbness and tingling in the thumb, index and long fingers, and radial half of the ring finger; aching and pain; and weakness with pinching and gripping tasks.

A wrist orthosis positioning the wrist in 0 to 15 degrees of extension can minimize compression of the median nerve by preventing a prolonged flexed posture of the wrist and reducing repetitive movement of the tendons in the carpal tunnel, allowing all inflamed structures to rest and heal. Clients may need further evaluation of symptoms, which may be aggravated by strong grasping motions. An orthosis that includes the metacarpophalangeal (MCP) joints can minimize movement of the lumbrical muscles into the carpal tunnel and reduce compression of the median nerve during repetitive grasping activities. Please refer to additional sources for information on contributing health risk factors for carpal tunnel syndrome.

Wearing Schedule

Depending on the severity of the client's symptoms, the wearing schedule for the client presenting with carpal tunnel symptoms may be full-time until numbness, tingling, and pain are resolved. Nighttime use is often prescribed for clients who have severe symptoms at night, causing them to waken with complete numbness in the affected fingers. Other clients might benefit from wearing the orthosis during activities that aggravate the symptoms. There is no one correct wearing schedule. Each client should be evaluated and prescribed an individualized wearing schedule that helps relieve his or her specific symptoms.

Evidence

Level I

- Huisstede, B. M., Fridén, J., Coert, J. H., Hoogvliet, P., & European HANDGUIDE Group. (2014). Carpal tunnel syndrome: Hand surgeons, hand therapists, and physical medicine and rehabilitation physicians agree on a multidisciplinary treatment guideline—Results from the European HANDGUIDE study. *Archives of Physical Medicine and Rehabilitation, 95*(12), 2254-2264.

  ○ The authors describe a Delphi consensus strategy where expert surgeons, physicians, and therapists meet and agree on the description, symptoms, and diagnosis of carpal tunnel syndrome and discuss the effectiveness of surgical and nonsurgical interventions. The experts agreed that patients with carpal tunnel syndrome should first be given home instructions to avoid certain wrist postures, instructions combined with splinting, corticosteroid injection, corticosteroid injections plus splinting, and, finally, surgery to alleviate symptoms. A relationship between the severity/duration and choice of therapy was found by the experts and reported in the guideline.

- Page, M. J., Massy-Westropp, N., O'Connor D., & Pitt V. (2012). Splinting for carpal tunnel syndrome. *Cochrane Database of Systematic Reviews, 7,* CD010004. doi:10.1002/14651858.CD010004

  ○ This systematic review examined the effectiveness of splinting for mild to moderate carpal tunnel syndrome compared with no other treatment, with a placebo, and with other nonsurgical interventions. Of the 19 studies included in this systematic review, most were of low quality with the risk of bias. It is difficult to determine from the evidence whether one splint design or wearing schedule is more effective than another, or if splinting is more effective than other nonsurgical interventions for carpal tunnel syndrome (e.g., exercises and oral steroids). The authors concluded that more research is needed to find out how effective and safe splinting is for people with carpal tunnel syndrome, particularly in the long term.

Level II

- Bardak, A. N., Alp, M., Erhan, B., Paker, N., Kaya, B., & Önal, A. E. (2009). Evaluation of the clinical efficacy of conservative treatment in the management of carpal tunnel syndrome. *Advances in Therapy, 26*(1), 107-116.

  ○ This study compared tendon and nerve-gliding exercises with splinting and injections in patients with carpal tunnel syndrome. A total of 111 patients with carpal tunnel syndrome were randomized into three treatment groups looking at different combinations of the above protocols. All patients reported improved symptoms after treatment, but patients receiving injections and splinting and tendon and nerve-gliding exercises (or without the additional exercises) improved better than patients performing only tendon and nerve-gliding exercises. The splint provided positioned the wrist in a neutral position and was worn for 3 weeks initially full-time, then at night only for the additional 4 weeks of the testing period.

- Celik, B., Paker, N., Celik, E. C., Bugdayci, D. S., Ones, K., & Ince, N. (2015). The effects of orthotic intervention on nerve conduction and functional outcome in carpal tunnel syndrome: A prospective follow-up study. *Journal of Hand Therapy, 28*(1), 44-48. doi:10.1016/jht.2014.07.008

  ○ These authors conducted a prospective comparative study examining the effectiveness of wearing a wrist immobilization orthosis for 6 consecutive weeks in treatment for mild to moderate carpal tunnel syndrome. Electromyography (EMG) studies and other outcome measures sensitive to carpal tunnel intervention were used. Results indicated improvement in EMG findings with orthotic use after 6 weeks, with no significant change in other outcome measures. The authors note that changes in EMG findings may be more sensitive than carpal tunnel syndrome outcome questionnaires. This study supports use of wrist orthoses for mild to moderate carpal tunnel syndrome.

WRIST SPRAINS

A wrist **sprain** is an injury to the ligaments in the wrist that connect the carpus to the forearm bones. Ligaments are especially important in maintaining the joint space between the carpal bones (arranged in proximal and distal rows) and the radius and ulna. Sprains can be classified as mild when ligaments are stretched or severe when ligaments are completely torn. Torn ligaments can lead to carpal bone instability, a common source of pain and decreased hand function. A wrist orthosis can help maintain the ligaments in their optimal position and alignment to facilitate healing and allow the client to use his or her injured hand for light activities of daily living (ADL).

Wearing Schedule

A client presenting with pain due to a ligament sprain or tear should wear a wrist immobilization orthosis full-time in order to alleviate symptoms and allow for healing of the injured structures, or as directed by the referring physician. More severe injuries may require surgical intervention. Wrist orthoses may be used following surgery to protect the repaired structures, optimize healing, and facilitate light use of the injured hand.

Evidence

There is a lack of current research to support the use of an orthosis with wrist sprains. However, the following two studies are cited.

Level II

- Rønning, R., Rønning, I., Gerner, T., & Engebretsen, L. (2001). The efficacy of wrist protectors in preventing snowboarding injuries. *American Journal of Sports Medicine, 29*(5), 581-585.

  ○ These authors conducted a randomized clinical trial of 5029 snowboarders to investigate the effect of wearing a wrist support during the activity to see if it was helpful at preventing injury. A total of 2515 participants of the study received a wrist support, and 2514 did not. The primary endpoint was fracture or sprain of the wrist with loss of range of motion (ROM) and pain of at least a 4-day duration. Eight wrist injuries occurred in the braced group, and 29 occurred in the control group. The wrist support used in the study was a commercially available wrist wrap with D-ring strapping and a volar-based formable aluminum support. The authors conclude that a wrist support can help prevent wrist injuries in a high-impact sport such as snowboarding, but they also determined that the support used in this study may have been too soft to absorb the necessary amount of energy to reduce the number of injuries of the wrist.

Level V

- Prosser, R., Herbert, R., & LaStayo, P. C. (2007). Current practice in the diagnosis and treatment of carpal instability: Results of a survey of Australian hand therapists. *Journal of Hand Therapy, 20*(4), 249-242.

  - The authors surveyed hand therapists in Australia regarding the treatment of carpal instabilities. Although patients with this diagnosis often have full ROM, functional ADL may be affected due to pain and decreased grip strength. Respondents reported that patient education and wrist splinting were the most commonly provided treatments. Use of wrist orthoses may help decrease pain and motion, contributing to healing and stability. Although this is a Level V paper and only reports the results of a survey, it does indicate current practice patterns and the use of orthoses as a therapeutic intervention.

WRIST FRACTURES

Fracture of any of the carpal bones (except the scaphoid, which typically requires immobilization of the wrist and first metacarpal bone) or the radius or ulna bones may be designated a wrist fracture, although the most commonly injured bone is the distal radius (Figure 4-2). Some wrist fractures may be treated with surgery involving volar or dorsal plating, external fixation, and/or K-wires; others are treated with immobilization using plaster casts or immobilized with the use of a removable orthosis. Often, after surgery or after the cast or external fixator has been removed, a wrist orthosis may be fabricated to support and position the healing structures and to allow the client to begin active wrist ROM, exercises, and light use of the injured hand.

Wearing Schedule

Following surgical procedures to stabilize a wrist fracture, a wrist orthosis may be used to protect and support healing structures. Clients should be instructed to wear the wrist immobilization orthosis full-time, except for exercises and hygiene for several weeks. Full healing of the bony structures will indicate when it is safe to discharge the orthosis. Nighttime wear and use during activities may continue for several additional weeks as an extra precaution.

Evidence

Level II

- Bong, M. R., Egol, K. A., Leibman, M., & Koval, K. J. (2006). A comparison of immediate post reduction splinting constructs for controlling initial displacement of fractures of the distal radius: A prospective randomized study of long-arm versus short-arm splinting. *Journal of Hand Surgery, 41*(5), 766-770.

  - These authors conducted a prospective, randomized, controlled trial comparing use of a plaster,

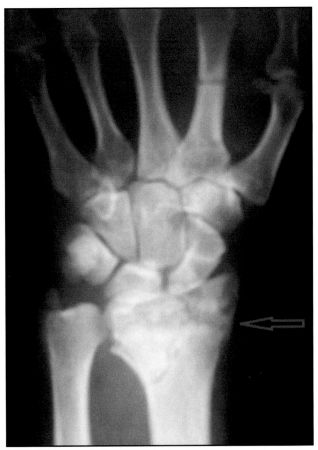

Figure 4-2. X-ray of a fracture to the distal radius.

long-arm, sugar tong splint and a short-arm, radial gutter splint in maintaining reduction following displaced distal radius fractures. Results indicated that both splints were effective at maintaining the initial fracture reduction, but patients in the short-arm group had significantly higher Disabilities of the Arm, Shoulder and Hand scores. This study used plaster splints in both groups, but findings support use of wrist immobilization orthoses/splints over long-arm orthoses for initial management of displaced distal radius fractures.

- Williams, K. G., Smith, G., Luhmann, S. J., Mao, J., Gunn, J. D., & Luhmann, J. D. (2014). A randomized controlled trial of cast versus splint for distal radial buckle fracture. *Pediatric Emergency Care, 29*(5), 555-559.

  - The authors conducted a randomized, controlled trial comparing casting verses splinting to treat distal radial buckle fractures in patients aged 2 to 17 years. Outcomes measured were parental and patient satisfaction, preference, convenience, and pain. Results support use of wrist splints for all variables except pain. Pain was higher in the splint group, but results were not statistically significant.

Figure 4-3. The lateral epicondyle is the origin for the wrist and digit extensor muscles: extensor carpi radialis brevis, extensor digitorum, extensor carpi ulnaris, and part of the extensor carpi radialis longus.

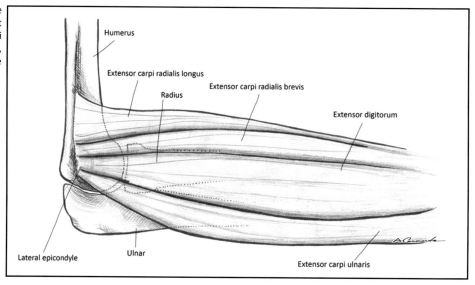

This study supports use of wrist orthoses for management of distal radial buckle fractures in the pediatric population.

TENDINITIS

Wrist **tendinitis** is a common condition caused by inflammation or irritation of any one or more of the tendons crossing the wrist (extensor carpi radialis longus, extensor carpi radialis brevis, extensor carpi ulnaris, flexor carpi radialis, or the flexor carpi ulnaris). The flexor digitorum superficialis and flexor digitorum profundus tendons may also be involved. The site of inflammation and pain may also arise from the involved muscle's origin at the elbow (medial and/or lateral epicondyle) and can be more pronounced with gripping tasks and wrist movement (Figure 4-3). A wrist orthosis can help maintain the wrist in a specific position to allow rest of the involved tendons and facilitate continued use of the affected hand in functional tasks.

Wearing Schedule

The orthosis is typically worn full-time initially to decrease symptoms. Tendinitis of the wrist muscles may take up to 6 weeks to resolve with rest and reduced activities, including immobilizing the involved tendon(s) in a wrist immobilization orthosis that limits or reduces strain on the tendon insertion site. For example, a wrist orthosis for treatment of tendinitis of the flexor carpi radialis tendon may be positioned in 10 degrees of flexion.

Evidence

Level II

- Garg, R. G., Adamson, G. J., Dawson, P. A., Shankwiler, J. A., & Pink, M. M. (2010). A prospective randomized study comparing a forearm strap brace versus a wrist splint for the treatment of lateral epicondylitis. *Journal of Shoulder and Elbow Surgery, 19*(4), 508-512.

  ○ The authors conducted a prospective randomized, controlled trial comparing the effectiveness of a wrist immobilization orthosis and a forearm counterforce brace for management of acute lateral epicondylitis. Pain was significantly less with use of the wrist orthosis, but both interventions were similar in all other clinical outcomes.

ARTHRITIS

Both **osteoarthritis (OA)** and RA can affect the wrist with decreased motion, pain, and weakness (Figure 4-4).

RA is an autoimmune disease that typically affects the wrist and small joints in the hand and often occurs on both sides of the body. The synovial tissue within joints and surrounding tendon sheaths is targeted by the body's immune system and can cause significant joint dysfunction (Table 4-1).

In contrast, OA is a wear-and-tear degenerative condition where the cartilage lining the articular joint surfaces is affected by repeated stress on the joints as a client ages or by past injury to the articulating surface(s) of the joint. The larger weightbearing joints, along with the shoulder, elbow, wrist, and small finger and thumb joints, are most commonly affected. OA can affect only one joint in the body, but it is more common to have the condition on both sides (see Table 4-1). A wrist orthosis can help with both RA and OA symptoms by supporting the wrist in a resting and comfortable position to reduce pain, facilitate grasp, release hand function, improve grip strength, and protect the wrist joints during ADL tasks.

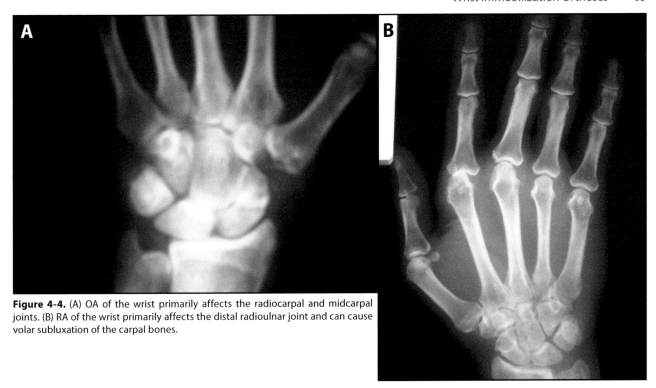

Figure 4-4. (A) OA of the wrist primarily affects the radiocarpal and midcarpal joints. (B) RA of the wrist primarily affects the distal radioulnar joint and can cause volar subluxation of the carpal bones.

Table 4-1

COMPARISON OF RHEUMATOID ARTHRITIS AND OSTEOARTHRITIS

	RHEUMATOID ARTHRITIS	OSTEOARTHRITIS
SYMPTOMS	Joints may be painful, swollen, and stiff. Frequent fatigue and a general feeling of being ill are typical.	Joints ache and may be tender but have little or no swelling. Whole-body symptoms are not usually present.
PATTERN OF PATHOLOGY	Often affects small and large joints on both sides of the body (symmetrical), such as both hands, both wrists and elbows, and the balls of both feet	Symptoms often begin on one side of the body and may spread to the other side. Symptoms begin gradually and are often limited to one set of joints, usually the finger joints closest to the fingernails or the thumbs, large weightbearing joints (hips, knees), or the spine.
SPEED OF ONSET	Relatively rapid, over weeks to months	Slow, over years
DISEASE ETIOLOGY	Autoimmune	Normal wear and tear/degenerative

Wearing Schedule for Rheumatoid Arthritis

Orthotic intervention for clients with RA can help with positioning, pain relief, and functional assistance. Depending on the individual needs of the client, orthoses can be worn full-time or on an as-needed basis to assist with specific tasks and activities. Clients with RA benefit from lightweight materials and noncumbersome designs. Specific attention should be paid to the strapping materials used to avoid pressure points and to make sure each client

has adequate pinch strength to pull the straps open and to close them. Additionally, it is important for the practitioner to be aware that immobilizing the wrist can place more stress on the MCP, proximal interphalangeal, and distal interphalangeal joints during hand use. Including the MCP joints may help if this is a concern.

Wearing Schedule for Osteoarthritis

Orthoses provide pain relief and support to joints affected by OA. Clients should be encouraged to wear these orthoses as needed for symptom reduction and assistance with ADL. Initially, full-time use of the wrist orthosis may reduce symptoms of pain enough to allow for a gradual decrease of orthotic use over time.

Evidence

Level I

- Valdes, K., & Marik, T. (2010). A systematic review of conservative interventions for osteoarthritis of the hand. *Journal of Hand Therapy, 24*(4), 444-451.

  ○ The authors conducted a systematic review looking at conservative treatments for the management of hand OA. Orthoses are a common intervention and cited in 11 of the 21 studies included in this review. The authors conclude that there is high to moderate evidence to support the use of wrist orthoses for this population.

- Egan, M., Brosseau, L., Farmer, M., Ouimet, M. A., Rees, S., Tugwell, P., & Wells, G. (2001). Splints and orthosis for treating rheumatoid arthritis. *Cochrane Database of Systematic Reviews, 4*, 1-26.

  ○ The authors sought to determine the effectiveness of splints/orthoses in relieving pain, decreasing swelling, and/or preventing deformity and to determine the effect of splints/orthoses on strength, mobility, and function in people with RA. They reviewed a total of 10 papers reporting on the use of working wrist splints (5), resting hand and wrist splints (2), and special shoes and insoles (4). They report that there is evidence that wearing wrist splints during work decreases grip strength and does not affect pain, morning stiffness, pinch grip, or quality of life after up to 6 months of regular wear. In addition, no evidence was found to suggest that resting wrist and hand splints change pain, grip strength, or number of swollen joints. However, participants reported that they preferred the use of orthoses to nonuse, and padded resting splints to unpadded ones. There is insufficient evidence to make firm conclusions about the effectiveness of working wrist splints in decreasing pain or increasing function for people with RA. Potential adverse effects, such as decreased ROM, do not seem to be an issue. Although resting hand and wrist splints do not seem to affect ROM or pain, participants report that they prefer wearing a resting splint to not wearing one.

ABNORMAL TONE

In the absence of disease or injury, muscles have resting tone, or resistance to passive stretch. This is created by connective tissues present in muscle, as well as input from the central and peripheral nervous systems. A common physical impairment in the upper extremity following brain trauma or stroke is development of abnormal muscle tone.

There are different terms used to describe abnormalities in tone. These include **flaccidity**, **hypertonicity**, **hypotonicity**, and **rigidity**. Flaccidity is characterized by absence of both muscle tone and deep tendon reflexes. No active movement in the extremity is observed. Flaccidity typically presents immediately following a traumatic injury or event in the brain or spinal cord. It can also occur following injury to a lower motor nerve or peripheral nerve. Hypertonicity typically develops a few weeks later but may also be present immediately following injury. In contrast to flaccidity, hypertonicity is an increase in muscle tone with resistance to active and passive movement. Injury to upper motor neurons in the brain or spinal cord interrupts the normal pathway between these neurons and the lower motor neurons. Stretch reflexes become hyperactive, resulting in increased muscle tone. In hypertonicity, changes can also occur in the connective tissue of the involved muscles and surrounding joints, resulting in soft tissue and/or joint contractures. Rigidity is also an increase in muscle tone, but muscles on both sides of a joint are affected, resulting in loss of voluntary movement in all directions that a joint moves. This is in contrast to hypertonicity, where muscle(s) on one side of a joint demonstrate increased tone, and muscle(s) on the other side become inactive, or weak. Hypotonicity, or less-than-normal muscle tone, is characterized by muscle weakness and impaired ability to resist the force of gravity during active movement. Wrist immobilization orthoses can help support hypotonic or flaccid muscles that cross the wrist to prevent overstretching, help prevent the development of joint stiffness and shortening of muscle fibers and tendons, and position the wrist for improved functioning of the fingers where there is some volitional muscle control.

Peripheral Nerve Injury

Following injury to one or more of the three peripheral nerves described hereafter, muscles that move the wrist and/or fingers can become paralyzed or weak due to loss of nerve impulses from the peripheral nerve to the muscle(s). Affected muscles have no or minimal muscle tone and lose their ability to contract normally to move joints. Figure 4-5A shows the classic wrist drop deformity associated with radial nerve palsy. Injury to the median and/or ulnar nerves can also create muscle imbalance across the wrist. Wrist orthoses can help support weak or paralyzed muscles, help to rebalance muscle forces across the wrist to improve finger and thumb function, and prevent overstretching or shortening of affected muscles. This is especially important for injuries involving the radial nerve where the wrist extensor muscles cannot contract strongly enough against the force of gravity to extend the wrist, creating significant muscle imbalance and loss of grip and prehensile function (Figure 4-5B). The wrist orthosis may also be used as a base for outriggers use in dynamic mobilization orthoses for radial nerve palsy. This advanced type of orthosis will be addressed in Chapter 10.

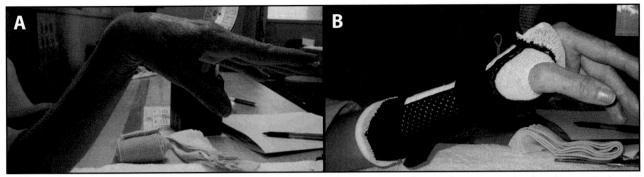

Figure 4-5. (A) Paralysis of the wrist and digit extensor muscles causes the wrist to drop into flexion. This is commonly referred to as *wrist drop*. (B) A wrist immobilization orthosis can help rebalance the muscle forces across the wrist and enable the client to perform grasp and release functions more easily.

Wearing Schedule for Muscle Paralysis or Altered Muscle Tone

Clients with muscle weakness, paralysis, or high tone should be instructed to wear the wrist orthosis as much as possible to prevent overstretching or shortening of affected soft tissues and minimize the risk of contracture development. The orthosis should be used as long as muscle imbalance persists or until recovery of sufficient muscle strength (at least a grade 4 muscle strength).

Evidence

Level V

- Hannah, S. D., & Hudak, P. L. (2001). Splinting and radial nerve palsy: A single-subject experiment. *Journal of Hand Therapy, 14*(4), 195-201.

   ◦ These authors describe a client with radial nerve palsy and three different orthoses provided for functional use during recovery. The authors assess the client's ability to function while wearing each of the three orthotic designs and make suggestions for this assessment.

- McKee, P., & Nguyen, C. (2007). Customized dynamic splinting: Orthoses that promote optimal function and recovery after radial nerve injury: A case report. *Journal of Hand Therapy, 20*(1), 74-88.

   ◦ The authors describe the complications associated with a radial nerve injury and chronicle the recovery of a client with this diagnosis and the orthotic management provided.

- Colditz, J. C. (1987). Splinting for radial nerve palsy. *Journal of Hand Therapy, 1*(1), 18-24.

   ◦ The author describes the etiology of the loss of radial nerve function and details different orthoses that assist in providing functionality to the injured extremity.

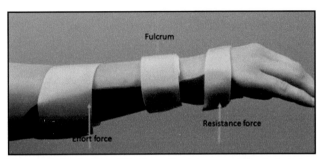

Figure 4-6. A wrist immobilization orthosis is an example of a first-class lever system: the wrist is the fulcrum, the forearm component the effort force, and the hand the resistance force.

Biomechanical Principles to Consider With Wrist Immobilization Orthoses

A wrist immobilization orthosis represents a first-class lever system. This means that the wrist is the fulcrum, or axis; the forearm component is the effort arm/force; and the entire hand is the resistance arm/force (Figure 4-6).

The width of the forearm component should span half the width of the forearm and wrist and cover two-fourths the length of the forearm. This will distribute forces over a large area and optimize security and comfort of the orthosis. These concepts are especially important for designs that are volarly or dorsally based. Circumferentially designed orthoses can potentially be shorter in length because more support is offered along the entire width of the forearm and wrist. A narrow orthosis that is not conformed well around the forearm may compromise wrist support, create pressure areas, and allow the orthosis to rotate or move on the extremity when worn (Figure 4-7).

Other important biomechanical concepts to consider include the following:

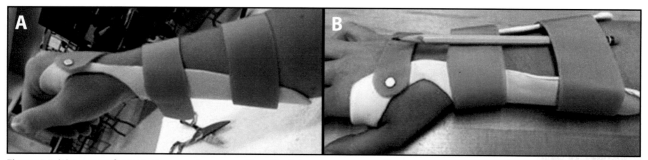

Figure 4-7. (A) A narrow forearm component can cause the orthosis to move unnecessarily, cause pressure areas, and compromise wrist support. (B) A wider-than-necessary forearm component does not conform well to the body and can cause unnecessary movement when the orthosis is worn.

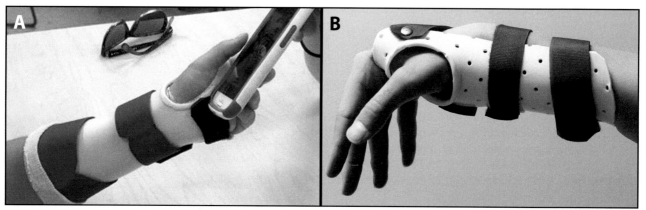

Figure 4-8. (A) Strategic placement of straps on a wrist immobilization orthosis helps to secure the orthosis on the extremity and optimizes fit and comfort. (B) Narrow straps may compromise support of the wrist and allow the orthosis to move unnecessarily when worn. Straps that are too wide can impede movement of uninvolved joints.

- Support of the proximal and distal transverse arches: the natural concavity formed by the distal carpal row and the bases of metacarpal bones in the palm should be fully supported, and the distal end of the orthosis should clear the MCP joints completely.

- Flare the proximal edge adequately, particularly if the orthosis is to be worn at night. Clients often flex their elbows while sleeping, and the proximal edge may create pressure on the tissues in the forearm.

- Strapping:
  - The dorsal aspect of the wrist, especially the ulnar head, may be subject to compressive forces from the wrist strap. Placing a pad on the inside of the strap over the ulnar head and flaring the low-temperature thermoplastic material (LTTM) away from this bony prominence will optimize comfort and security of the orthosis.
  - The straps should be strategically placed to provide optimal support: one directly over the wrist (this is critical for **volar** and **dorsal designs**, less so for circumferential designs), one on the proximal end, and one on the distal end of the orthosis.

  - The straps should be as wide as possible to distribute the forces over a large area (Figure 4-8).

- All edges should be smooth and all corners rounded to prevent pressure areas and sharp points. The distal edges of the wrist orthosis (just proximal to the distal palmar crease) must be sufficiently flared to prevent unwanted compressive and shear forces in the palm during finger flexion/gripping. The proximal edge should also be flared.

- All bony prominences should be free of unwanted forces. Specifically, avoid compressive and/or shear forces at the ulnar head and/or radial styloid. Ensure that the LTTM is flared away from these bony prominences. Padding can be added after the material has been flared away for comfort if needed (Figure 4-9).

- All corners of the orthosis should be flared and rounded to prevent pressure areas and optimize comfort.

- The orthosis should not block full thumb movement or opposition to the second and third digits. The orthosis should cover most of the thenar eminence crease to support the wrist, but the thenar muscles should be free to contract. Make sure the client is able to make a full, comfortable fist (Figure 4-10).

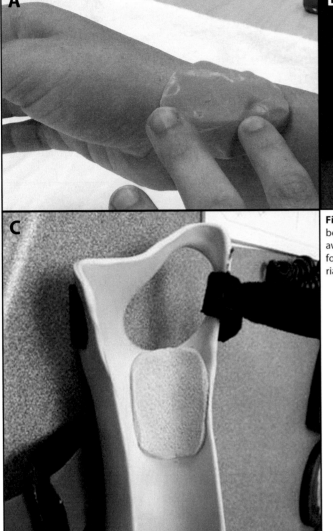

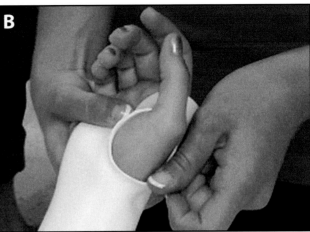

Figure 4-9. (A) Judicious use of padding on bony prominences applied before molding can help to prevent pressure areas. (B) Flaring the LTTM away from the body prominence after molding can prevent compressive forces on the tissues. (C) Padding can be applied after flaring the material away from the tissues to optimize comfort.

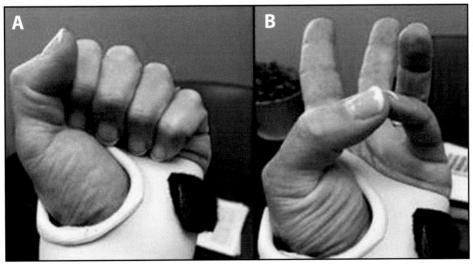

Figure 4-10. (A) The client should be able to make a full fist in the orthosis and (B) oppose his or her thumb to their second, third, and forth digits easily.

Table 4-2

WRIST ORTHOSES DESIGNS

	VOLAR DESIGN	DORSAL DESIGN	THUMB HOLE DESIGN	CIRCUMFERENTIAL DESIGN
ADVANTAGES AND DISADVANTAGES	Provides light support through the first web and covers the volar wrist Blocks sensory input to palm	Allows exposure of the palm for sensory input and increased functional use of the hand	Provides strong radial support around the thumb for larger hands, edema or low tone	Offers compressive forces on volar and dorsal forearm Good for edema management and the addition of outriggers May be difficult to don and doff
CLINICAL CONDITIONS	Can be used for all wrist conditions	Especially helpful with wrist drop and increased wrist tone	Can be used for all wrist conditions	Especially for wrist fractures and carpal instability
RECOMMENDED MATERIAL THICKNESS FOR ADULTS	1/12 to 1/8 inch	1/12 to 1/8 inch	1/12 to 1/8 inch	1/16 to 4/42 inch or 1/12 inch
MATERIAL CHARACTERISTICS	Moderate drapability	Moderate rigidity	Moderate drapability	Coated material

Wrist Immobilization Orthotic Designs

There are four commonly used wrist designs: volar, dorsal, thumb hole, and circumferential (Table 4-2). A common name of these orthoses collectively is the **wrist cock-up** orthosis. The practitioner may also choose a radial- or ulnar-based wrist design if support is needed specifically on the ulnar or radial aspect of the forearm and wrist. These wrist orthoses are known as *radial* and *ulnar gutter orthoses* and are only mentioned here as alternative designs. Each orthosis should be easy for the client to put on and take off. Strapping should also be straightforward and secure the orthosis snugly around the hand, wrist, and forearm. The practitioner must specifically consider the anatomy of the forearm and wrist when fabricating a wrist orthosis. Knowledge of the clinical condition and the affected anatomy will help the practitioner understand how the orthosis will influence these structures and assist him or her in determining the most appropriate orthosis design.

The following sections review each design, its main uses, and its advantages and disadvantages.

VOLAR DESIGN

The volar-based wrist immobilization orthosis rests on the volar surface of the wrist and forearm, with a narrow strip of LTTM through the first web space (Figure 4-11). This design is most suited for conditions where light support is needed, such as night use with carpal tunnel syndrome or for clients with smaller hands because there is less LTTM around the thumb. This design uses an important strap across the dorsal aspect of the wrist that plays a critical role in stabilizing the wrist in the orthosis. This strap may not be adequate for the support of heavy hands, such as with flaccidity or those with spasticity or edema. In these instances, a circumferential, thumb hole, or dorsal design is more suitable because they provide support that is more rigid.

Fabrication Tip

Let gravity assist with this design. Place the client's elbow on the table and let the forearm be unsupported in supination so that the muscles are not flattened against the table.

Gently help the material conform to the arches and the thenar eminence. Do not place pressure anywhere on the surface of the orthosis and use broad, smooth hand strokes to conform the LTTM. Ensure that there is no pressure over the radial styloid or ulnar head.

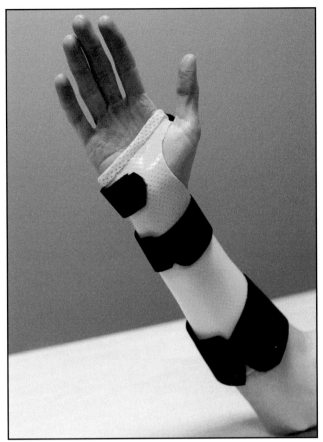

Figure 4-11. The volar design sits on the volar aspect of the hand, wrist, and forearm and has a strip of LTTM through the web space.

THUMB HOLE DESIGN

The thumb hole design also rests on the volar surfaces of the wrist and forearm (Figure 4-12). Instead of a strip of LTTM coming volarly through the first web space, the LTTM surrounds the thumb on all sides, thus creating a hole for the thumb, and offers adequate placement for the dorsal-based strap across the metacarpals. This design offers more support for the wrist than the volar design but can be more challenging to fabricate. For example, the practitioner must be careful and prevent excessive wrinkling of the material around the thumb on the dorsal surface during fabrication to prevent uneven pressure distribution under the LTTM.

Fabrication Tip

Make sure to cut the thumb hole the correct size. It should not be so large that the entire radial side of the wrist slides through it, but also ensure that it clears the thenar eminence so these muscles can contract normally and the thumb can move freely.

DORSAL DESIGN

The dorsal-based wrist immobilization orthosis rests on the dorsal aspect of the metacarpals, wrist, and forearm, with

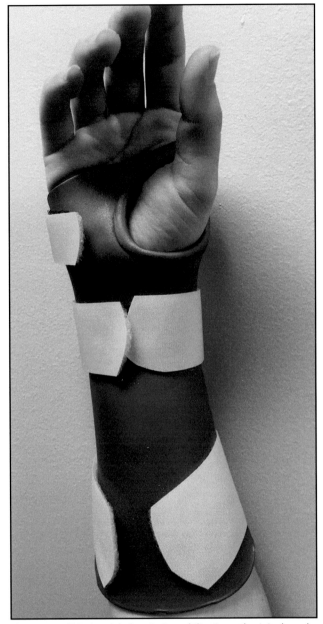

Figure 4-12. This thumb hole wrist immobilization orthosis is also volar based and has LTTM surrounding the thumb, creating a hole through which the thumb can go.

a palmar thermoplastic bar for added support (Figure 4-13). This design is often considered to be more functional than the traditional volar design because the volar forearm, wrist, and proximal palm are free of LTTM. This allows the client to receive more sensory input while using his or her hand in the orthosis, and it is less restrictive than the volar design. In the dorsal design, a small thermoplastic palmar bar lies across the palm just below the distal palmar crease and is used to secure the wrist in the orthosis. With this design, the practitioner can also choose to use strapping material across the palm; however, strapping offers less support than the LTTM. This design can also be used as a base for mobilization orthoses.

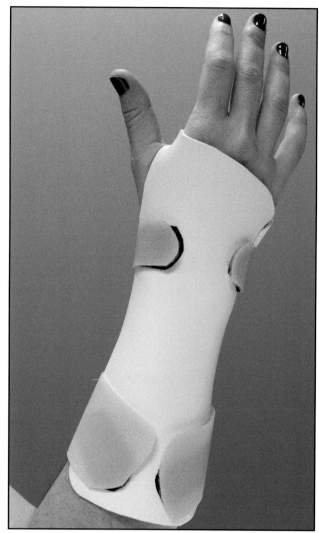

Figure 4-13. The dorsal-based wrist immobilization orthosis rests on the dorsal aspect of the hand, wrist, and forearm.

Fabrication Tip

Have the client rotate the forearm slightly in pronation as the material starts to harden. The ulnar head is most prominent in pronation, and this allows the material over the ulnar head to conform well and create enough space for this prominence.

CIRCUMFERENTIAL DESIGN

The circumferential wrist immobilization orthosis encompasses the volar and dorsal aspects of the forearm, wrist, and metacarpals (Figure 4-14). This design offers the most support and protection. It is most suited for conditions requiring more rigid support, such as forearm and wrist fractures, ligament and nerve injuries, burns, muscle paralysis, and significant hand and wrist traumatic injuries. Because of its circumferential design, it is also well suited for managing edema and as a base for mobilization orthoses because this design is typically more stable on the

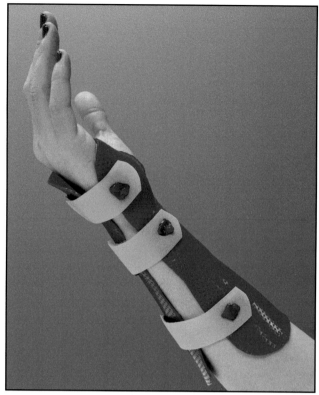

Figure 4-14. The circumferential wrist immobilization orthosis encompasses the volar and dorsal aspects of the hand, wrist, and forearm.

forearm and does not migrate distally with hand use. The circumferential design, although the most supportive, can be more difficult for clients to take on and off and is more challenging to fabricate as compared with the volar or dorsal designs.

Fabrication Tips

As with the dorsal design, have the client rotate the forearm slightly in pronation as the material starts to harden. The ulnar head is most prominent in pronation, and this allows the material over the ulnar head to conform well and create enough space for this prominence.

Make sure to use a coated product and wait for the material to harden sufficiently before popping open and removing the orthosis.

Orthotic Fabrication Steps

Please also see the demonstration videos for more information.

1. Pattern making
   ○ Wrist immobilization orthosis: volar design (Figure 4-15)
   ○ Wrist immobilization orthosis: dorsal design (Figure 4-16)

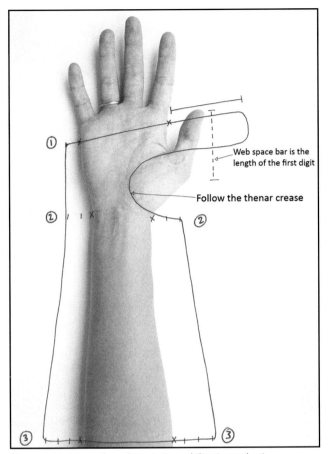

Web space bar is the length of the first digit

Follow the thenar crease

Figure 4-15. Pattern for volar wrist immobilization orthosis.

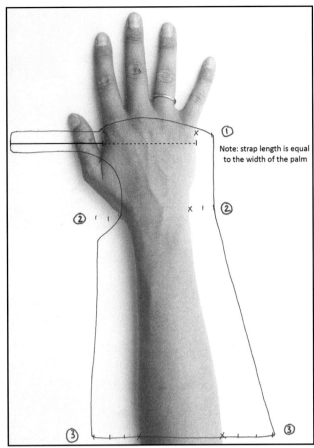

Note: strap length is equal to the width of the palm

Figure 4-16. Pattern for dorsal wrist immobilization orthosis.

- ○ Wrist immobilization orthosis: thumb hole design (Figure 4-17)
- ○ Wrist immobilization orthosis: circumferential design (Figure 4-18)
2. Material selection (Table 4-3)
3. Client positioning
4. Molding techniques
5. Finishing techniques: edges and strapping
   - ○ Strapping must always be matched to the size of the client. For most adults, straps should be 1.5 inches wide at the wrist and proximal forearm to optimize security of the orthosis and assist in force distribution. Proximal strapping should be angled to accommodate the muscles of the forearm. This is especially true when using the volar design. Straps placed circumferentially at the wrist optimize wrist support and security. The 1-inch distal strap should come just proximal to the metacarpal heads and align correctly (higher on the radial side, lower on the ulnar side of the hand). The adhesive Velcro (Velcro BVBA) hook should be covered completely with the strapping material. This will avoid the Velcro from snagging on clothing or blankets and

will make the straps more secure. Be sure to round strap and Velcro hook corners.
6. Orthosis check-out
   - ○ Can the client fully flex and extend his or her fingers?

     If no, adjust the distal edge of the orthosis so it clears the distal palmar crease. Remember that the orthosis will be higher on the radial side of the hand.
   - ○ Can the client oppose his or her thumb to the index and long fingers easily?

     If no, adjust the size of the thumb opening or the edge over the thenar crease so the thenar muscles are clear to contract.
   - ○ Can the client flex his or her elbow without the orthosis migrating distally?

     If no, the orthosis is too long or the proximal edge is not flared adequately.
   - ○ Does the client complain of discomfort when moving his or her hand in the orthosis?

     If yes, locate the area(s) of discomfort. Some possible solutions include the following:

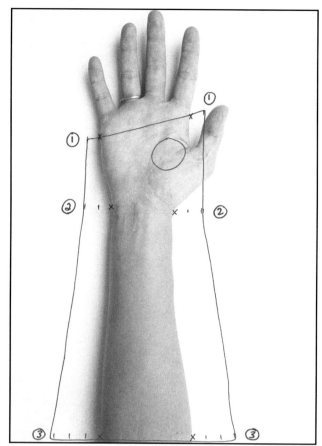

Figure 4-17. Pattern for thumb hole wrist immobilization orthosis.

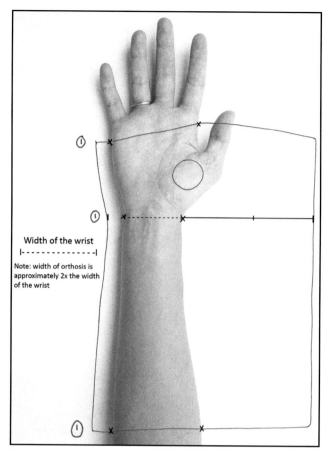

Width of the wrist

|- - - - - - - - - - - - -|

Note: width of orthosis is approximately 2x the width of the wrist

Figure 4-18. Pattern for circumferential wrist immobilization orthosis.

- *Flare more over the bony prominences and add padding if necessary (remember to do this AFTER the material has been moved away from the body).*
- *Flare the distal edge and be sure it clears the distal palmar crease.*
- *Flare around the thumb more to ensure that it can move freely.*
- *Smooth and round all rough edges.*
- *Reposition straps to secure the hand in the orthosis, especially the wrist strap.*

○ Are the corners of the orthosis rounded and smooth?

If no, round and smooth all corners of the orthosis.

○ Are the straps secure and edges rounded?

If no, adjust the straps: the wrist strap should go in a circumferential fashion around the wrist; the ends should meet together. No Velcro should be exposed. The proximal strap should be angled on the orthosis so it sits flat on the forearm. The distal strap should stabilize the distal metacarpals during finger movement.

○ Is the wrist strap positioned over the ulnar head? Is there padding to avoid pressure?

If no, reposition the strap so it is directly over the wrist and ulnar head. Place a doughnut pad directly over the ulnar head and secure it to the undersurface of the strap (see demonstration video).

○ Is the forearm strap angled to accommodate for the shape of the forearm?

If no, reposition the strap so it lies flat against the muscle bulk of the proximal forearm.

○ Is the distal strap secure?

If no, lengthen the strap and corresponding Velcro (longer strapping material and Velcro increases security). Use rivets to fasten one end of the strap if there is not enough surface area to secure it with Velcro.

○ Are all indentations and pattern marks removed?

If no, use a heat gun to smooth thermoplastic material. Rubbing alcohol can be used to remove wax pencil marks. Ink cannot be removed, so refrain from using this when drawing your pattern on the LTTM.

○ Remove the orthosis after 5 to 10 minutes and observe the skin. Are there any reddened areas?

If yes, adjust the orthosis by flaring and smoothing edges and/or flaring material away from bony prominences.

Table 4-3

LTTM CHOICES FOR WRIST IMMOBILIZATION ORTHOSES

MATERIAL CONSIDERATIONS	VOLAR DESIGN	DORSAL DESIGN	THUMB HOLE DESIGN	CIRCUMFERENTIAL DESIGN
Thickness	For adults, use 1/8-inch thickness. Use 3/32 or 1/12 inch for children or smaller hands/wrists.	For adults, use 1/8-inch thickness, especially if used to attach mobilization components.	For adults, use 1/8-inch thickness. Use 3/32 or 1/12 inch for children or smaller hands/wrists.	Use 3/32 or 1/12 inch. Thinner materials can be used due to the circumferential design.
Conformability	Select a material that will support the wrist and hand arches. Intimate conformability is not necessary.	Select a material that will support the wrist and hand arches. Intimate conformability is not necessary.	Select a material that will support the wrist and hand arches. Intimate conformability is not necessary.	Select a material that will conform well around the forearm muscles and the hand arches. One with minimal to moderate resistance to stretch is recommended.
Elasticity	Products with moderate resistance to stretch	Products with moderate resistance to stretch	Products with moderate resistance to stretch recommended	Products with moderate to low resistance to stretch are recommended to allow the material to conform well around the wrist and forearm.
Memory	Choose a product with high memory if frequent adjustments are anticipated.	Choose a product with high memory if frequent adjustments are necessary.	Choose a product with memory if frequent adjustments are necessary.	Choose a product with memory if frequent adjustments are necessary.

○ Review the purpose and care of the wrist orthosis with the client. Does he or she understand the following?:

- The purpose of the orthosis
- The daily wearing schedule
- How to take care of the orthosis
- How to don and doff correctly

If no, discuss the wearing schedule and care of the orthosis with the client before he or she leaves the clinic and provide clear written instructions to take home with him or her (refer to the Appendix at the end of Chapter 3). Take a photo of the orthosis correctly positioned using a smart phone and send it to your client for reference along with written instructions on the wearing schedule. Document all of your instructions to the client and maintain a copy of these in the client's chart.

SPECIAL CONSIDERATIONS

Pediatric Clients

- Consider using colored LTTM and/or colored straps to appeal to younger clients. Allow them to choose decorations like stickers or add thermoplastic designs to their orthoses to help them to feel that they are part of the process.

- Consider using creative strapping techniques such as shoelaces or other devices that require two hands to prevent removal by younger children who may not understand the need to wear the orthosis. Sometimes it is recommended to cover the orthosis with a sleeve or long stockinette to prevent a young client from taking it off (Figure 4-19).

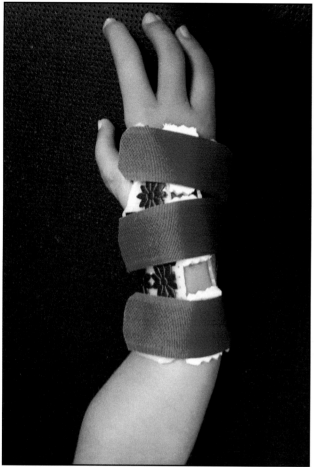

Figure 4-19. Orthoses can be customized to meet the needs of pediatric clients. (Reprinted with permission from Anna Ovsyannikova.)

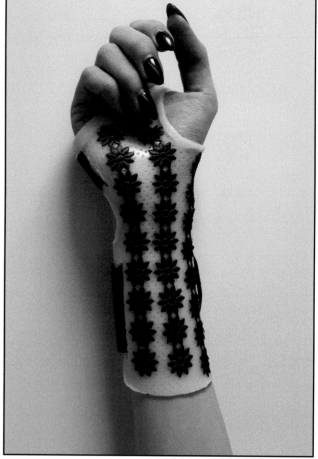

Figure 4-20. A personalized orthosis for a geriatric client. (Reprinted with permission from Anna Ovsyannikova.)

Geriatric Clients

- Consider using contrasting colored materials and straps for visually impaired clients.
- Straps can be attached directly to the thermoplastic material by the use of dry heat or a rivet so that elderly clients do not lose the straps at night.
- Clients with fragile skin may require additional skin protection through the use of padding, extra layers of stockinette, lightweight LTTM, and special soft straps (Figure 4-20).

Each client is an individual, and the selected wrist orthosis must match the client's needs (Figure 4-21). Please see the additional helpful hints in Box 4-2.

Summary

- Knowledge of the key anatomical structures affected by a wrist orthosis will help the practitioner understand how the orthosis will influence these structures and assist him or her in determining the most appropriate orthotic design and wearing schedule.
- The goals of a wrist immobilization orthosis and the specifics of each individual wearing schedule will vary depending on the client's needs and the diagnosis.
- A wrist immobilization orthosis represents a first-class lever system.
- A wrist immobilization orthosis can be fabricated using a volar, dorsal, thumb hole, or circumferential design. The design chosen depends on the client's clinical condition, his or her current functional needs, the specific indications requested by the referring physician, and practitioner's preference.
- Special populations such as pediatric and geriatric clients may require specific orthotic designs or adaptations to achieve the best outcomes with orthoses.
- Each orthosis must be molded to the individual anatomy for the best fit. Post-fabrication critique and check-out help identify areas for modification and optimize client comfort.

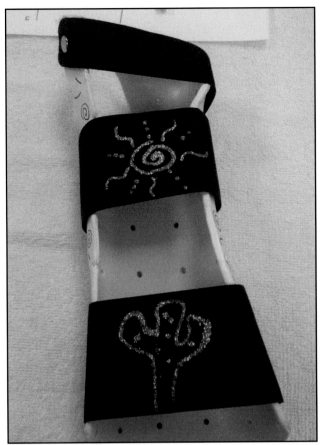

Figure 4-21. Each client can personalize his or her orthosis to make it meaningful to him or her.

In Your Client's Shoes

As an occupational therapy practitioner, it is very important to appreciate the impact that an orthosis will have on your client's daily occupations. The orthosis can potentially interfere with many if not all of your client's daily activities. You should experience how it feels to wear an orthosis for an extended period of time. This experience will enable you to be client centered when using orthoses as an intervention strategy in your practice. You must consider how to instruct your client on the importance of the wearing schedule and the benefits of compliance for maximum benefits (see Figure 4-17).

Suggested Reading

Amini, D. (2011). Occupational therapy interventions for work-related injuries and conditions of the forearm, wrist, and hand: A systematic review. *American Journal of Occupational Therapy, 65*(1), 29-46. doi:10.5014/ajot.2011.09186

Bardak, A. N., Alp, M., Erhan, B., Paker, N., Kaya, B., & Önal, A. E. (2009). Evaluation of the clinical efficacy of conservative treatment in the management of carpal tunnel syndrome. *Advances in Therapy, 26*(1), 107-116.

Box 4-2. Helpful Hints

- A circumferential wrist design offers increased rigidity. Clients needing more wrist support may benefit from this design, thicker materials, and/or longer orthoses. Thinner materials can be used for these orthoses, which will make the orthosis lighter, less bulky, and easier for the client to don and doff.

- Perforated materials are appropriate for clients in warmer climates, those with open wounds, or those who need more ventilation.

- LTTM with memory is important when frequent readjustments of the wrist orthosis are required (e.g., clients with edema or tendon injury). This makes remolding the orthosis easier and is cost efficient.

Beasley, J. (2012). Osteoarthritis and rheumatoid arthritis: Conservative therapeutic management. *Journal of Hand Therapy, 25*(2), 163-171.

Bong, M. R., Egol, K. A., Leibman, M., & Koval, K. J. (2006). A comparison of immediate postreduction splinting constructs for controlling initial displacement of fractures of the distal radius: A prospective randomized study of long-arm versus short-arm splinting. *Journal of Hand Surgery, 31*(5), 766-770.

Celik, B., Paker, N., Celik, E. C., Bugdayci, D. S., Ones, K., & Ince, N. (2015). The effects of orthotic intervention on nerve conduction and functional outcome in carpal tunnel syndrome: A prospective follow-up study. *Journal of Hand Therapy, 28*(1), 44-48. doi:10.1016/jht.2014.07.008

Colditz, J. C. (1987). Splinting for radial nerve palsy. *Journal of Hand Therapy, 1*(1), 18-24.

Coppard, B. M., & Lohman, H. (2014). *Introduction to orthotics: A clinical reasoning and problem-solving approach* (4th ed.). St. Louis, MO: Elsevier Mosby.

Egan, M., Brosseau, L., Farmer, M., Ouimet, M. A., Rees, S., Tugwell, P., & Wells, G. (2001). Splints and orthosis for treating rheumatoid arthritis. *Cochrane Database of Systematic Reviews, 4*, 1-26

Fedorczyk, J. M. (2012). Tendinopathies of the elbow, wrist, and hand: Histopathology and clinical considerations. *Journal of Hand Therapy, 25*(2), 191-200.

Garg, R. G., Adamson, G. J., Dawson, P. A., Shankwiler, J. A., & Pink, M. M. (2010). A prospective randomized study comparing a forearm strap brace versus a wrist splint for the treatment of lateral epicondylitis. *Journal of Shoulder and Elbow Surgery, 19*(4), 508-512.

Hall, B., Lee, H. C., Fitzgerald, H., Byrne, B., Barton, A., & Lee, A. H. (2014). Investigating the effectiveness of full-time wrist splinting and education in the treatment of carpal tunnel syndrome: A randomized controlled trial. *American Journal of Occupational Therapy, 67*(4), 448-459.

Hannah, S. D., & Hudak, P. L. (2001). Splinting and radial nerve palsy: A single-subject experiment. *Journal of Hand Therapy, 14*(4), 195-201.

Huisstede, B. M., Fridén, J., Coert, J. H., Hoogvliet, P., & European HANDGUIDE Group. (2014). Carpal tunnel syndrome: Hand surgeons, hand therapists, and physical medicine and rehabilitation physicians agree on a multidisciplinary treatment guideline—Results from the European HANDGUIDE study. *Archives of Physical Medicine and Rehabilitation, 95*(12), 2254-2264.

Jacobs, M. A., & Austin, N. M. (2014). *Orthotic intervention for the hand and upper extremity* (2nd ed.). Baltimore, MD: Lippincott Williams & Wilkins.

Kinnear, B. Z., Lannin, N. A., Cusick, A., Harvey, L. A., & Rawicki, B. (2014). Rehabilitation therapies after botulinum toxin-A injection to manage limb spasticity: A systematic review. *Physical Therapy, 94*(11), 1569-1581.

Lannin, N., Lannin, N. A., & Ada. L. (2011). Neurorehabilitation splinting: Theory and principles of clinical use. *NeuroRehabilitation, 28*(1), 21-28. doi:10.3233/NRE-2011-0628

McKee, P., & Nguyen, C. (2007). Customized dynamic splinting: orthoses that promote optimal function and recovery after radial nerve injury: A case report. *Journal of Hand Therapy, 20*(1), 74-88.

O'Conner, D., Mullet, H., Doyle, M., Mofidi, A., Kutty, M., & O'Sullivan, M. (2003). Minimally displaced Colles' fractures: A prospective randomized trial of treatment with a wrist splint or a plaster cast. *Journal of Hand Surgery, 28*(1), 50-53.

Özgen, M., Güngen, G., Sarsan, A., Ardıç, F., Çalışkan, S., Sabir, N., … Baydemir, C. (2011). Determination of the position on which the median nerve compression is at the lowest in carpal tunnel syndrome and clinical effectiveness of custom splint application. *Rheumatology International, 31*(8), 1031-1036.

Page, M. J., Massy-Westropp, N., O'Connor, D., & Pitt, V. (2012). Splinting for carpal tunnel syndrome. *Cochrane Database of Systematic Reviews, 7*, CD010003.

Prosser, R., Herbert, R., & LaStayo, P. C. (2007). Current practice in the diagnosis and treatment of carpal instability: Results of a survey of Australian hand therapists. *Journal of Hand Therapy, 20*(3), 239-243. doi:10.1197/j.jht.2007.04.006

Rønning, R., Rønning, I., Gerner, T., & Engebretsen, L. (2001). The efficacy of wrist protectors in preventing snowboarding injuries. *American Journal of Sports Medicine, 29*(5), 581-585.

Valdes, K., & Marik, T. (2010). A systematic review of conservative interventions for osteoarthritis of the hand. *Journal of Hand Therapy, 23*(4), 334-350.

Williams, K. G., Smith, G., Luhmann, S. J., Mao, J., Gunn, J. D., & Luhmann, J. D. (2013). A randomized controlled trial of cast versus splint for distal radial buckle fracture: An evaluation of satisfaction, convenience, and preference. *Pediatric Emergency Care, 29*(5), 555-559.

Test Your Knowledge

SHORT ANSWER

1. Identify the anatomical landmarks associated with a wrist immobilization orthosis.

2. Describe the biomechanical principles that apply to a wrist immobilization orthosis.

3. List the movements that a client should be able to perform without difficulty when wearing a wrist immobilization orthosis.

4. Describe four different wrist immobilization designs and discuss the rationale for each.

5. List the appropriate orthotic design and LTTM suitable for the following:

   a. A 45-year-old woman with carpal tunnel syndrome where the orthosis is worn at night only.

   b. A 6-year-old boy with a stable, nondisplaced distal radius fracture.

   c. A 45-year-old man with a distal radius and ulna fracture.

   d. An 80-year-old woman with RA.

MULTIPLE CHOICE

6. What type of lever system does a wrist immobilization orthosis represent?

   a. A third-class lever system

   b. A first-class lever system

   c. A second-class lever system

   d. A fourth-class lever system

7. What will occur if the lever system represented by a wrist immobilization orthosis is not balanced?

   a. The wrist will not be sufficiently supported in the orthosis.

   b. The fingers will not be able to move fully.

   c. The elbow will not be able to flex fully.

   d. The thumb will not move freely.

8. Which of the following landmarks do not apply to a wrist immobilization orthosis?

   a. The olecranon

   b. The pisiform

   c. The ulnar styloid

   d. The radial styloid

9. What is the recommended method of preventing pressure on a bony prominence when fabricating a wrist immobilization orthosis?

   a. Pad the area after molding the orthosis.

   b. Flare the LTTM away from the area after molding the orthosis.

   c. Pad the area prior to molding the orthosis.

   d. Make the forearm component of the orthosis as long as possible.

10. How should the wrist be positioned in a wrist immobilization orthosis to optimize grasp?

    a. 0 degrees

    b. 10 to 40 degrees of extension

    c. 45 degrees of extension

    d. 20 degrees of flexion

11. Why is it important to clear the distal palmar crease completely when fabricating a wrist immobilization orthosis?

    a. This allows for full thumb mobility in the orthosis.

    b. This allows for full proximal interphalangeal and distal interphalangeal joint mobility in the orthosis.

    c. This allows for full elbow mobility in the orthosis.

    d. This allows for full digit flexion and gripping in the orthosis.

12. What is the primary advantage of the dorsal wrist immobilization orthosis design?

    a. It allows for more sensory input in the palm.

    b. It allows for more digit mobility.

    c. It allows for more thumb mobility.

    d. It is easier to fabricate than the volar or circumferential designs.

13. When might a practitioner choose a circumferential wrist immobilization design over a volar or dorsal design?

    a. When a client needs more rigid support.

    b. When a client has difficulty putting the orthosis on.

    c. When a client needs light support.

    d. When a client needs to wear the orthosis only at night.

CASE STUDIES

Case Study 1

Linda is a 72-year-old, right-hand–dominant female who fractured her right distal radius following a fall while walking her dog 4 days ago. She was seen by an orthopedic surgeon, but because her fracture was stable, no surgical intervention was needed.

She presents for therapy with a prescription that reads:

Right distal radius fracture:

1. *Evaluate and treat.*

2. *Provide wrist orthosis.*

3. *Edema management and ROM: shoulder, elbow, and digits.*

Your assessment:

Linda presents in therapy for her first visit in a temporary plaster splint secured on her hand and wrist with an ACE bandage (3M). The right wrist shows considerable bruising and swelling, especially in the hand and all four digits. Wrist circumference is measured as 8.6 cm on the right and 8.0 cm on the left. Linda states that she has a lot of pain with shoulder, elbow, and digit motion. Composite digit flexion is limited; average distance from the tips of the digits to the distal palmar crease is 4 to 5 cm. Manual muscle testing and grip strength testing was deferred due to recent fracture. Linda's pain was evaluated using the visual analog scale and rated as 8 to 9 of 10 with movement on the right, and 5/10 at rest. Linda is anxious to remove the temporary splint because it is very heavy and uncomfortable. Linda appears agitated and distressed. She states that she lives alone with no family members in the area. She admits to being anxious about taking care of her dog and her apartment.

Using different clinical reasoning approaches, answer the following questions about this client and the prescribed orthosis.

Procedural Reasoning

1. What client factors are important to consider when determining the most suitable orthotic design for this client?

2. Which wrist immobilization orthotic design would be most appropriate for this client? Why?

3. What LTTM properties are important to consider?

4. Describe the instructions you would give this client on:

    ◦ How to care for the orthosis

    ◦ Wearing schedule

    ◦ Precautions

    ◦ Exercises/activities

Pragmatic Reasoning

5. What resources are available to fabricate this orthosis (time, materials, expertise)?

6. Are you able to clearly document the need for this orthosis?

7. Does evidence-based practice support the use of this orthosis for this client's diagnosis?

Interactive Reasoning

8. What are the client's goals and valued occupations?

9. What impact will the client's injury and use of the orthosis have on her ADL?

Conditional Reasoning

10. What factors will influence this client's compliance to the wearing schedule of this orthosis?

Narrative Reasoning

11. How does this injury and, more specifically, this orthotic intervention, affect this client's valued occupations?

12. What activities is this client the most concerned about?

Ethical Reasoning

13. Does the client understand the need for the orthosis?

14. Does the client have the resources to be able to pay for the orthosis (as applicable)?

15. What other options are available to this client if she lacks the resources necessary to pay for the orthosis?

16. Write one short-term goal (1 to 2 weeks) and one long-term goal (6 to 8 weeks) for this client.

Case Study 2

Kayla is a 32-year-old woman with a 2-week history of tingling and numbness in her right dominant hand. Her symptoms are more pronounced at night and when she uses her computer keyboard for long periods. She is concerned that she may be developing carpal tunnel syndrome and is eager to begin treatment. She is married with two young children and reports having "normal" pregnancies.

She presents for therapy with a prescription that reads:
Right carpal tunnel syndrome:

1. *Occupational therapy evaluation and treatment*

2. *Right wrist immobilization orthosis*

3. *Client education on work station set-up and home program*

Your assessment:

Kayla demonstrates no impairment in mobility for both upper extremities, and her grip and pinch strength are within normal limits bilaterally. She does have mild sensory impairment in her right thumb and second and third digits (3.22 mg with Semmes-Weinstein monofilaments). No impairment was noted in two-point discrimination of all fingertips and thumb in the right hand. Phalen's maneuver is positive on the right with complaints of paresthesia in her right hand after 10 to 20 seconds. She is independent in all ADL but notices that it is harder for her to use her computer keyboard toward the end of her work day, and she occasionally wakes up with marked numbness in her right hand. She enjoys going to the park with her kids, doing yoga and pilates, and cooking with her family.

Using different clinical reasoning approaches, answer the following questions about this client and the prescribed orthosis.

Procedural Reasoning

1. What client factors are important to consider when determining the most suitable orthotic design for this client?

2. Which wrist immobilization orthotic design would be most appropriate for this client? Why?

3. What LTTM properties are important to consider?

4. Describe the instructions you would give this client on:
   - How to care for the orthosis
   - Wearing schedule
   - Precautions
   - Exercises/activities

Pragmatic Reasoning

5. What resources are available to fabricate this orthosis (time, materials, expertise)?

6. Are you able to clearly document the need for this orthosis?

7. Does evidence-based practice support the use of this orthosis for this client's diagnosis?

Interactive Reasoning

8. What are the client's goals and valued occupations?

9. What impact will the client's injury and use of the orthosis have on her ADL?

Conditional Reasoning

10. What factors will influence this client's compliance to the wearing schedule of this orthosis?

Narrative Reasoning

11. How does orthotic intervention affect this client's valued occupations?

12. What activities is this client the most concerned about?

Ethical Reasoning

13. Does the client understand the need for the orthosis?

14. Does the client have the resources to be able to pay for the orthosis (as applicable)?

15. What other options are available to this client if she lacks the resources necessary to pay for the orthosis?

16. Write one short-term goal (1 to 2 weeks) and one long-term goal (6 to 8 weeks) for this client.

Appendix

STUDENT ASSIGNMENTS

1. Define all of the key terms used in this chapter.

2. As an occupational therapy practitioner, you must provide your client with detailed instructions for wearing and caring for his or her orthosis. This document must be required for the client's official records and insurance payments. Select one of the wrist orthotic designs from this chapter and prepare a client-centered handout for wearing this orthosis. Base your client description on the case study in this chapter. Include the following in the handout:
   - A description/name of the orthosis
   - An outline of the wearing schedule (remember this will vary depending on the client's condition)
   - A description of how to clean and care for the orthosis

- Instructions on what the client should be aware of when wearing the orthosis (e.g., red areas on skin, pain, increased swelling)
- Contact information and follow-up instructions

3. Prepare a case study of a client requiring a wrist immobilization orthosis. Use one of the evidence-based resources cited in the chapter to support your orthotic intervention. Summarize the research and explain the outcomes of the study.

4. As an occupational therapy practitioner, it will be interesting and informative for you to spend an extended period wearing an orthosis to appreciate the effect that an orthosis will have on your client's daily occupations. Wear a wrist immobilization orthosis designed by your lab partner for a 24-hour period. Take note of how it feels to have one body part immobilized. Elaborate in paragraphs on the following:

- Describe the orthosis, material used, positioning, and typical diagnosis for this particular orthosis.
- Comfort and ease of use: Is the orthosis easy to take on and off? Does the orthosis fit under clothing? Are there any pressure areas? What needs to be modified and how?
- Personal and public image: Does the orthosis attract attention in public? Does the orthosis attract attention in your family? How did this make you feel, even as a class assignment?
- Functionality: How were you able to function with the orthosis? Was the position helpful or harmful? What would the typical wearing schedule be for a client with the typical need for this orthosis? What instructions should be given to the typical client with the need for this orthosis?
- How does this change your appreciation of what your clients are experiencing with their orthoses?

5. Complete the check-out form on the next page.

Multiple Choice Answer Key

6. b
7. a
8. a
9. c
10. b
11. d
12. a
13. a

Wrist Orthosis Check-Out Form

(This can be used for faculty to evaluate students' completed orthoses,
as well as for students to reference when evaluating their own completed orthosis.)

Fabricate one of the orthotic designs for a wrist immobilization orthosis on your classmate and complete the following check-out form:

Name of Orthosis:

Purpose of Orthosis:

Design/Function

_____ The wrist is positioned correctly for condition.

_____ The thenar area is cleared adequately.

_____ The distal palmar crease is clear/full MCP joint motion is observed.

_____ The orthosis is half the width of the forearm.

_____ The orthosis is two-fourths the length of the forearm.

_____ The hand arches are supported: distal and proximal transverse arches, longitudinal arch.

_____ Full thumb-to-fingertip opposition is observed.

_____ The orthosis does not migrate distally with elbow flexion.

_____ The orthosis does not cause impingement or pressure areas.

_____ The orthosis clears all bony prominences.

Straps/Orthosis Appearance

_____ The straps are in the correct position: wrist, forearm, and hand.

_____ The straps are secure and corners rounded.

_____ The orthosis edges are smooth and corners rounded.

_____ The proximal edge is flared.

_____ The orthosis is free of fingerprints, pattern marks, or indentations.

CHAPTER 5

Wrist and Hand
Immobilization Orthoses

Key Terms

Antideformity position
Ball design
Brachial plexus palsy
Close-packed position
Cone design
Erb's palsy

Functional hand position
Intrinsic plus position
Open-packed position/position
   of deformity
Palmar abduction

Position of safe immobilization (POSI)
Radial deficiency
Subluxation
Tenodesis effect
Zig-zag deformity

Learning Outcomes

Upon completion of this chapter, you will be able to:

1. Describe three to five common clinical conditions and goals for a wrist and hand immobilization orthosis.

2. Identify pertinent anatomical structures and biomechanical principles involved in a wrist and hand immobilization orthosis and apply these concepts to orthotic design and fabrication.

3. Identify the four most commonly selected orthotic designs and describe the rationale for choosing one design over another.

4. Design suitable patterns for the four common types of wrist and hand immobilization orthoses and identify the pertinent anatomical landmarks.

5. Outline the steps involved in the fabrication of a wrist and hand immobilization orthosis.

6. Complete the molding and finishing of a wrist and hand immobilization orthosis.

7. Evaluate the fit and function of a completed wrist and hand immobilization orthosis and identify and address all areas needing adjustment.

8. Identify elements of a client education program following provision of a wrist and hand immobilization orthosis.

9. Describe special considerations of wrist and hand orthotic design and fabrication.

Schofield, K., & Schwartz, D. *Orthotic Design and Fabrication*
for the Upper Extremity: A Practical Guide (pp 81-99).
© 2019 Taylor & Francis Group.

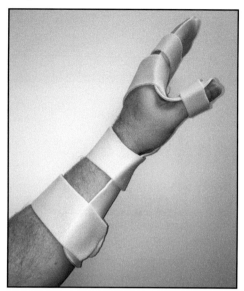

Figure 5-1. This is the position used to immobilize the wrist and hand following injury to prevent development of joint and/or soft tissue contractures. (Reprinted with permission from Chad Royer.)

Introduction

Immobilization of the wrist and hand is necessary for treatment of certain conditions. Traumatic injuries that involve multiple joints and soft tissues may cause significant edema and pain and require immobilization of the entire hand and wrist. Painful arthritic episodes may also require immobilization of the wrist and hand. Other situations may arise where a client has little volitional control of the distal upper extremity (UE) and may also benefit from an orthosis that immobilizes the wrist and hand, often described as a wrist and hand immobilization orthosis. Such situations include multiple sclerosis, cerebral vascular accidents, traumatic brain injuries, and spinal cord injuries. Children with a wide range of congenital conditions, such as juvenile rheumatoid arthritis (RA), radial club hand, **brachial plexus palsy**, cerebral palsy, and others, may need the support of a wrist hand immobilization orthosis at various stages in their development.

Proper hand and wrist positioning in a wrist and hand immobilization orthosis is critical for healing of involved structures and preventing contractures of the involved joints and shortening of the tissues. In the absence of disease or injury, the hand and wrist assume a typical resting, or functional, position. This position, often referred to as the *functional resting hand position*, is characterized by wrist extension, metacarpophalangeal (MCP) joint flexion, slight proximal interphalangeal (PIP) and distal interphalangeal (DIP) joint flexion, and thumb abduction (Figure 5-1). When the digit and thumb flexor muscles are relaxed (flexor digitorum superficialis, flexor digitorum profundus, and flexor pollicis longus), this is the natural

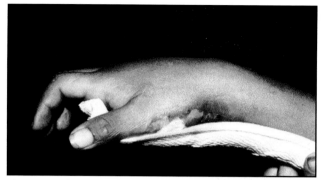

Figure 5-2. The open-packed position, or position of deformity, can encourage development of joint and/or soft tissue contractures.

position that the digits and thumb assume when the wrist extends. This is known as the **tenodesis effect**. Following injury, the hand often assumes an **open-packed position**, or **position of deformity** (Figure 5-2). This is a position where the articular surfaces of a joint are in minimal contact with each other and the collateral ligaments and joint capsule are lax, or loose. This is opposed to the **close-packed position**, where the articular surfaces of the joint are in maximum contact with each other and the joint capsule and collateral ligaments are taut, or tight. The hand often assumes the open-packed position following injury due to pain and development of edema. This position is characterized by wrist slight flexion, extension of the MCP joints, flexion of the PIP and DIP joints, and adduction of the thumb web space. This can lead to development of joint and soft tissue contractures if not corrected early. The two most common positions used for wrist and hand orthoses are the resting hand position (or **functional hand position**) and the **antideformity position**, also known as the **intrinsic plus position** (Figure 5-3). Some clinicians refer to this as the **position of safe immobilization (POSI)**. A summary of the different hand positions is shown in Box 5-1.

The position chosen for the orthosis will depend on the client's condition and goals of the orthosis.

Wrist and hand immobilization orthoses are used for a wide variety of diagnoses and conditions. It is important to design and mold these orthoses properly so that they fit each individual client appropriately. The basic design for the wrist and hand orthosis takes into account the client's clinical condition, his or her functional needs, specifications set by the referring physician, and the most appropriate low-temperature thermoplastic material (LTTM). Some examples include the following:

- When a client presents with severe edema of the involved extremity, it is preferable to select an LTTM with full memory because the orthosis may need to be remolded when the client's edema decreases over time.

- If the client's hand is large and presents with increased tone, the LTTM must have enough rigidity to support the weight of the involved extremity.

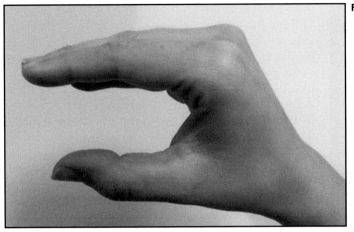

Figure 5-3. Intrinsic plus, or antideformity position.

Box 5-1. Hand and Wrist Positions

OPEN-PACKED POSITION/POSITION OF DEFORMITY

- Wrist: 10 to 20 degrees of flexion
- MCP joints: extension
- PIP and DIP joints: flexion
- Thumb: adduction

RESTING HAND POSITION

- Wrist: 10 to 20 degrees of extension
- MCP joints: 50 to 55 degrees of flexion
- PIP and DIP joints: 10 to 20 degrees of flexion
- Thumb: full palmar abduction (perpendicular to the second digit)

CLOSE-PACKED/ANTIDEFORMITY POSITION/ POSI

- Wrist: 20 to 30 degrees of extension
- MCP joints: 70 to 90 degrees of flexion
- PIP and DIP joints: full extension, or 0 degrees
- Thumb: full palmar abduction (perpendicular to the second digit)

Box 5-2. Common Goals of Wrist and Hand Immobilization Orthoses

PROTECTION

- Support and position the wrist, hand, digits, and thumb following surgery, trauma, or injury to protect and rest injured structures.
- Support and position the wrist, hand, digits, and thumb to provide pain relief.
- Provide joint protection for arthritic joints and minimize further joint deformity.

RESTING HAND POSITION

- Prevent joint and soft tissue contractures following surgery, trauma, or injury to the hand and wrist.
- Prevent contractures during healing following burn or other injuries.
- Position the wrist and hand to prevent shortening of muscles and tendons due to changes in muscle tone.
- Position the wrist and hand to maintain or achieve best joint alignment for function.

- If the client is elderly and frail, a lightweight, less rigid, and highly moldable LTTM may conform best to the anatomy and be less heavy for the client to support.

- When working with a pediatric client, it is important to consider that children grow at times more rapidly than at other times. The orthosis must be checked regularly for proper fit, especially if the child complains of pain or discomfort due to the orthosis suddenly becoming too tight or too small.

Goals for Use of a Wrist and Hand Immobilization Orthosis

The goals of a wrist and hand immobilization orthosis will vary depending on the individual client and his or her condition. The most common goals of wrist and hand immobilization orthoses are presented in Box 5-2.

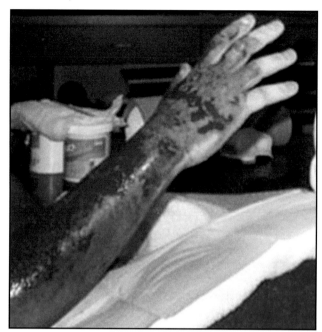

Figure 5-4. Injuries such as burns can cause the hand to assume an open-packed position due to pain and edema on the dorsal aspect of the hand.

When fabricating a wrist and hand immobilization orthosis, the practitioner must have a thorough understanding of the specific clinical condition or diagnosis and the expected outcome following orthotic use. It is important that the practitioner use sound clinical reasoning when selecting the most appropriate design and material to meet the client's particular needs.

Clinical Conditions and Wearing Schedules

This section describes common clinical conditions where a wrist and hand immobilization orthosis is often prescribed. Readers are encouraged to review the references provided for additional details regarding each clinical condition. Current evidence available supporting the use of wrist and hand orthoses as an intervention strategy is also discussed.

BURNS

Orthotic intervention plays a critical role in preventing contractures and maintaining length of tissues in the burned hand. Immediately following a burn injury, it is common for the hand and wrist to assume an open-packed position due to pain and edema formation, particularly on the dorsal aspect of the metacarpals (Figure 5-4). The wrist and hand immobilization orthosis is typically used, but the positioning of the hand may vary from the normal resting

hand position to the antideformity position (see Box 5-1). This involves placing the wrist in 30 to 50 degrees of extension, the MCP joints in 70 to 90 degrees of flexion, and the PIP and DIP joints in full extension; this is referred to as the *intrinsic plus position*, or *antideformity position*, as mentioned previously. The thumb is placed in full **palmar abduction** due to the risk of adduction contractures of the first web space. This orthosis may be used immediately following a burn injury, ideally during the inflammatory and fibroplastic phases of wound healing (0 to 6 weeks), to prevent development of joint or soft tissue contractures as the burn scar heals and matures. The skin, scar tissue, and orthosis must be periodically checked for proper fit and adjustments. When allowed, active range of motion (ROM) is initiated and encouraged.

Evidence

Level IV

- Fufa, D., Chuang, S., & Yang, J. (2015). Post burn contractures of the hand. *Journal of Hand Surgery America, 39*(9), 1869-1876. doi:10.1016/j.jhsa.2015.03.018

  ○ These authors describe current surgical and therapeutic intervention strategies following burn injuries to the hand and wrist. Principles of acute burn care include use of resting hand orthoses in an intrinsic-plus or antideformity position to prevent or minimize joint and skin contractures. Following hand burn reconstructive surgery, similar orthotic principles are employed to maintain proper joint positioning.

Level V

- Dewey, W. S., Richard, R. L., & Parry, I. S. (2011). Positioning, splinting, and contracture management. *Physical Medicine and Rehabilitation Clinics North America, 22*, 229-257.

  ○ In this narrative review, the authors recommend use of resting hand immobilization orthoses in all stages of burn rehabilitation (acute, intermediate, and long term) for maintenance of functional hand joint positioning, prevention of tissue shortening due to scar tissue deposition, skin graft protection and positioning, and correction of existing joint and/or soft tissue contractures. Hand position recommended is 15 to 25 degrees of wrist extension, 60 to 70 degrees of MCP joint flexion, full PIP and DIP joint extension, and thumb palmar abduction.

MULTIPLE FRACTURES AND TRAUMA

Crush and compression injuries and multiple fractures of any of the carpal bones, the radius and/or ulna at the wrist, the metacarpals, and the phalanges may require a wrist and hand immobilization orthosis for support, protection, and positioning. The positioning of the wrist and

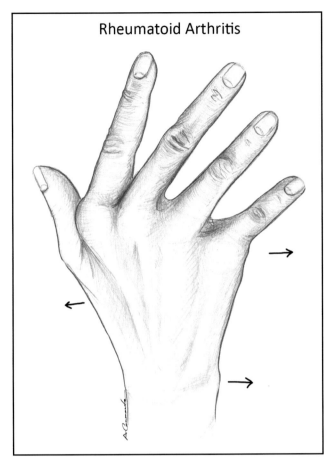

Figure 5-5. Zig-zag deformity is often associated with RA.

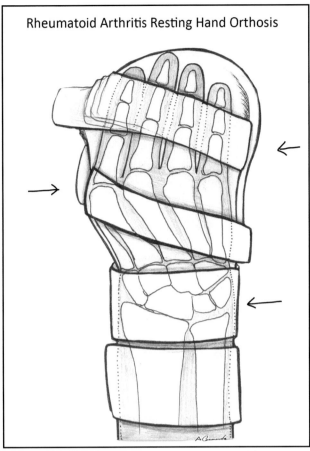

Figure 5-6. An orthosis can help reposition the wrist and digits to minimize further deformity.

hand in this orthosis may be in the functional hand or antideformity position depending on the injury itself, the extent of the edema, the wounds, and the overall pain level.

ARTHRITIS

Both osteoarthritis (OA) and RA can affect the wrist and hand by causing impaired motion, pain, and weakness. RA typically affects the UE joints symmetrically, and the wrist, MCP joints, and PIP joints are commonly involved. Deformities include ulnar deviation of the wrist and volar **subluxation** of the carpus, along with associated ulnar drift and volar subluxation of the MCP joints, resulting in what is commonly referred to as **zig-zag deformity** (Figures 5-5 and 5-6).

OA typically affects the wrist, PIP and/or DIP joints, and MCP joint of the thumb. The MCP joints of the digits are rarely affected. Wrist and hand immobilization orthoses can help decrease both RA and OA symptoms by supporting the wrist and hand in a resting and comfortable position to reduce pain, which can secondarily help prevent further deformity and improve hand function (see Figure 5-6).

Evidence

Level V

- Beasley, J. (2012). Osteoarthritis and rheumatoid arthritis: Conservative therapeutic management. *Journal of Hand Therapy, 25*(2), 163-172. doi:10.1016/jht.2011.11.001

  ○ Use of wrist and hand immobilization orthoses for RA patients can help reduce pain and reduce joint deformity. Care should be taken to address all involved joints if the client presents with zig-zag deformity, specifically the carpometacarpal joints of the digits. Positioning the MCP joints in an anti-ulnar drift position can worsen the radial deviation deformity seen at the carpometacarpal joints and metacarpals.

- Chim, H. W., Reese, S. K., Toomey, S. N., & Moran, S. L. (2015). Update on the surgical treatment for rheumatoid arthritis of the wrist and hand. *Journal of Hand Therapy, 27*(2), 134-142. doi:10.1016/j.jht.2013.12.002

  ○ Use of wrist and hand immobilization orthoses following MCP joint arthroplasty surgery rather than a dynamic MCP joint extension orthotic design is

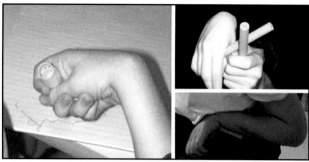

Figure 5-7. Following brain trauma or stroke, clients can develop abnormalities in muscle tone, such as hypertonicity.

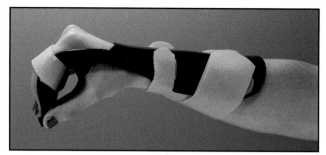

Figure 5-8. A wrist and hand immobilization orthosis can help to position the hand and wrist to minimize the development of joint and/or soft tissue contractures.

now recommended for clients with RA. The authors note that compliance is improved with these orthoses and clients have an easier time donning and doffing the orthosis during the rehabilitation phase.

ABNORMAL TONE

In the absence of disease or injury, muscles have resting tone, or resistance to passive stretch. This is created by connective tissues present in muscle, as well as input from the central and peripheral nervous systems. A common physical impairment in the UE following brain trauma or stroke is the development of abnormal muscle tone. There are different terms used to describe abnormalities in tone. These include *flaccidity, hypertonicity, hypotonicity,* and *rigidity.* Flaccidity is characterized by absence of both muscle tone and deep tendon reflexes. No active movement in the extremity is observed. Flaccidity typically presents immediately following a traumatic injury or event in the brain or spinal cord. It can also occur following injury to a lower motor nerve or peripheral nerve. Hypertonicity typically develops a few weeks later but may also be present immediately following injury. In contrast to flaccidity, hypertonicity is an increase in muscle tone with resistance to active and passive movement. Injury to upper motor neurons in the brain or spinal cord interrupts the normal pathway between these neurons and the lower motor neurons. Stretch reflexes become hyperactive, resulting in increased muscle tone. In hypertonicity, changes can also occur in the connective tissue of the involved muscles and surrounding joints, resulting in soft tissue and joint contractures. Rigidity is also an increase in muscle tone, but muscles on both sides of a joint are affected, resulting in loss of voluntary movement in all directions that a joint moves. This is in contrast to hypertonicity, where muscles on one side of a joint demonstrate increased tone and muscles on the other side become inactive, or weak. Hypotonicity, or less-than-normal muscle tone, is characterized by muscle weakness and impaired ability to resist the force of gravity during active movement. Wrist and hand immobilization orthoses can help support hypotonic or flaccid muscles, help prevent the development of joint and soft tissue contractures, and

temporarily reduce hypertonicity of the wrist and digit flexor muscles (Figures 5-7 and 5-8).

Evidence

Level I

- Ivy, C. C., Smith, S. M., & Materi, M. M. (2015). Upper extremity orthoses use in amyotrophic lateral sclerosis/motor neuron disease: A systematic review. *International Journal of Physical Medicine & Rehabilitation, 3*(2), 264.

  ∘ These authors examined the current literature to determine common orthotic interventions for individuals with amyotrophic lateral sclerosis/motor neuron disease. Available evidence to support orthotic intervention for this population is limited to Level IV (case reports) and Level V (expert opinions). Such evidence suggests that wrist and hand immobilization orthoses can help reduce pain, provide rest to fatigued musculature, and prevent development of joint and soft tissue contractures.

Level II

- Copley, J., Kuipers, K., Fleming, J., & Rassafiani, M. (2013). Individualized resting hand splints for adults with acquired brain injury: A randomized, single blinded, single case design. *Neurorehabilitation, 32*(5), 885-898.

  ∘ These authors investigated the effects of a wrist and hand immobilization orthosis on wrist and digit spasticity following brain injury in adults using a randomized, single-blinded, single-case design. Results support use of orthotic intervention in positively influencing wrist and digit flexor spasticity, tissue stiffness, and passive digit motion in individuals without joint or soft tissue contractures.

Level III

- Pizzi, A., Carlucci, G., Falsimi, C., & Verdesca, S. (2005). Application of a volar static splint in post-stroke spasticity of the upper limb. *Archives of Physical Medicine and Rehabilitation, 86,* 1855-1859.

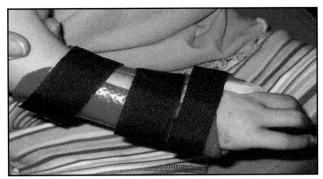

Figure 5-9. This orthosis illustrates centralization of the wrist on the forearm and hand following surgery to transfer the second digit to the thumb (the child has radial deficiency and absence of a thumb).

- ○ These authors conducted a pretest-posttest trial study to assess the effectiveness of a volar-based resting hand immobilization orthosis on spasticity, wrist and elbow passive ROM, pain, and spasms in clients with post-stroke upper limb spasticity. Wrist and elbow pain, passive ROM, and flexor carpi radialis spasticity were positively affected by use of an orthosis for 90 minutes per day for 3 months. The orthosis was well tolerated by the study participants.

PEDIATRIC CONDITIONS

Children may benefit from wrist and hand immobilization orthoses for conditions such as **radial deficiencies** and brachial plexus palsy. A brief overview of these conditions is provided here. Radial deficiencies (Figure 5-9) refer to all congenital hand anomalies with failure of formation along the radial border of the UE. Orthotic intervention may be started immediately after birth. A program of passive stretching along with orthotic intervention is introduced. A wrist and hand immobilization orthosis can help centralize the hand, maintain digital alignment, and prevent flexion contractures of the digits. The orthosis may be worn full-time until the baby begins to use the hands. Particular attention must be addressed to the increased prominence of the ulnar styloid. The LTTM can be carefully formed so as to not put pressure on this bony prominence.

Evidence

Level V

- Takagi, T., Seki, A., Takayama, S., & Watanabe, M. (2017). Current concepts in radial club hand. *The Open Orthopaedics Journal, 11*, 369-377.
  - ○ These authors provide an overview of current treatment considerations for radial club hand. Use of orthoses is recommended soon after birth and should continue for at least 6 months, with the goal of stretching tight soft tissues and aligning the hand and wrist with the ulna. The authors also recommend inclusion of the elbow due to the small size of

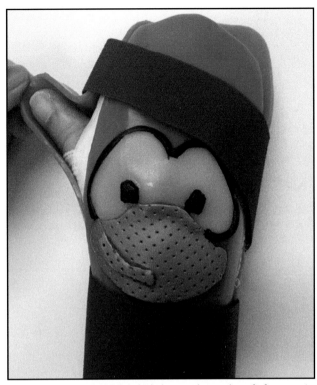

Figure 5-10. A child with brachial plexus palsy can benefit from a wrist and hand immobilization orthosis. (Reprinted with permission from Maria Candida Miranda Luzo.)

the arm. Continued use of orthoses combined with stretching is advised until 2 to 3 years of age.

Brachial plexus palsy is an injury to the brachial plexus that occurs at birth. **Erb's palsy**, injury to the C5-C6 nerve roots of the brachial plexus, is the most common injury of this type. Many children with this condition will recover spontaneously within the first 2 months of life. Children who do not exhibit recovery by 3 months of age may have permanent impairments, which may include limited ROM, decreased strength, and a smaller UE. Initial treatment may include passive stretching of every joint and orthotic intervention. The typical posturing of the UE in brachial plexus palsy is an extended elbow, pronated forearm, flexion of the wrist and digits, and the thumb adducted into the palm. A wrist and hand immobilization orthosis is important for proper positioning to maintain joint alignment and to prevent deformities and or contractures (Figure 5-10).

Wrist and Hand Immobilization Orthotic Designs

The practitioner should create a customized design when fabricating a wrist and hand immobilization orthosis for each individual client. The most common designs are volar, volar/dorsal, design for hypertonicity, and design for RA. The specific design should depend on the client's

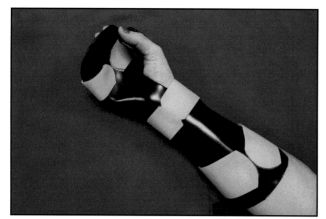

Figure 5-11. A volar design covers the volar surfaces of the hand, wrist, and forearm.

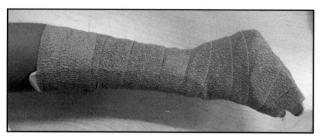

Figure 5-12. This wrist and hand immobilization orthosis can be used following a burn injury.

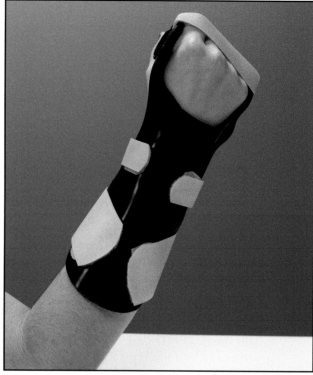

Figure 5-13. A volar/dorsal design may be better suited for situations where it is contraindicated to have thermoplastic material over wounds, pins, or skin grafts.

clinical condition, indications requested by the referring physician, and practitioner clinical reasoning. This section reviews each of the four most common designs, the main applications, and the advantages and disadvantages of each design.

VOLAR DESIGN

The volar-based wrist and hand immobilization orthosis covers the volar surfaces of the hand, wrist, and forearm and extends to the tips of the digits and thumb (Figure 5-11). In the resting hand position, the wrist is in 20 to 30 degrees of extension, the digit MCP joints in 50 to 55 degrees of flexion, the PIP and DIP joints in slight flexion, and the thumb supported in abduction and slight flexion (see Box 5-1). In the intrinsic plus position, or antideformity position, the digit MCP joints are immobilized in 70 degrees of flexion; the digit PIP and DIP joints in full extension, or 0 degrees; and the thumb in palmar abduction to maintain the web space (see Box 5-1). As discussed previously, the intrinsic plus position is most commonly used following a burn injury to the hand but can be applied to other conditions where the client is at risk for development of severe scarring and contractures. The orthosis may be secured initially with light elastic bandage such as Coban wrap (3M), cotton bandages, or an Ace bandage (3M) to accommodate for edema, wounds, and exudate (Figure 5-12). A key strap across the

dorsal aspect of the wrist plays a critical role in stabilizing the wrist in this design. Additional strapping supports the forearm, hand, digits, and thumb.

VOLAR/DORSAL DESIGN

The volar/dorsal-based wrist and hand immobilization orthosis design may be more suitable for conditions that present with hypertonicity in the wrist and digit flexor muscles, or for situations where it is contraindicated to have LTTM over fragile wounds, pins, or skin grafts (Figure 5-13). In this design, the forearm component is placed on the dorsal aspect of the forearm and wrist and the palmar component on the volar aspect of the palm and digits. Gravity assists with the positioning of the forearm and wrist, but the material must be maintained at all times under the palm. This design positions the wrist in extension by the lever created by the dorsal forearm component, thereby eliminating the need for a strap to secure the wrist in the orthosis.

DESIGN FOR HYPERTONICITY

The wrist and hand immobilization orthosis for hypertonicity design positions the digits in abduction and the thumb in extension. This position may assist in temporarily reducing muscle tone in the wrist and digit flexor

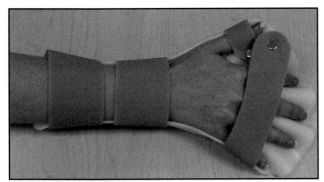

Figure 5-14. Digit abduction and thumb extension in a wrist and hand immobilization orthosis design.

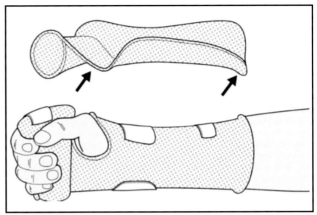

Figure 5-15. The cone design can be used for clients with hypertonicity. (Reprinted with permission from Orfit Industries.)

muscles (Figure 5-14). Other options include the **cone** or **ball designs**. The cone orthosis positions the digits around a conical form (Figure 5-15).

The ball design orthosis specifies an orthosis fashioned over a ball during fabrication where the practitioner can separate each digit into its own space. This is done by using a tool or the practitioner's digits to form a space from underneath the material, separating each digit into its own compartment in the palmar portion of the material.

DESIGN FOR RHEUMATOID ARTHRITIS

The wrist and hand immobilization orthosis design for individuals with RA offers protection and rest for the wrist and digits during periods of inflammation known as *flare-ups*. This design protects the wrist and positions the digit MCP joints in normal joint alignment and 10 to 20 degrees of flexion but leaves the PIP and DIP joints and thumb joints free to move (Figure 5-16).

See Table 5-1 for a comparison of the most common wrist and hand immobilization orthotic designs.

The following are important considerations (Figure 5-17):

- The distal transverse arch: The metacarpal heads should be supported fully, with care taken to accommodate the difference in length of the metacarpal bones. The arch is naturally higher on the radial side of the hand.

- The proximal transverse arch: The natural concavity formed by the distal carpal row and the bases of metacarpal bones should be fully supported.

- The longitudinal arch: This arch should be fully maintained in the orthosis, including the metacarpals and proximal, middle, and distal phalanges. The orthosis should conform to the natural concavity of this arch, unless the antideformity position is being used.

- The web space: The thumb must be positioned in palmar abduction and the LTTM conformed to match the web space. This will help to maintain tissue length and minimize the development of a first web space contracture (Figure 5-18).

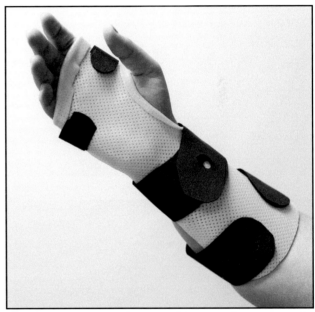

Figure 5-16. This wrist and hand immobilization orthosis supports the wrist and MCP joints for individuals with RA but leaves the PIP and DIP joints free, along with the thumb.

- Bony prominences: The dorsal aspect of the MCP, PIP, and DIP joints, as well as the thumb MCP and interphalangeal (IP) joints, may be subject to compressive forces from the straps. Padding these areas inside the straps will optimize comfort and security of the orthosis.

- Hand edema: As discussed in Chapter 2, the relative laxity of the skin on the dorsal aspect of the hand encourages development of edema in this area following injury. As a result, the hand typically falls into a position of comfort: MCP joint extension, PIP and DIP joint flexion, thumb adduction, and wrist flexion. The practitioner must take care to accommodate for the edema and position the hand and wrist correctly to prevent joint and soft tissue contractures

Table 5-1

COMPARISON OF THE MOST COMMON WRIST AND HAND IMMOBILIZATION ORTHOTIC DESIGNS

	TYPICAL POSITION OF FABRICATION	ADVANTAGES OF DESIGN	DISADVANTAGES OF DESIGN
VOLAR	Forearm in supination	Allows for visualization of arches, web space, and other anatomical landmarks; gravity assists placement	May be difficult for positioning in the first web space while maintaining the MCP joints in flexion
VOLAR/ DORSAL	Forearm in pronation when clients cannot supinate the forearm	Allows for practitioner's control of multiple joints; no surface contact on flexor muscle bellies (contact might increase tone)	Must work against gravity while forming palmar component
CONE DESIGN	Forearm in supination or pronation	Allows for client's digits to grasp around material during wear	Need to wrap material around cone and prevent it from sticking
RA	Forearm in pronation	Leaves the fingers free to move at the PIP and DIP joints	Does not prevent contractures of the PIP and DIP joints or maintain length of the digits in proper alignment
BALL DESIGN	Forearm in pronation, palm placed over LTTM over ball	Allows for separation of each digit into its own space	May be challenging to separate each individual finger while also molding material around forearm and wrist

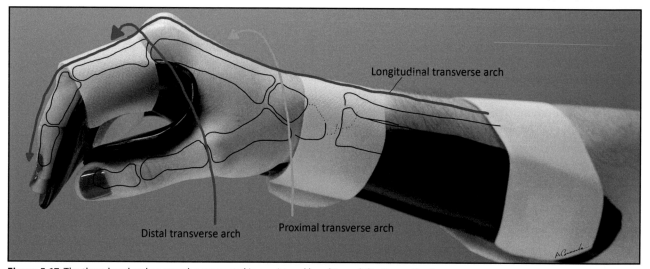

Figure 5-17. The three hand arches must be supported in a wrist and hand immobilization orthosis.

(antideformity or resting hand position) when fabricating a wrist and hand immobilization orthosis. The strapping may constrict the tissues underneath and cause edema to collect between the straps if placed too tightly. Light elastic bandage such as Coban wrap, cotton bandages, or an Ace bandage can be used to secure the orthosis until the edema subsides.

Biomechanical Principles to Consider With Wrist and Hand Immobilization Orthoses

Similar to many orthoses that immobilize a single joint or a series of joints, a wrist and hand immobilization

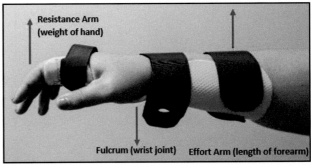

Figure 5-19. A wrist and hand immobilization orthosis represents a first-class lever system.

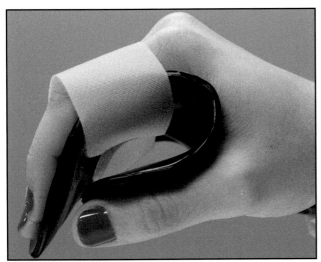

Figure 5-18. The thumb component of a wrist and hand immobilization orthosis must fully support the first web space and position the thumb in palmar abduction.

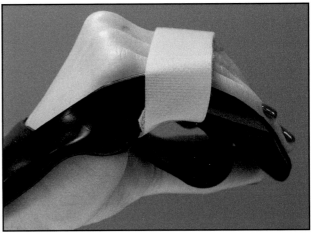

Figure 5-20. The digits need to be fully supported in the hand portion of the orthosis.

orthosis represents a first-class lever system. This means that the wrist is the fulcrum, or axis; the forearm trough is the effort arm/force, and the entire hand is the resistance arm/force (Figure 5-19).

To ensure that the orthosis supports the hand and wrist adequately, the forearm portion should be at least two-thirds the length of the forearm. This is especially important because this orthosis must support the weight of the wrist, digits, and thumb. Other important fabrication points to consider include the following:

- Flare the proximal edge adequately, particularly if the orthosis is to be worn at night. Clients often flex their elbows while sleeping, and the proximal edge may create pressure.

- Support the digits in the pan portion of the orthosis (Figure 5-20). Troughs on the radial and ulnar sides prevent the digits from slipping off the sides. The tips of the digits should not extend past the distal edge.

- Support the thumb in wide abduction and slight flexion and place in front of the index finger.

Orthotic Fabrication Steps

Please also see the demonstration videos for more information.

1. Pattern making
   - Wrist and hand immobilization orthosis: resting hand orthosis (Figure 5-21)
   - Wrist and hand immobilization orthosis: volar/dorsal design (Figure 5-22)
   - Wrist hand immobilization orthosis: design for RA (Figure 5-23)

2. Material selection
   - LTTM choices for wrist and hand immobilization orthoses are described in Table 5-2.

3. Client positioning

4. Molding techniques

5. Finishing techniques: edges and strapping

6. Orthosis check-out
   - Can the client flex his or her elbow without the orthosis migrating distally?

     If no, the orthosis is too long or the proximal edge is not flared adequately.

   - Does the client complain of discomfort while resting his or her hand in the orthosis?

     If yes, locate the area(s) of discomfort. Some possible solutions include the following:

     - *Flare more space around the bony prominences. Padding may be added, but this needs to be done after the LTTM is flared away.*

     - *Smooth and round all rough edges.*

     - *Reposition straps to secure the hand in the orthosis, especially the wrist strap.*

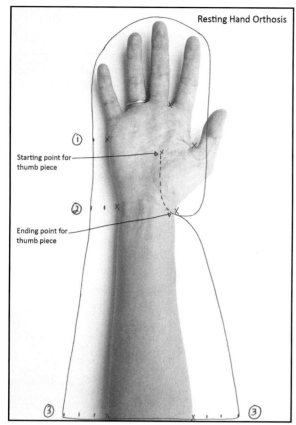

Figure 5-21. Volar wrist and hand immobilization orthosis pattern design.

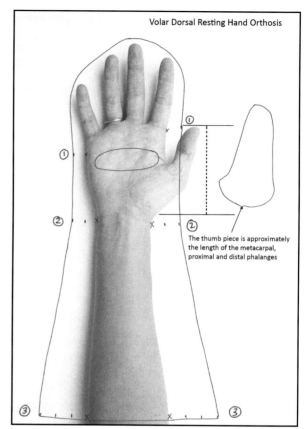

Figure 5-22. Volar/dorsal wrist and hand immobilization orthosis pattern design.

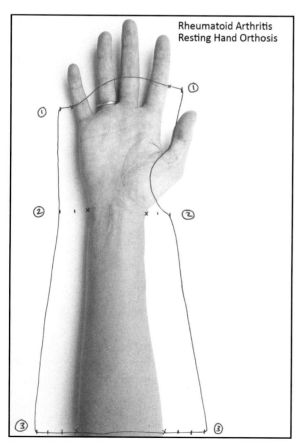

Figure 5-23. Design for RA.

- Are the corners of the orthosis rounded and smooth?

  If no, round and smooth all corners of the orthosis.

- Are the straps secure and edges rounded?

  If no, adjust the straps: The wrist strap should go in a circumferential fashion around the wrist; the ends should meet together. No Velcro should be exposed. The proximal strap should be angled on the orthosis so it sits flat on the forearm. The distal strap should stabilize the proximal phalanges comfortably.

- Is the wrist strap positioned over the ulnar head? Is there padding to avoid pressure?

  If no, reposition the strap so it is directly over the wrist and ulnar head. Place a doughnut pad directly over the ulnar head and secure it to the undersurface of the strap.

- Is the forearm strap angled to accommodate for the shape of the forearm?

  If no, reposition the strap so it lies flat against the muscle bulk of the proximal forearm.

- Are all of the distal straps secure?

  If no, lengthen the strap and corresponding Velcro (longer strapping material and Velcro increases security).

Table 5-2

LTTM Choices for Wrist and Hand Immobilization Orthoses

MATERIAL CONSIDERATIONS	RESTING HAND ORTHOSIS	VOLAR/DORSAL DESIGN	DESIGN FOR RHEUMATOID ARTHRITIS
Thickness	For adults, use 1/8-inch thickness. For children, use 1/12 or 3/32 inch.	For adults and children, use 1/8-inch thickness (to support, counteract spasticity/hypertonicity).	3/32-inch thickness or 1/8 inch perforated (ensure that the material is as lightweight as possible).
Drapability	Select a material that will support the wrist and hand arches. Intimate conformability is not necessary.	Select a material that will support the wrist and hand arches. Intimate conformability is not necessary.	Select a material that will conform well in the palm and digits and over enlarged bony prominences such as the ulnar head.
Elasticity	Products with high resistance to stretch recommended.	Products with high resistance to stretch recommended.	Products with moderate resistance to stretch recommended. Avoid overly rigid materials.
Memory	Choose a product with high memory if frequent adjustments are anticipated.	Choose a product with high memory if frequent adjustments are necessary.	Choose a product with memory if frequent adjustments are necessary (e.g., if the client experiences multiple flare-ups).

∘ Are all indentations and pattern marks removed?

If no, use a heat gun to smooth the LTTM. Rubbing alcohol can be used to remove wax pencil marks. Ink cannot be removed, so refrain from using this when drawing your pattern on the LTTM.

∘ Remove the orthosis after 5 to 10 minutes and observe the skin. Are there any reddened areas?

If yes, adjust the orthosis by flaring and smoothing edges and/or flaring material away from bony prominences.

∘ Review the purpose and care of the resting hand immobilization orthosis with the client. Does he or she understand the following?:

■ The purpose of the orthosis

■ The daily wearing schedule

■ How to take care of the orthosis

■ How to don and doff correctly

If no, discuss the wearing schedule and care of the orthosis with the client before he or she leaves the clinic, and provide clear written instructions to take home with him or her (refer to the Appendix at the end of the chapter). Take a photo of the orthosis correctly positioned using a smart phone and send it to your client for reference along with written

instructions on the wearing schedule. Document all of your instructions to the client and maintain a copy of these in the client's chart.

See Box 5-3 for additional information and tips on orthotic fabrication for various clinical conditions.

Summary

• The goals of a wrist and hand immobilization orthosis and wearing schedule will vary depending on the client's needs and the diagnosis.

• A wrist and hand immobilization orthosis represents a first-class lever system.

• Common positioning for a wrist and hand immobilization orthosis is in the resting hand position or antideformity position.

• Each client may require a specific orthotic design or adaptation to achieve the best outcome with his or her orthosis.

• Each orthosis must be molded to the individual anatomy for the best fit.

• Post-fabrication critique and check-out helps identify areas for modification and optimize client comfort.

Box 5-3. Helpful Hints

- *Burns*: Clients with severe burns may require frequent dressing changes and wound care. The orthosis must be easy to take off and on with minimal movement required by the client. Choose dark-colored material to hide dirt and stains from medications or wounds. Consider securing the orthosis with cotton, inelastic bandages to avoid excessive compression on healing wounds.

- *Trauma and clients with significant edema*: Clients with edema will require frequent orthosis checkups to make sure the fit and positioning remain correct. Choose materials with memory for ease with remolding, and consider alternate methods to secure the orthosis such as Coban wrap, cotton, or Ace bandages. Consider cotton bandages in the early stages to avoid excessive pressure on the tissues from the dressings.

- *Arthritis*: Clients with OA or RA may tolerate lighter-weight materials that offer a little flexibility better than rigid supports. Consider appropriate padding for sensitive and fragile skin. To ensure that the straps are easy to handle when clients have limited pinch strength/dexterity, consider lengthening them or incorporating a loop on one end of the strap.

- *Spasticity*: Clients with high tone need well-fitting but rigid supportive orthoses to maintain positioning and provide tone-inhibiting counterpressure. Additional help with positioning may be needed from another practitioner to assist with positioning. Consider the volar/dorsal design, which acts as a lever while donning and is thus easier to put on. In rare instances, it may be necessary to mold the orthosis on another individual with a similar-sized hand and wrist and then fit to the client if he or she cannot tolerate the molding process.

- *Flaccidity*: Clients with flaccidity may have loss of muscle tone throughout the UE and may require a sling or other supportive device in addition to the wrist and hand immobilization orthosis. Frequent evaluation of orthosis fit and comfort by the practitioner is also an important consideration because these clients may have impaired sensory awareness of the extremity and be unable to provide feedback when he or she is wearing the orthosis.

- *Geriatrics*: You may want to choose colorful materials to make it easier to locate the orthosis. That said, this may have the possible disadvantage of also making the wearing of the orthosis more apparent. Number the straps to make donning and doffing the orthosis easy, and provide photos of proper wear as required. Consider using lightweight materials and padding the orthosis edges to optimize comfort and prevent skin breakdown.

- *Pediatrics*: Choose colorful materials and decorate to enhance compliance. Calm the child with soft music or by telling a story. Position the child in a comfortable position to reduce muscle tone if hypertonicity is an issue. Try to prevent sudden movements and loud noises that can startle. Speak calmly and slowly and handle the child's extremity firmly. The lever arm(s) may need to be extended to secure the orthosis on the hand properly (e.g., the elbow may need to be secured in the orthosis to prevent distal migration). Consider making a similar orthosis on a doll or stuffed animal, naming the orthosis to personalize it, or using decorations from a favorite toy figure.

In Your Client's Shoes

Using a wrist and hand immobilization orthosis will significantly impact your client's daily occupations. Depending on the diagnosis, some clients may require this orthosis be worn 24 hours per day, whereas others may use a 2 hours on/2 hours off schedule. Others may need the orthosis only at night. Can you determine which schedule matches each diagnosis described in this chapter?

You should experience how it feels to wear this type of orthosis for one of the schedules listed previously: either a full 24-hour period or 2 hours on/2 hours off daytime routine. This experience will enable you to be client centered when using orthoses as an intervention strategy in your practice. You must consider how to instruct your client on the importance of the wearing schedule and the benefits of compliance for maximum benefits.

Suggested Reading

Beasley, J. (2012). Osteoarthritis and rheumatoid arthritis: Conservative therapeutic management. *Journal of Hand Therapy, 25*(2), 163-172. doi:10.1016/jht.2011.11.001

Botte, M. J., Kivirahk, D. L., Kinoshita, Y. O., Thompson, M. A., Pacelli L. L., & Meyer, R. S. (2011). Hemiplegia. In T. M. Skirven, A. L. Osterman, J. M. Fedorczyk, & P. C. Amadio (Eds.), *Rehabilitation of the hand and upper extremity* (6th ed., pp. 1659-1683). Philadelphia, PA: Elsevier Mosby.

Callinan, N., Mathiowetz, V., Haskett, S., Backman, C., Porter, B., Goyert, J., & Palejko, G. (2005). Soft versus hard resting hand splints in rheumatoid arthritis: Pain relief, preference, and compliance. *Arthritis and Rheumatism (Arthritis Care and Research), 51*(5), 792-799.

Chim, H. W., Reese, S. K., Toomey, S. N., & Moran, S. L. (2015). Update on the surgical treatment for rheumatoid arthritis of the wrist and hand. *Journal of Hand Therapy, 27*(2), 134-142. doi:10.1016/j.jht.2013.12.002

Choi, J. S., Mun, J. H., Lee, J. Y., Jeon, J. H., Jung, Y. J., Soe, C. H., & Jang, K. U. (2011). Effects of modified dynamic metacarpophalangeal joint flexion orthoses after hand burn. *Annuals of Rehabilitation Medicine, 35*(6), 800-866.

Coppard, B. (2015). Hand immobilization orthoses. In B. M. Coppard & H. Lohman (Eds.), *Introduction to orthotics: A clinical reasoning & problem-solving approach* (5th ed., pp. 195-224). St. Louis, MO: Mosby Elsevier.

Copley, J., Kuipers, K., Fleming, J., & Rassafiani, M. (2013). Individualized resting hand splints for adults with acquired brain injury: A randomized, single blinded, single case design. *Neurorehabilitation, 32*(5), 885-898.

DeBoer, I. G., Peeters, A. J., Ronday, H., Mertens B. J., Breedveld, F., & Vlieland, T. (2008). The usage of functional wrist orthoses in patients with rheumatoid arthritis. *Disability and Rehabilitation, 30*(5), 286-295.

Dewey, W. S., Richard, R. L., & Parry, I. S. (2011). Positioning, splinting, and contracture management. *Physical Medicine and Rehabilitation Clinics North America, 22*, 229-257.

Egan, M., Brosseau, L., Farmer, M., Oiumet, M. A., Rees, S., Wells, G., & Tugwell, P. (2003). Splints/orthoses in the treatment of rheumatoid arthritis. *Cochrane Database of Systematic Reviews, 1*, CD004018.

Feinberg, J., & Brandt, K. D. (1981). Use of resting hand splints by patients with rheumatoid arthritis. *American Journal of Occupational Therapy, 35*(3), 173-178.

Fufa, D., Chuang, S., & Yang, J. (2015). Postburn contractures of the hand. *Journal of Hand Surgery America, 39*(9), 1869-1876.

Jacobs, M., & Austin, N. (2015). *Orthotic intervention for the hand and upper extremity: Splinting principles and process* (2nd ed.). Baltimore, MD: Lippincott Williams & Wilkins.

Ivy, C. C., Smith, S. M., & Materi, M. M. (2015). Upper extremity orthoses use in amyotrophic lateral sclerosis/motor neuron disease: A systematic review. *International Journal of Medical Rehabilitation, 3*, 264. doi:10.4172/2329-9096.1000264

McKee, P., & Rivard, A. (2005). Orthoses as enablers of occupation: Client-centered splinting for better outcomes. *Canadian Journal of Occupational Therapy, 71*(5), 306-315.

McPherson, J. J., Kreimeyer, D., Aalderks, M., & Gallagher, T. (1982). A comparison of dorsal and volar resting hand splints in the reduction of hypertonus. *American Journal of Occupational Therapy, 36*(10), 665-670.

Pizzi, A., Carlucci, G., Falsimi, C., & Verdesca, S. (2005). Application of a volar static splint in poststroke spasticity of the upper limb. *Archives of Physical Medicine and Rehabilitation, 86*, 1855-1859.

Skirven, T. M., Osterman, A. L., Fedorczyk, J. M., & Amadio, P. C. (Eds.). (2011). *Rehabilitation of the hand and upper extremity* (6th ed.). Philadelphia, PA: Elsevier.

Takagi, T., Seki, A., Takayama, S., & Watanabe, M. (2017). Current concepts in radial club hand. *The Open Orthopaedics Journal, 11*, 369-377. doi:10.2174/1874325001711010369

Test Your Knowledge

SHORT ANSWER

1. Identify all anatomical landmarks associated with a wrist and hand immobilization orthosis.

2. Describe the biomechanical principles that apply to a wrist and hand immobilization orthosis and outline one element that differs from a wrist immobilization orthosis.

3. Identify and describe the two common hand positions used with a wrist and hand immobilization orthosis.

4. Describe the five different wrist and hand immobilization orthoses designs and discuss the rationale for each.

5. List the appropriate orthotic design and LTTM suitable for the following:
   - A 60-year-old woman with longstanding RA.
   - A 20-year-old man with multiple metacarpal and digital fractures.
   - A 6-year-old young boy with hand and wrist paralysis from a severe brachial plexus injury.
   - A 15-year-old teenage girl with dorsal hand, wrist, and forearm burns.

MULTIPLE CHOICE

6. How should the thumb be positioned in a wrist and hand immobilization orthosis?
   a. Extension
   b. Palmar abduction
   c. Flexion
   d. Opposition

7. What is the antideformity position?
   a. Wrist extension, 70 degrees of MCP joint flexion, 0 degrees of PIP and DIP joint extension, thumb palmar abduction.
   b. Wrist extension, 50 degrees of MCP joint flexion, PIP and DIP joints in slight flexion, thumb in palmar abduction.
   c. Wrist extension, digit MCP and IP joint extension, thumb extension.
   d. Wrist extension, MCP joint extension, PIP and DIP joints and thumb not included in orthosis.

8. What is the resting, or functional, hand position?
   a. Wrist extension, 50 degrees of MCP joint flexion, PIP and DIP joints in slight flexion, thumb in palmar abduction.
   b. Wrist extension, 70 degrees of MCP joint flexion, 0 degrees of PIP and DIP joint extension, thumb palmar abduction.
   c. Wrist extension, digit MCP and PIP and DIP joint extension, thumb extension.
   d. Wrist extension, MCP joint extension, PIP and DIP joints and thumb not included in orthosis.

9. Which of the following conditions include a wrist and hand immobilization orthosis as an intervention strategy?

    a. Carpal tunnel syndrome

    b. Distal radius fracture

    c. Wrist OA

    d. Wrist and digit flexor spasticity

10. Which wrist and hand immobilization orthosis design is recommended for treatment of hand burns?

    a. Volar/dorsal design

    b. Volar design with the PIP and DIP joints and thumb out of the orthosis

    c. Volar design in an antideformity position

    d. Volar design in a resting, or functional, hand position

11. What material characteristic is recommended when fabricating a wrist and hand immobilization orthosis?

    a. Moderate resistance to stretch

    b. 1/16 inch thickness

    c. No perforations

    d. Translucent materials

12. What material characteristic is recommended when fabricating a wrist and hand immobilization orthosis for hand burns?

    a. Perforations

    b. 1/8 inch thickness

    c. Maximum flexibility/low rigidity

    d. Lack of memory

13. What type of lever system does a wrist and hand immobilization orthosis represent?

    a. Third class

    b. Second class

    c. First class

14. What joint(s) must be stabilized in a wrist and hand immobilization orthosis to maintain proper hand positioning?

    a. The thumb MCP joint

    b. The PIP joints

    c. The wrist

    d. The DIP joints

15. Which hand arch is important to support in a wrist and hand immobilization orthosis?

    a. The volar transverse arch

    b. The longitudinal arch

    c. The dorsal transverse arch

    d. The middle transverse arch

CASE STUDIES

Case Study 1

John is an 81-year-old right-hand–dominant male who suffered a major stroke several days ago. He is presently awaiting discharge to a rehabilitation hospital but is still in the acute care unit of the hospital. The attending physician has sent a prescription that reads:

Right cardiovascular accident

1. *Evaluate and treat.*

2. *Provide wrist hand immobilization orthosis.*

3. *Contracture management and ROM: shoulder, elbow, wrist and digits.*

Your assessment:

John is seen bedside for his first inpatient therapy appointment. He is still relatively unsteady walking around the room and has been referred to physical therapy for balance and gait training. The left hand and wrist are flaccid with little voluntary control of the digits. Wrist circumference is measured as 8.0 cm on the right and 10.0 cm on the left. There is pain with shoulder, elbow, and digital motion. Manual muscle testing and grip strength testing are deferred due to lack of voluntary control. Pain is evaluated using the visual analog scale and rated as 9/10 with movement on the left and 3/10 at rest. John is anxious and uncomfortable throughout the exam and is accompanied by his wife, who will be his primary caretaker. She is concerned about his ability to walk independently and remarks that John is an avid gardener and photographer.

Using different clinical reasoning approaches, answer the following questions about this client and the prescribed orthosis:

Procedural Reasoning

1. What client factors are important to consider when determining the most suitable orthotic design for this client?

2. Which positioning in the wrist and hand immobilization orthosis would be most appropriate for this client? Why?

3. What LTTM properties are important to consider?

4. Describe the instructions you would give this client on:

    ◦ How to care for the orthosis

    ◦ Wearing schedule

    ◦ Precautions

    ◦ Exercises/activities

Pragmatic Reasoning

5. What resources are available to fabricate this orthosis (time, materials, expertise)?

6. Are you able to clearly document the need for this orthosis?

7. Does evidence-based practice support the use of this orthosis for this client's diagnosis?

Interactive Reasoning

8. What are the client's goals and valued occupations?

9. What effect will the client's injury and use of the orthosis have on his activities of daily living?

Conditional Reasoning

10. What factors will influence this client's compliance to the wearing schedule of this orthosis?

Narrative Reasoning

11. How does this injury and, more specifically, this orthotic intervention affect this client's valued occupations?

12. What activities is this client the most concerned about?

Ethical Reasoning

13. Does the client understand the need for the orthosis?

14. Does the client have the resources to be able to pay for the orthosis (as applicable)?

15. What other options are available to this client if he lacks the resources necessary to pay for the orthosis?

16. Write one short-term goal (1 to 2 weeks) and one long-term goal (6 to 8 weeks) for this client.

Case Study 2

Jeffrey is a 35-year-old, right-hand–dominant roofer who presents with second- and third-degree dorsal forearm and hand burns on his right UE. He was seen in the emergency room several days ago after accidentally spilling hot tar onto his arm while working. The emergency room physician treated Jeffrey by debriding of the dead tissue, cleaning the wounds, and lightly wrapping the arm with dressings and gauze. Jeffrey now presents for therapy with a prescription that reads:

Right forearm, wrist and hand burn: second and third degree:

1. *Evaluate and treat.*
2. *Provide orthosis.*
3. *Wound care and dressing changes.*
4. *Active ROM and functional activities.*

Your assessment:

The right dorsal forearm and wrist are red and slightly swollen in comparison to the left. Wrist circumference is measured as 8.2 cm on the right and 7.3 cm on the left. After removal of the gauze and wrappings, the extent of the burn is evident. Part of the skin is reddened, blistering, and oozing clear fluid. Other parts are charred looking, white, and waxy.

The entire forearm, wrist, and dorsal hand are tender to palpation, and there is pain reported on the dorsal aspect of the hand, especially with digital motion. Active wrist and digital motion are significantly limited. Manual muscle testing and grip strength testing are deferred at this time. Pain is evaluated using the visual analog scale and rated as 10/10 with wrist and digital movement and 5/10 at rest. Jeffrey reports loss of sensation on the dorsal forearm and wrist but denies any numbness, tingling, or other sensory symptoms in his palmar right hand and digits.

Jeffrey is married with one small toddler son. He is eager to return to work and to his valued leisure occupations: playing sports with friends, visiting with his family, and playing with his son.

Using different clinical reasoning approaches, consider the following questions about this client and the prescribed orthosis. Some questions may be directed more toward the client, and some questions may be directed more toward you as the practitioner for reflection.

Procedural Reasoning

1. What client factors are important to consider when determining the most suitable positioning in a wrist and hand immobilization orthosis for this client?

2. What thermoplastic material properties are important to consider?

3. Describe the instructions you would give this client on:
   - How to care for the orthosis
   - Wearing schedule
   - Precautions
   - Exercises/activities

Pragmatic Reasoning

4. What resources are available to fabricate this orthosis (time, materials, expertise)?

5. Are you able to clearly document the need for this orthosis?

6. Does evidence-based practice support the use of this orthosis for this client's diagnosis?

Interactive Reasoning

7. What are the client's goals and valued occupations?

8. What effect will the client's injury, and use of the orthosis, have on his activities of daily living?

Conditional Reasoning

9. What factors will influence this client's compliance to the wearing schedule of this orthosis?

Narrative Reasoning

10. How does this injury and, more specifically, this orthotic intervention affect this client's valued occupations?

11. What activities is this client most concerned about?

Ethical Reasoning

12. Does the client understand the need for the orthosis?

13. Does the client have the resources to be able to pay for the orthosis (as applicable)?

14. What other options are available to this client if he lacks the resources necessary to pay for the orthosis?

15. Write one short-term goal (1 to 2 weeks) and one long-term goal (6 to 8 weeks) for this client.

Appendix

STUDENT ASSIGNMENTS

1. Define all the key terms used in this chapter.

2. As an occupational therapy practitioner, you must provide your client with detailed instructions for wearing and caring for his or her orthosis. This document must be required for the client's official records and insurance payments. Select one of the wrist and hand immobilization orthosis designs from this chapter and prepare a client-centered handout for wearing this orthosis. Base your client description on one of the two case studies in this chapter. Include the following in the handout:

   ° A description/name of the orthosis

   ° An outline of the wearing schedule (remember that this will vary depending on the client's condition)

   ° A description of how to clean and care for the orthosis

   ° Instructions on what the client should be aware of when wearing the orthosis (e.g., red areas on skin, pain, swelling)

   ° Contact information and follow-up instructions

3. Prepare a case study of a client requiring a wrist and hand immobilization orthosis. Use one of the cited resources in the chapter to support your orthotic intervention. Summarize the research and explain the outcomes of the study.

4. As an occupational therapy practitioner, it will be interesting and informative for you to spend an extended period wearing an orthosis to appreciate the effect that an orthosis will have on your client's daily occupations. Wear a wrist and hand immobilization orthosis designed by your lab partner for a 12-hour period, preferably through the night. Take note of how it feels to have one body part completely immobilized. Elaborate in paragraphs on the following:

   ° Describe the orthosis, material used, positioning, and typical diagnosis for this orthosis.

   ° Comfort and ease of use: Is it easy to take on and off? Are there any pressure areas that caused discomfort? What areas need to be modified? How would you do this?

   ° Personal and public image: Did the orthosis attract attention to your family members, roommates, children, and/or parents?

   ° Functionality: How was your function affected by this orthosis? Was the position helpful or harmful? What would the typical wearing schedule be for this type of orthosis?

   ° How does this change your appreciation of what your clients are experiencing with their orthosis?

5. Complete the check-out form on the next page.

Multiple Choice Answer Key

6. b

7. a

8. a

9. d

10. c

11. a

12. a

13. d

14. c

15. b

Wrist and Hand Orthosis Check-Out Form

*(This can be used for faculty to evaluate students' completed orthoses,
as well as for students to reference when evaluating their own completed orthosis.)*

Fabricate one of the orthotic designs for a wrist and hand immobilization orthosis on your classmate and complete the following check-out form.

Name of Orthosis:

Purpose of Orthosis:

Design/Function

____ **Functional Position**

____ **Antideformity Position**

____ The wrist is positioned in extension.

____ The MCP joints are positioned in flexion (degree of flexion matches purpose of orthosis).

____ The PIP joints are positioned correctly.

____ The DIP joints are positioned correctly.

____ The thumb is positioned correctly in palmar abduction and slight flexion.

____ The pan portion supports all of the digits.

____ The orthosis is half the width of the forearm.

____ The orthosis is at least two-thirds the length of the forearm.

____ The hand arches are supported: distal and proximal transverse arches, longitudinal arch.

____ The orthosis does not migrate distally with elbow flexion.

____ The orthosis does not cause impingement or pressure areas.

____ The orthosis clears all bony prominences.

____ The orthosis completely immobilizes the wrist, thumb, and digits.

Straps/Orthosis Appearance

____ The straps are in the correct position: forearm, wrist, digits, and thumb.

____ The straps are secure and corners rounded.

____ The orthosis edges are smooth and corners rounded.

____ The proximal edge is flared.

____ The orthosis is free of fingerprints, pattern marks, or indentations.

CHAPTER 6

Forearm- and Hand-Based Thumb Orthoses

Key Terms

Ape hand deformity	Metacarpophalangeal (MCP) joint	Thumb boutonniere deformity
Carpometacarpal (CMC) joint	Neoprene orthoses	Thumb-in-palm deformity
de Quervain's tenosynovitis	Radial collateral ligament	Thumb spica
Gamekeeper's thumb	Scaphoid fracture	Thumb swan neck deformity
Interphalangeal (IP) joint	Short opponens	Ulnar collateral ligament
Long opponens	Skier's thumb	

Learning Outcomes

Upon completion of this chapter, you will be able to:

1. Describe the clinical conditions and goals for prescribing a forearm-based thumb orthosis.

2. Describe the clinical conditions and goals for prescribing a hand-based thumb orthosis.

3. Identify pertinent anatomical structures and biomechanical principles involved in forearm- and/or hand-based thumb orthoses and apply these concepts to orthotic design and fabrication.

4. Identify the most commonly selected orthotic designs and describe the rationale for choosing one design over another.

5. After reviewing the instructional videos:

    a. Outline the steps involved in the fabrication of forearm- and hand-based thumb orthoses.

    b. Complete the molding and finishing of forearm and hand-based thumb orthoses.

    c. Evaluate the fit and function of completed forearm- and hand-based thumb orthoses and identify and address all areas needing adjustment.

6. Design suitable patterns for the three common types of forearm- and hand-based thumb orthoses and identify the pertinent anatomical landmarks.

7. Identify elements of a client education program following provision of forearm- and hand-based thumb orthoses.

8. Describe special considerations of forearm- and hand-based thumb orthotic designs and fabrication for pediatric and geriatric clients.

Schofield, K., & Schwartz, D. *Orthotic Design and Fabrication for the Upper Extremity: A Practical Guide* (pp 101-123).
© 2019 Taylor & Francis Group.

Box 6-1. Common Goals of Forearm- and Hand-Based Thumb Orthoses

PROTECTION

- Support and protect the thumb CMC, MCP, and/or IP joints following surgical repair of structures.
- Support and protect the thumb after a fracture or ligament injury.
- Offer relief and joint protection from a painful tendinitis or arthritis.

POSITIONING

- Position the thumb to maintain the web space to prevent contracture.

IMPROVE FUNCTION

- Support and position the thumb in abduction and opposition to improve prehensile hand function due to muscle paralysis or weakness.
- Use the thumb orthosis as a base for outrigger attachments to create mobilization orthoses or adaptive equipment.

Introduction

The thumb is a key component of hand function. When a clinical condition affects the thumb, an orthosis for immobilization may be important for stability and/or pain relief. Orthoses for the thumb may include the wrist or may be designed to keep the wrist free.

There are several different design options for these orthoses. The design chosen will depend on multiple factors, including the client's clinical condition, his or her functional needs, and specifications set by the referring physician.

GOALS FOR USE OF FOREARM- AND HAND-BASED THUMB ORTHOSES

The goals of forearm- and hand-based thumb orthoses will vary depending on the individual client's needs and clinical condition. Box 6-1 reviews common goals.

When fabricating forearm- and hand-based thumb orthoses, the practitioner must consider each client's specific clinical condition or diagnosis, the expected clinical outcome following orthotic use, and use of sound clinical reasoning to select the most appropriate design for the client. As discussed, the particular design chosen depends on multiple factors. A forearm-based thumb orthosis (also called a **long opponens** or long **thumb spica**) immobilizes the wrist, **carpometacarpal (CMC) joint**, and/or the

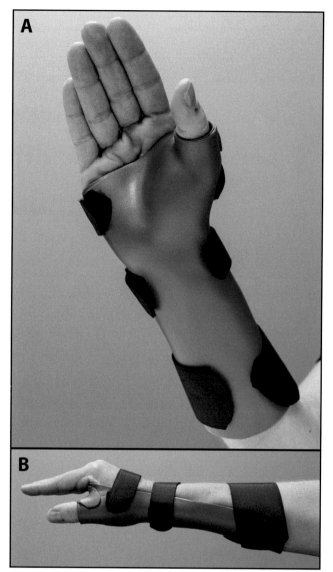

Figure 6-1. (A) Volar view and (B) radial view of an orthosis including the forearm, wrist, and thumb known as a *long opponens orthosis*.

metacarpophalangeal (MCP) and **interphalangeal (IP) joints** (Figure 6-1).

A hand-based thumb orthosis (also called a **short opponens** or short thumb spica) immobilizes the CMC joint and most often includes the MCP joint as well. The thumb IP joint may also be included if this joint is involved (Figure 6-2).

Practitioners treating clients with arthritis of the thumb joint(s), fractures, sprains, ligament injuries, or other pathologies recognize the benefits that orthoses can offer their clients. These benefits include pain relief, stability, prevention or correction of deformity, positioning during healing, and improved functional ability. It is critical to perform an ongoing assessment of the client's current status, particularly in relation to his or her functional ability during the time the orthosis is part of the intervention. Custom-made thumb orthoses may require adaptations to

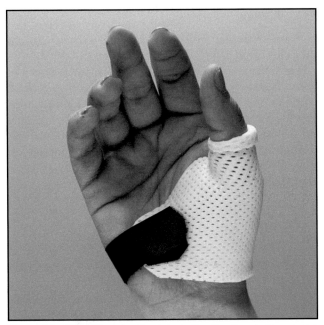

Figure 6-2. A hand-based orthosis including the thumb, known as a *short opponens orthosis*.

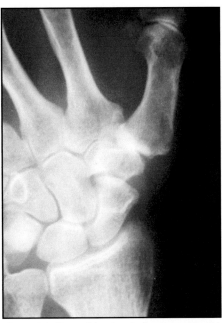

Figure 6-3. X-ray of the thumb demonstrating OA of the CMC joint.

meet the client's changing needs. Inflamed or injured swollen joints require rest and protection; however, prolonged immobilization may lead to loss of range of motion (ROM) due to joint stiffness. Use of orthoses may help prevent the development of soft tissue and/or joint contractures and may improve function, allowing the client to maintain independence.

Clinical Conditions and Wearing Schedules

The following section describes common clinical conditions where a thumb orthosis is prescribed and the current evidence supporting this orthosis as an appropriate intervention strategy. Readers are encouraged to review the references provided for additional details regarding each clinical condition and search current research databases for updated evidence as it becomes available.

RHEUMATOID ARTHRITIS AND OSTEOARTHRITIS

Both rheumatoid arthritis (RA) and osteoarthritis (OA) can affect the thumb with decreased motion, pain, joint instability, and weakness. Radiographic evidence of both OA and RA demonstrates significant changes in bony alignment and structure (Figure 6-3).

As discussed in Chapter 4, RA is an autoimmune disease that commonly affects the wrist and small joints in the hand and usually occurs bilaterally (Figure 6-4).

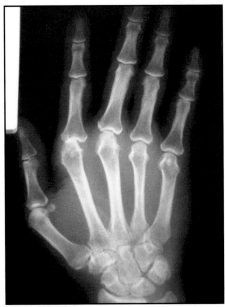

Figure 6-4. X-ray of the thumb demonstrating RA of the CMC and MCP joints.

The thumb CMC and MCP joints are often affected in clients with RA, and the most commonly seen thumb deformities are **thumb boutonniere deformity**, which is MCP joint flexion with IP joint hyperextension, and **thumb swan neck deformity**, which is MCP joint hyperextension with or without IP joint flexion (Figure 6-5). Both deformities can affect a client's prehensile function.

In addition to the thumb joint pathology, clients with RA will likely have multiple joint pathologies that affect both the wrist and digit MCP joints, necessitating orthoses that address these joints as well.

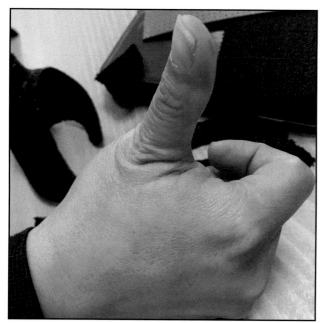

Figure 6-5. Photograph of a client with RA of the thumb highlighting instability or subluxation of the MCP joint.

OA is a wear-and-tear degenerative condition where the cartilage lining the articular joint surfaces is affected by repeated stresses placed on it due to age, repetitive activities, and past injury. The most common site of OA in the hand is the first CMC joint. This joint is subject to considerable stress during prehensile tasks, which can lead to degenerative changes with aging. OA is a common condition, affecting up to 20% of men and women over the age of 40 years. A family history of OA, postmenopausal women, hypermobility of the CMC joint, and history of repetitive grasping and resistive pinching activities predispose individuals to this condition. With time, the repetitive pinching forces and strong pull of the adductor pollicis and intrinsic thumb muscles causes the base of the first metacarpal to sublux dorsally and radially on the trapezium. This causes considerable pain, instability, and loss of prehensile function. OA may affect only one joint in the body, but it is more common to have the condition on both sides.

Forearm- and hand-based thumb orthoses can alleviate symptoms of both RA and OA by supporting the wrist (forearm-based orthosis) and thumb in a resting and comfortable position to reduce pain, facilitate pinch-and-release thumb function, improve pinch strength, provide joint stability, and protect the thumb joints during activities of daily living (ADL). For clients with OA of the first CMC joint, orthoses are the mainstay in conservative management. The specific goals of an orthosis for this condition are pain reduction, joint protection during ADL, optimization of functional use of the affected hand by stabilizing the thumb, and prevention of adduction contractures of the first web space.

Wearing Schedule

A recommended wearing schedule for a thumb orthosis for a client with arthritis is to wear it as needed during periods of inflammation, swelling, and pain. The client can be encouraged to remove the orthosis periodically to perform gentle ROM exercises and hygiene. When the inflammatory episode has resolved or diminished, the client can reduce orthosis use. For some clients, wearing the orthosis only during activities or only at night may be the appropriate schedule. Use clinical reasoning and discussion with the client to develop an individual treatment plan.

Evidence

Level I

- Valdes, K., & Marik, T. (2010). A systematic review of conservative interventions for osteoarthritis of the hand. *Journal of Hand Therapy, 23*, 334-351.

  ○ This systematic review of conservative treatments for OA of the hand found 11 studies that described orthotic intervention. The studies indicated that a thumb-based orthosis can improve function and decrease pain. Moderate to high evidence exists to support this intervention.

- Amini, D. (2011). Occupational therapy interventions for work-related injuries and conditions of the forearm, wrist, and hand: A systematic review. *American Journal of Occupational Therapy, 65*, 2936. doi:10.5014/ajot.2011.09186

  ○ This systematic review of interventions therapists use to treat work-related injuries found that orthotic intervention for thumb-based pain due to OA is an effective intervention regardless of specific design.

Level II

- Bani, M. A., Arazpour, M., Kashani, R. V., Mousavi, M. E., & Hutchins, S. W. (2013). Comparison of custom-made and prefabricated neoprene splinting in patients with the first carpometacarpal joint osteoarthritis. *Disability and Rehabilitation: Assistive Technology, 8*(3), 232-237.

  ○ This crossover design study compared the use of custom-made orthoses with neoprene prefabricated orthoses for immobilization of the base of the thumb in patients with CMC OA. Key outcome measures were pain, function, grip strength, and pinch strength. The authors found that custom-made orthoses were better at pain reduction.

- Cantero-Téllez, R., Valdes, K., Schwartz, D. A., Medina-Porqueres, I., Arias, J. C., & Villafañe, J. H. (2018). Necessity of immobilizing the metacarpophalangeal joint in carpometacarpal osteoarthritis: Short-term effect. *Hand (N Y), 13*(4), 412-417.

○ In this study conducted on the use of orthotic intervention for the conservative management of CMC joint OA, the authors note that different types of orthoses have been used to improve patients' symptoms. However, there are no guidelines specifying if inclusion of the thumb MCP in an orthosis is required in the treatment of thumb CMC joint OA. The main objective of this study was to determine the effectiveness of two different thumb CMC joint orthotic designs on pain reduction and improved hand function: one design immobilized both the MCP joint and the CMC joint, and the other design immobilized only the CMC joint. A total of 66 patients were included in the study. One group of 33 patients received a short thumb orthosis with the MCP joint excluded, and the other group of 33 patients received a short thumb orthosis with the MCP joint included. Outcomes measures included the visual analog scale for pain and the Quick Disabilities of the Arm, Shoulder and Hand (Spanish version) for function. In both patient groups, the orthoses contributed to decreased pain levels and improved functional abilities. However, there was no significant difference between the two groups regarding pain or improvement in daily activities. The authors concluded that there are benefits of either thumb orthotic design on pain reduction and functional improvement, even after 1 week of using the orthoses as the sole conservative treatment.

Level V

- Beasley, J. (2012). Osteoarthritis and rheumatoid arthritis: Conservative therapeutic management. *Journal of Hand Therapy, 25*, 163-172.

  ○ This paper presents conservative treatment options for managing arthritis. Orthoses are a method of providing stability to weakened structures of the thumb and help maintain joint alignment. Patients prefer a hand-based short thumb orthosis, and nighttime use appears to help relieve symptoms and decrease disability after wear for 12 months.

DE QUERVAIN'S TENOSYNOVITIS

De Quervain's tenosynovitis, also called *de Quervain's disease* and *de Quervain's syndrome*, is a condition that involves the two tendons of the first dorsal compartment of the wrist (refer to the extensor tendon compartments in Chapter 2), the abductor pollicis longus and extensor pollicis brevis. These tendons run in a small compartment along the radial aspect of the wrist and thumb and are subject to repetitive stress with movement of the wrist and thumb together, such as wringing a towel, opening jars, and cutting with scissors. This condition is more commonly seen in women, and symptoms often appear in the early

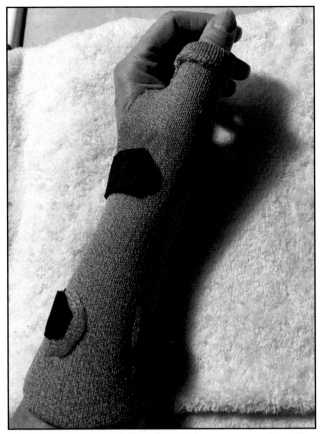

Figure 6-6. A long opponens orthosis to limit movement for a client with de Quervain's tenosynovitis.

postpartum period (6 to 9 months after delivery). Swelling of the abductor pollicis longus and extensor pollicis brevis tendons and their tendon sheath causes pain on the radial side of the wrist near the radial styloid and is often aggravated with movement of the thumb. An orthosis that immobilizes the wrist and thumb CMC and MCP joints minimizes movement of the abductor pollicis longus and extensor pollicis brevis tendons, which can help reduce inflammation and pain during functional tasks (Figure 6-6).

Wearing Schedule

For a client presenting with symptoms of de Quervain's tenosynovitis, an appropriate wearing schedule for the forearm-based thumb immobilization orthosis is full-time for a period of 4 to 6 weeks or until symptoms have diminished considerably or resolved.

Evidence

Level I

- Cavaleri, R., Schabrun, S. M., Te, M., & Chipchase, L. S. (2016). Hand therapy versus corticosteroid injections in the treatment of de Quervain's disease: A systematic review and meta-analysis. *Journal of Hand Therapy, 29*(1), 3-11.

○ Although corticosteroid injections are often cited as the best conservative treatment intervention for clients with symptoms of de Quervain's disease, there are no reviews that have compared their effectiveness with other interventions commonly used in hand therapy clinics. The purpose of this systematic review was to compare the effectiveness of corticosteroid injections with that of hand therapy interventions alone and also with a combined hand therapy/corticosteroid injection approach in the treatment of de Quervain's disease. The authors conducted a search of key databases to identify experimental studies published between January 1950 and November 2014. Outcome measures included treatment success, pain, quality of life, and function. Results: Both corticosteroid injections and hand therapy interventions were shown to improve pain and function from baseline, but the between-group differences were not significant (across six studies). However, significantly more participants were treated successfully when a combined approach was used, including an orthosis, corticosteroid injection, and hand therapy, compared with either just orthoses or just injections alone.

Level II

- Menendez, M. E., Thornton, E., Kent, S., Kalajian, T., & Ring, D. (2015). A prospective randomized clinical trial of prescription of full-time versus as-desired splint wear for de Quervain tendinopathy. *International Orthopaedics, 39*(8), 1563-1569.

  ○ The authors tested whether patients with a diagnosis of de Quervain's tendinopathy wearing a splint full-time did better, worse, or the same as patients who wore their splint when they chose to do so. Because many authors feel that complete rest of the involved tendons will aid in healing, it is important to determine the best wearing schedule of the long opponens splint used to treat this condition. The authors conducted this randomized clinical trial of 8 weeks of full-time splint wear versus wearing the splint when desired. The authors found no significant difference in symptoms between the two groups. However, at the end of the trial, only 70% of the patients were contacted for final outcomes, and there was no clear method to determine patient compliance with the splinting protocol.

- Smith, M. (2009). Literature review: Splinting and education in the treatment of de Quervains disease: Effect and practability. *Irish Journal of Occupational Therapy, 37*(1), 38-46.

  ○ The authors reviewed studies on different treatment strategies for de Quervain's disease and concluded that splinting is effective for mild cases and for patients post-pregnancy; splinting with injections can reduce symptoms; splinting the wrist in neutral may be effective, yet there is no reported optimum thumb position; and there is no specific splint wearing schedule, but 2 to 6 weeks of wear is suggested.

- Cavaleri, R., Schabrun, S. M., Te, M., & Chipchase, L. S. (2016). Hand therapy versus corticosteroid injections in the treatment of de Quervain's disease: A systematic review and meta-analysis. *Journal of Hand Therapy, 29*(1), 3-11.

  ○ The authors reviewed the evidence to determine the best treatment options for de Quervain's disease, considered a work-related upper limb disorder, and included six studies in this systematic review. The included studies evaluated the effectiveness of hand therapy treatment and corticosteroid injections and also looked at the effectiveness of either treatment alone. Three studies compared corticosteroid injections with wrist/thumb orthoses, three studies compared a combined orthosis/corticosteroid injection approach with orthoses or injections alone, and one study compared acupuncture with corticosteroid injections. The authors concluded that splinting is effective when combined with corticosteroid injections as compared with splinting alone as a treatment.

- Huisstede, B. M., Coert, J. H., Fridén, J., & Hoogvliet, P. (2014). Consensus on multidisciplinary treatment guideline for de Quervain disease: Results from the European HANDGUIDE study. *Physical Therapy, 94*(8), 1095-1190.

  ○ A Delphi consensus strategy was used to determine the best multidisciplinary treatment guidelines for patients with de Quervain's disease. A systematic review of surgical and nonsurgical interventions was published, and 35 experts in the field (surgery and rehabilitation) from participating European countries participated in the discussions. Patient instructions with other interventions such as nonsteroidal anti-inflammatory drugs and splinting or injections and splinting were considered suitable treatment options. Splinting choices should be either a long, lower arm–based (wrist immobilized) splint including the IP joint of the thumb or a long, lower arm–based (wrist immobilized) splint excluding the IP joint of the thumb. The recommended wearing schedule dictated that the splint should be worn for 3 to 8 weeks, 24 hours per day, excluding grooming and except for brief periods of pain-free ROM.

ULNAR COLLATERAL AND RADIAL COLLATERAL LIGAMENT SPRAIN/INJURY

An **ulnar collateral ligament** sprain is an injury to the ligaments supporting the thumb MCP joint (Figure 6-7).

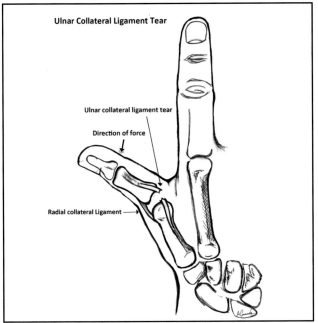

Figure 6-7. Ulnar collateral ligament tear/avulsion (gamekeeper's/skier's thumb).

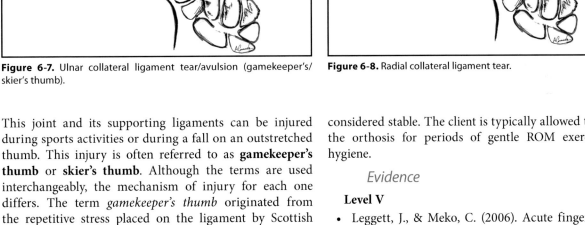

Figure 6-8. Radial collateral ligament tear.

This joint and its supporting ligaments can be injured during sports activities or during a fall on an outstretched thumb. This injury is often referred to as **gamekeeper's thumb** or **skier's thumb**. Although the terms are used interchangeably, the mechanism of injury for each one differs. The term *gamekeeper's thumb* originated from the repetitive stress placed on the ligament by Scottish gamekeepers as they euthanized rabbits. Skier's thumb, in contrast, is a more acute injury to the ligament resulting from a fall that forces a ski pole from the hand, rupturing the ligament. In addition, a small piece of bone can avulse off the thumb metacarpal head along with the ligament. Consequently, the thumb MCP joint becomes unstable, and pinching and other prehensile tasks become difficult to perform. A hand-based thumb orthosis can help maintain the ligament/bony fragment in a position for healing and stabilize the thumb MCP joint.

The **radial collateral ligament** can also be injured during sports activities or following a fall on an outstretched thumb (Figure 6-8). This type of injury is much less common than the ulnar collateral ligament injury. A hand-based thumb orthosis can help maintain the radial-based ligaments in a position for healing. A hand-based thumb orthosis can protect and stabilize the thumb MCP joint to facilitate healing after joint injury.

Wearing Schedule

The appropriate wearing schedule for a hand-based thumb orthosis for a client with ulnar or radial collateral ligament injuries is to wear it full-time as protection and support until the ligaments have healed and the joint is considered stable. The client is typically allowed to remove the orthosis for periods of gentle ROM exercises and hygiene.

Evidence

Level V

- Leggett, J., & Meko, C. (2006). Acute finger injuries: Part II. Fractures, dislocations, and thumb injuries. *American Family Physician, 73*(5), 827-834.

  ○ The authors discuss various finger and joint injuries and appropriate treatment and interventions. Stable ulnar collateral ligament injuries are treated with a thumb orthosis or cast. If a fracture dislocation or Stenar lesion is suspected, then surgery is required. A Stenar lesion occurs when part of the ulnar collateral ligament is trapped outside of the adductor aponeurosis and constitutes a more serious injury.

- Michaud, E. J., Flinn, S., & Seitz, W. H. (2010). Treatment of grade III thumb metacarpophalangeal ulnar collateral ligament injuries with early controlled motion using a hinged splint. *Journal of Hand Therapy, 23*(1), 77-82.

  ○ The authors of this article suggest an alternative design for a custom-made hinged thumb orthosis to allow early motion in the healing ulnar collateral ligament injury. They base their suggestion on evidence pointing to the use of custom-made hand-based orthoses for thumb ulnar collateral ligament injuries of the MCP joint and the fact that 85% to 90% of patients achieve good to satisfactory results with an early active motion home program.

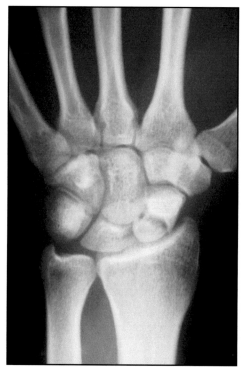

Figure 6-9. X-ray of the carpal bones highlighting a scaphoid fracture.

THUMB FRACTURE

Fractures can occur in any of the thumb bones (meta-carpal, proximal, or distal phalanges). Use of a custom-fabricated forearm- or hand-based thumb orthosis is often prescribed to stabilize and protect the bone(s) during the healing process, either with conservative management or following surgery. An orthosis is also commonly prescribed following cast removal to provide protection while the client works on regaining joint mobility.

Although not considered a bone of the thumb, fractures involving the scaphoid require immobilization of the wrist, thumb CMC, MCP, and perhaps the IP joint. The scaphoid is the most commonly fractured carpal bone and accounts for 60% to 70% of all carpal fractures and 11% of all hand fractures. Most **scaphoid fractures** occur in the middle of the bone, or waist, followed by the proximal pole and tubercle (Figure 6-9). The vascularity of the scaphoid significantly affects the outcome of these fractures. Up to 90% of the blood vessels that supply the scaphoid are distal to the waist, or middle of the bone. Consequently, these fractures frequently require a longer period of immobilization, as long as 3 to 6 months. Forearm-based thumb orthoses are often prescribed following cast removal for protection or initially to immobilize and protect the fracture.

Wearing Schedule

The appropriate wearing schedule for a thumb orthosis for a client with thumb fractures is to wear it full-time for protection and support until the fracture has healed. An orthosis is also commonly used following cast removal and is worn for protection while the client regains wrist and thumb mobility. The client may be permitted to remove the orthosis for periods of gentle ROM exercises and hygiene if the fracture is stable.

Evidence

Level I

- Doornberg, J. N., Buijze, G. A., Ham, S. J., Ring, D., Bhandari, M., & Poolman, R. W. (2011). Nonoperative treatment for acute scaphoid fractures: A systematic review and meta-analysis of randomized controlled trials. *Journal of Trauma and Acute Care Surgery, 71*(4), 1073-1081.

  ○ The authors completed a systematic review of the literature from 1966 to 2010 looking at studies involving nonoperative management of acute scaphoid injuries to determine the best treatment. In total, 523 patients were included in four trials, including two evaluating below-elbow casting versus above-elbow casting; one trial comparing below-elbow casting including the thumb versus excluding the thumb; and one trial comparing fractures with a below-elbow cast with the wrist in 20 degrees of flexion to 20 degrees of extension, with both types excluding the thumb. There were no significant differences in union rate, pain, grip strength, time to union, or osteonecrosis for the various nonoperative treatment methods. The authors concluded that no specific casting or immobilization method exists that is better than others.

Level II

- Mallee, W. H., Doornberg, J. N., Ring, D., Maas, M., Muhl, M., van Dijk, C. N., & Goslings, J. C. (2014). Computed tomography for suspected scaphoid fractures: Comparison of reformations in the plane of the wrist versus the long axis of the scaphoid. *Hand (N Y), 9*(1), 117-121.

  ○ The authors conducted a multicentered, single-blind, randomized, controlled, clinical trial comparing outcomes in patients given one of two forms of immobilization: with the thumb included or without the thumb included. Computed tomography 10 weeks after injury revealed that when immobilization had excluded the thumb, 85% of scaphoid fractures had healed, but when immobilization had included the thumb, 70% of such fractures had healed. Differences in wrist motion; grip strength; or arm, shoulder, or hand disability between the two patient groups were insignificant. Other authors have also concluded that immobilization including the thumb does not offer a clear advantage over immobilization excluding the thumb.

- Lawton, J. N., Nicholls, M. A., & Charoglu, C. P. (2007). Immobilization for scaphoid fracture: Forearm rotation in long arm thumb-spica versus Munster thumb-spica casts. *Orthopedics, 30*(8), 612-614.

- The authors report on a study demonstrating healing of scaphoid fractures in 9.5 weeks versus 12.7 weeks with conservative management of a nondisplaced scaphoid fracture when treatment was initiated with a long arm thumb spica cast that includes the elbow. The reported advantage to a long arm cast is a decrease in the shearing motion of the volar radiocarpal ligaments accompanying forearm rotation. A disadvantage of using a long arm cast to immobilize a patient with a scaphoid fracture is the additional potential for elbow joint stiffness and muscle atrophy that can occur during the required period of immobilization.

Level V

- Mulligan, J., & Amblum, J. (2014). Diagnosis and treatment of scaphoid fracture. *Emergency Nurse, 22*(3), 18-23.

  - The authors provide a literature review of manuscripts describing evaluation techniques for determining if a scaphoid fracture is present. They also examine the description of different methods of immobilization, including the usage of above-elbow versus below-elbow casts and the position of the wrist inside the cast. In studies that compared the use of above-below casting with the thumb included versus below-elbow casting without the thumb, there do not appear to be significant differences in healing rates or nonunion rates. Variables to consider in immobilization for management of scaphoid fractures include above- versus below-elbow, the inclusion or exclusion of the thumb, and the wrist positioned in extension versus flexion.

- Hart, R. G., Kleinert, H. E., & Lyons, K. (2005). A modified thumb spica for thumb injuries in the emergency department. *American Journal of Emergency Medicine, 23*(6), 777-781.

  - The authors describe the various injuries to the thumb seen in the emergency room of a hospital that require immediate immobilization. Although an orthosis applied in the emergency room is typically fabricated from plaster, the information provided in this article discusses the different diagnoses involving the thumb that are typically seen, including fractures, ulnar collateral ligament injuries, and general trauma to the thumb. Positioning in the immobilization splint is described in detail.

- Carlsen, B. T., & Moran, S. L. (2009). Thumb trauma: Bennett fractures, Rolando fractures, and ulnar collateral ligament injuries. *Journal of Hand Surgery, 34*(5), 945-952.

  - This Level V background article provides relevant information on a variety of diagnoses involving

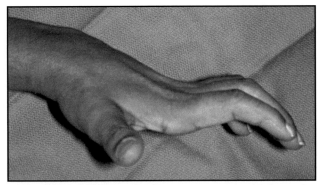

Figure 6-10. A client with a deformity known as *ape hand deformity* due to injury of the median and ulnar nerves.

the thumb. It does not include specific information on the provision of orthoses but may be helpful at describing the different diagnoses and the anatomical structures involved in each case.

MEDIAN NERVE INJURY/PALSY

Injury to the median nerve can occur proximally in the forearm or more distally at the level of the wrist. Clients present with significant motor and sensory deficits. The loss of sensation can be very debilitating due to the absence of sensory input from the thumb, index, and long fingers with prehensile tasks. Injury to the median nerve near the wrist presents with muscle weakness or paralysis in the majority of the thenar muscles (abductor pollicis brevis, superficial head of the flexor pollicis brevis, and opponens pollicis), along with the lumbrical muscles to the index and long fingers. This affects digit MCP flexion and thumb opposition, flexion, and abduction. This posture is commonly referred to as **ape hand deformity** because of the inability to abduct and oppose the thumb (Figure 6-10).

A more proximal injury to the median nerve in the forearm will also affect the flexor digitorum superficialis, index and long flexor digitorum profundus, and flexor carpi radialis. Inability to actively position the thumb makes it very difficult for clients to grasp and manipulate objects with their thumb and radial digits. A hand-based orthosis can position the thumb to facilitate prehensile function and prevent adduction and extension posturing of the thumb and contracture of the web space (Figure 6-11).

Wearing Schedule

The appropriate wearing schedule for a hand-based thumb orthosis for a client with median nerve palsy is to wear it full-time as protection and support until the affected muscles are able to support and mobilize the thumb. Without an orthosis for support, the first web space may develop a contracture, and tightening of the thumb muscles and joint ligaments may occur. The client is allowed to remove the orthosis for periods of gentle ROM exercises and hygiene.

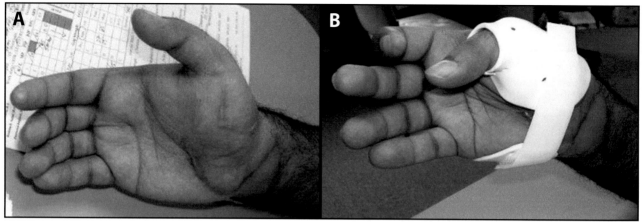

Figure 6-11. (A) Photograph of a client with median nerve palsy following a laceration to the wrist. (B) Photograph of the same client wearing a short opponens thumb orthosis to position the thumb for function.

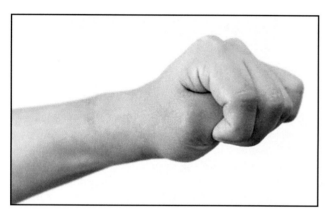

Figure 6-12. Thumb-in-palm deformity.

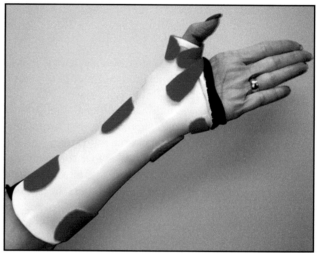

Figure 6-13. Forearm-based thumb and wrist or long opponens orthosis. (Reprinted with permission from Chad Royer.)

Evidence

Level V

- Chan, R. K. (2002). Splinting for peripheral nerve injury in upper limb. *Hand Surgery, 7*(2), 251-259.
  - This Level V paper offers suggestions for orthotic designs for patients with median nerve palsy. The importance of positioning the thumb in a functional position and maintaining the wide first web space is emphasized.

SPASTICITY/ADDUCTED THUMB IN CEREBRAL PALSY

A common pattern of spasticity is **thumb-in-palm deformity**, where the thumb is adducted tightly into the palm (Figure 6-12). The condition is common in children with cerebral palsy due to the increased tone of the adductor pollicis muscle. Placing the thumb in opposition and abduction with an orthosis can facilitate prehensile function and temporarily reduce spasticity. This posture is frequently associated with spasticity of the wrist and digital flexor muscles; a forearm-based orthosis that includes the wrist and thumb may be more suitable for controlling tendon length when the wrist and thumb are both involved (Figure 6-13).

Wearing Schedule

The appropriate wearing schedule for a thumb orthosis for a child with adducted thumbs is to it wear full-time for positioning and maintaining length of involved soft tissue structures. The client is allowed to remove the orthosis for periods of gentle ROM exercises and hygiene.

Evidence

Level II

- Ten Berge, S. R., Boonstra, A. M., Dijkstra, P. U., Hadders-Algra, M., Haga, N., & Maathuis, C. G. (2012). A systematic evaluation of the effect of thumb opponens splints on hand function in children with unilateral spastic cerebral palsy. *Clinical Rehabilitation, 26*(4), 362-371.

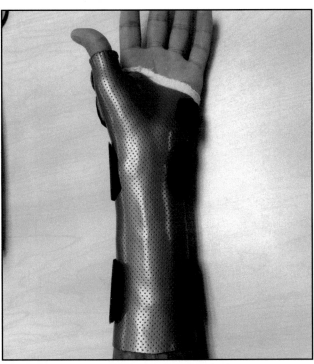

Figure 6-14. A thumb orthosis placed on the volar forearm.

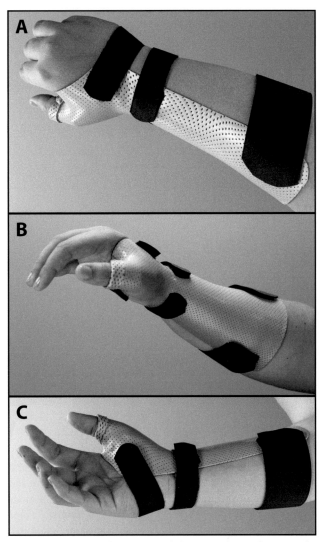

Figure 6-15. (A) Dorsal view, (B) radial view, and (C) volar view of a thumb orthosis placed on the radial forearm.

○ This small study evaluated the use of a short opponens orthosis in children with cerebral palsy. Overall hand functioning was improved even after removal of the orthosis. The orthosis used in the study was a prefabricated neoprene design reinforced with low-temperature thermoplastic material (LTTM). However, there may be implications here for custom-made thermoplastic orthoses.

Forearm- and Hand-Based Thumb Orthotic Designs

Many different designs exist for fabricating forearm- and hand-based thumb orthoses. The specific design will depend on the individual client's clinical condition, current functional needs, specific indications requested by the referring physician, and practitioner preference. The practitioner must consider the anatomy of the forearm, wrist, and thumb and how an orthosis will influence these structures when determining the most appropriate orthosis design. Other factors to consider include the specific joint(s) involved (wrist, thumb CMC, MCP, and/or IP joints); the client's size; the materials available; and whether a volar, radial-based, or circumferential design is the best option. This section reviews each design, its main uses, and its advantages and disadvantages.

FOREARM-BASED THUMB ORTHOSES

Common designs for the forearm-based thumb orthosis include the volar, radial gutter, and or circumferential designs (Box 6-2).

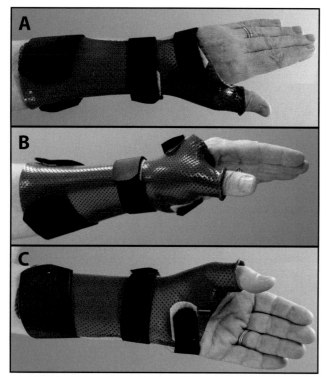

Figure 6-16. (A) Dorsal view, (B) volar view, and (C) radial view of a circumferential forearm-based thumb immobilization orthosis.

Volar Design

An orthosis with a volar design immobilizes the thumb CMC, MCP, and/or IP joint and the wrist and covers the volar aspect of the hand/palm, wrist, and forearm. Proper strapping keeps the orthosis correctly positioned and helps to prevent movement. This design is commonly used following scaphoid and/or trapezium fractures, CMC arthroplasty, thumb extensor tendon repairs, and de Quervain's tenosynovitis (see Figure 6-14).

Radial Gutter Design

The radial gutter design immobilizes the wrist, thumb CMC, MCP, and/or IP joint and covers the radial aspect of the thumb, wrist, and forearm (see Figure 6-15). This design can also be used to rest and protect inflamed tendons that cross the radial aspect of the wrist and thumb (de Quervain's tenosynovitis), protect and stabilize thumb metacarpal fractures, or protect and stabilize the thumb MCP joint following thumb ligament injuries (skier's or gamekeeper's thumb). This design may be more comfortable and less restrictive than the volar design due to the absence of LTTM on the ulnar aspect of the hand, wrist, and forearm.

Circumferential Design

The circumferential orthotic design immobilizes the wrist, thumb CMC, MCP, and/or IP joints and covers all aspects of the hand, wrist, and forearm, including the volar

Box 6-3. Hand-Based Thumb Orthosis Designs

VOLAR DESIGN
- Figure 6-17

CMC-ONLY DESIGN
- Figure 6-18

RADIAL-BASED DESIGN
- Figure 6-19

DORSAL DESIGN
- Figure 6-20

CONE DESIGN
- Figure 6-21

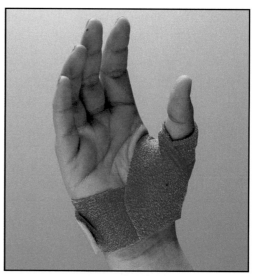

Figure 6-17. A volar-design orthosis for the thumb that includes the CMC and MCP joints.

and dorsal parts. This design provides the most support and protection due to its circumferential design and is well suited following scaphoid fractures, thumb extensor tendon repairs, and other conditions that require rigid support (see Figure 6-16).

HAND-BASED THUMB ORTHOSES

A variety of different designs are available for fabricating hand-based thumb orthoses. The design chosen depends on the client's clinical condition, current functional needs, specific indications requested by the referring physician, and practitioner preference. Orthotic designs vary depending on which joint(s) are included (thumb CMC, MCP, and/or IP joints) and whether the orthosis is volar based, dorsal based, or a simple cone design (Box 6-3).

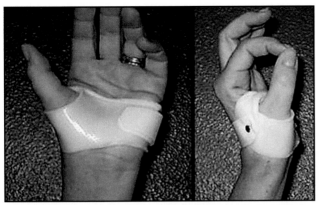

Figure 6-18. An orthosis for the thumb that includes only the CMC joint.

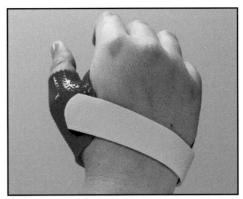

Figure 6-19. A radially based thumb orthosis is positioned on the radial surface of the hand.

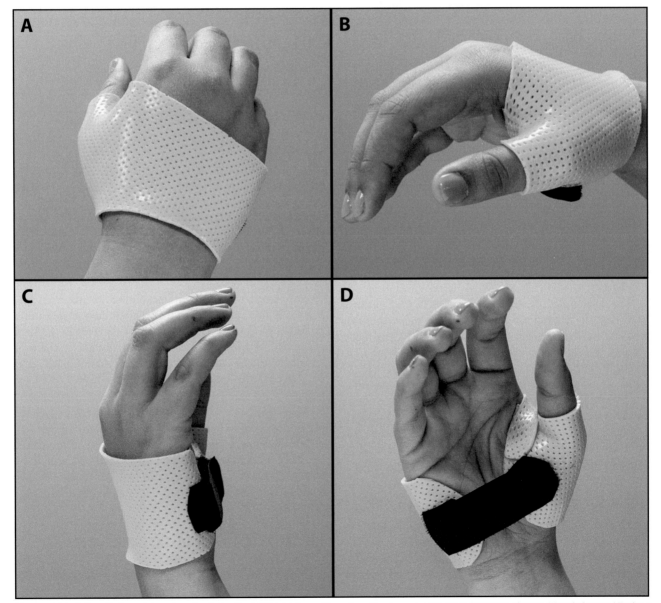

Figure 6-20. A dorsally based thumb orthosis for the CMC joint is positioned on the dorsum of the hand. (A) Dorsal view, (B) radial view, (C) ulnar view, and (D) volar view.

Figure 6-21. A thumb orthosis for the CMC joint known simply as the cone orthosis because it is shaped like a cone.

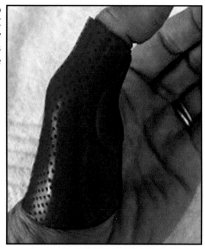

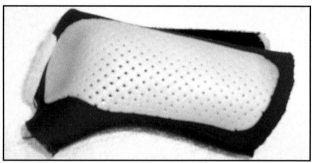

Figure 6-22. Neoprene thumb orthosis reinforced with thermoplastic material.

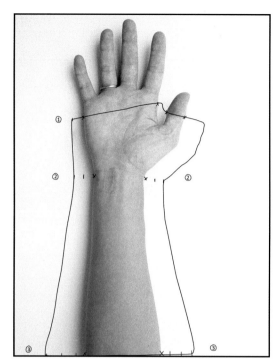

Figure 6-23. Forearm-based volar thumb design pattern.

Volar Designs

Thumb CMC and MCP Joint Orthosis

The volar-based thumb CMC and MCP joint orthosis positions the thumb in mid-abduction and opposition to allow for unrestricted lateral pinch. The LTTM incorporates the first, second, and fifth metacarpals and fits through the palm with a strap on the dorsal aspect of the hand. This design is commonly used to protect and stabilize a painful thumb CMC and/or MCP joint. The orthosis can also be molded on the dorsal aspect of the hand, leaving the palm free for sensory feedback. This design may be more functional for some clients, depending on their occupational demands (see Figure 6-17).

Thumb CMC Joint Orthosis

The thumb CMC joint orthosis is similar to the thumb CMC and MCP joint orthosis but does not include the thumb MCP joint. This orthosis, when molded well, stabilizes the base of the first metacarpal, thereby preventing dorsal subluxation of the first metacarpal base and adduction of the metacarpal during pinch that commonly occurs with arthritis of the first CMC joint (see Figure 6-18).

Dorsal Design

The dorsal-based thumb orthosis rests on the dorsal aspects of the metacarpals, with a palmar LTTM piece supporting the thenar muscles. This design is often considered to be more functional than the traditional volar design because the volar palm is relatively free of LTTM and only has a small strap from radial to ulnar borders. This allows clients to receive more sensory input while using their hands in the orthosis (see Figure 6-20).

Cone Design

The cone orthotic design immobilizes the thumb CMC and MCP joints and covers the thenar eminence and thumb proximal phalanx only (see Figure 6-21). This is the least restrictive of all hand-based thumb designs because it encompasses the thenar eminence and thumb CMC and MCP joints only and may be suitable for mild CMC joint OA.

More advanced designs may incorporate **neoprene** into the orthosis, either by itself or with the addition of thermoplastic components for rigidity. Neoprene can be purchased in different thicknesses and offers a less rigid yet very comfortable alternative for clients who may desire less stability but some support in their thumb joints (Figure 6-22).

Orthotic Fabrication Steps

Please also see the demonstration videos for more information.

1. Pattern making

   ◦ Pattern for forearm-based thumb orthosis (Figure 6-23)

   ◦ Pattern for hand-based thumb orthosis (Figure 6-24)

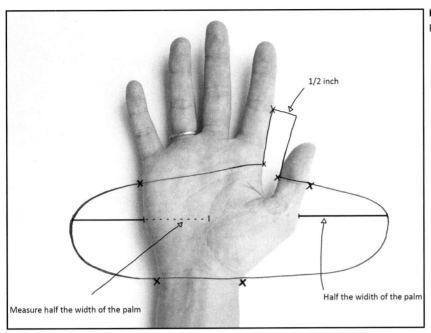

Figure 6-24. Hand-based volar thumb design pattern.

Table 6-1		
LTTM CHOICES FOR FOREARM- AND HAND-BASED THUMB ORTHOSES		
MATERIAL CONSIDERATIONS	**FOREARM BASED**	**HAND BASED**
Thickness	For adults, use 1/8-inch thickness. For children, use 1/12 or 3/32 inch.	For adults, use 3/32- or 1/12-inch thickness. For children, use 1/16 inch.
Drapability	Select a material that will conform well around the thenar muscles.	Select a material that will conform well around the thenar muscles.
Elasticity	Products with high elasticity should be stretched for best fit.	Products with high elasticity should be stretched for best fit.
Memory	Choose a product with high memory if you will need to redo the orthosis several times (e.g., as edema subsides).	Choose a product with high memory if you will need to redo the orthosis several times (e.g., as edema subsides).

2. Material selection
   ◦ Thermoplastic material choices for both forearm- and hand-based thumb orthoses are described in Table 6-1.
3. Client positioning
4. Molding techniques
5. Finishing techniques: edges and strapping
6. Orthosis check-out
   ◦ Can the client fully flex and extend his or her fingers?

   If no, adjust the distal edge of the orthosis so it clears the distal palmar crease. Remember that the orthosis will be higher on the radial side of the hand.

   ◦ Is the client's thumb positioned to enable him or her to laterally pinch?

   If no, remold the orthosis to position the thumb in lateral pinch.

   ◦ Can the client move his or her wrist in all directions without the orthosis interfering with this motion (for hand-based designs)?

   If no, the orthosis is too long or the proximal edge is not flared adequately.

   ◦ Does the client complain of discomfort when moving his or her hand in the orthosis?

   If yes, locate the area(s) of discomfort. Some possible solutions:

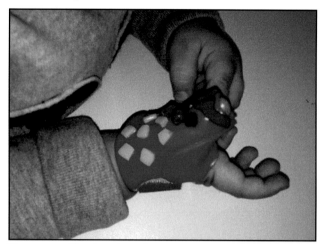

Figure 6-25. Thumb orthosis for a special pediatric client. (Reprinted with permission from Maria Candida Miranda Luzo.)

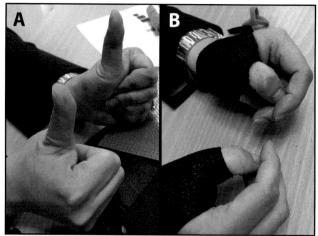

Figure 6-26. Bilateral thumb MCP joint instability (A) with hyperextension. (B) Short opponens orthoses provide MCP joint stability.

- *Flare the distal edge and be sure it clears the distal palmar crease.*
- *Flare around the thumb IP joint more to ensure that it can move freely.*
- *Smooth and round all rough edges.*
- *Bump out the area over the pisiform and apply padding.*

○ Are the corners of the orthosis rounded and smooth?

If no, round and smooth all corners of the orthosis.

○ Are the straps secure and edges rounded?

If no, adjust the straps. For forearm-based orthoses, the wrist strap should go in a circumferential fashion around the wrist; the ends should meet together. No Velcro (Velcro BVBA) should be exposed. The proximal strap should be angled on the orthosis so it sits flat on the forearm. The strap over the metacarpals should secure the orthosis on the hand.

○ Are all indentations and pattern marks removed?

If no, use heat gun to smooth the LTTM. Rubbing alcohol can be used to remove wax pencil marks. Ink cannot be removed, so refrain from using this when drawing your pattern on the LTTM.

○ Remove orthosis after 5 to 10 minutes and observe the skin. Are there any reddened areas?

If yes, adjust the orthosis by flaring and smoothing edges and/or flaring material away from bony prominences.

○ Review the purpose and care of the thumb orthosis with the client. Does the client understand why he or she is wearing it? When he or she should wear it? How to take care of it?

If no, discuss the wearing schedule and care of the orthosis with the client before he or she leaves the clinic, and provide clear written instructions to take

home with him or her (refer to the Appendix at the end of the chapter).

SPECIAL CONSIDERATIONS

Pediatric Clients

- Consider using colored LTTM and straps to appeal to younger clients. Allow them to choose decorations like stickers or add thermoplastic designs to their orthoses to help them to feel that they are part of the process (Figure 6-25).
- Consider using creative strapping techniques such as shoelaces or other devices that require two hands to prevent removal by younger children who may not understand the need to wear the orthosis. Sometimes it is recommended to cover the orthosis with a sleeve or a long stockinette to prevent a young client from taking it off.

Geriatric Clients

- Consider using contrasting-colored materials and straps for visually impaired clients.
- Straps can be attached directly to the LTTM by the use of dry heat so that elderly clients do not lose the straps at night.
- Clients with fragile skin may require additional skin protection through the use of padding, extra layers of stockinette, lightweight LTTM, and special soft straps.
- Adult clients may benefit from simple orthotic solutions to stabilize thumb joints with a minimum of material (Figures 6-26 and 6-27).
- Everyone will enjoy having a personally decorated orthosis (Figures 6-28 and 6-29).

Each client is an individual, and the selected hand-based thumb orthosis must match the individual's needs, size, and functional demands. Please see the additional helpful hints in Box 6-4.

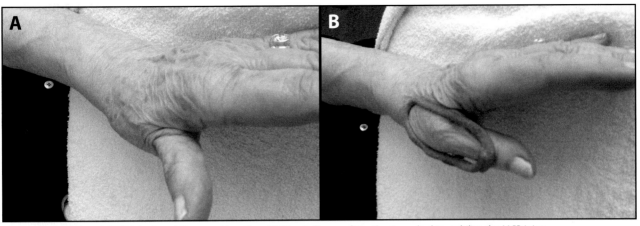

Figure 6-27. (A) Thumb MCP joint instability or subluxation. (B) Simple figure-of-8 orthosis applied to stabilize the MCP joint.

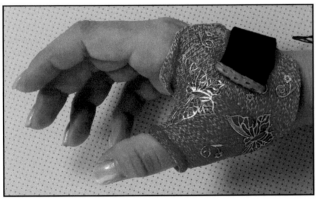

Figure 6-28. Decorating the orthosis to increase client compliance. (Reprinted with permission from Anna Ovsyannikova.)

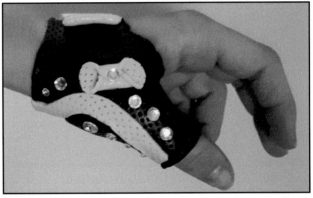

Figure 6-29. Decorating an orthosis to increase client compliance. (Reprinted with permission from Anna Ovsyannikova.)

Summary

- Knowledge of the key anatomical structures affected by forearm- and hand-based thumb orthoses will help the practitioner understand how the orthoses will influence these structures and will assist him or her in determining the most appropriate orthotic design and wearing schedule.

- The goals of forearm- or hand-based thumb orthosis and the specifics of each individual wearing schedule will vary depending on the client's needs and the diagnosis.

- Forearm- and hand-based thumb orthoses represent first-class lever systems.

- Thumb orthoses can be fabricated using a volar, dorsal, cone, or circumferential design. The design chosen depends on the client's clinical condition, current functional needs, specific indications requested by the referring physician, and practitioner preference.

- Special populations such as pediatric and geriatric clients may require specific orthotic designs or adaptations to achieve the best outcomes with orthoses.

Box 6-4. Helpful Hints

- Perforated materials are appropriate for warmer climates, clients with open wounds, or clients who need more ventilation.

- LTTM with memory is important when frequent readjustments of the short thumb opponens orthosis are required (e.g., clients with edema or tendon injury). This makes remolding the orthosis easier and is cost efficient.

- Clients needing increased thumb and wrist support may require a forearm-based thumb orthosis, even if the diagnosis has been described in this chapter.

- Each orthosis must be molded to the individual anatomy for the best fit. Post-fabrication critique and checkout helps identify areas for modification and optimize client comfort.

In Your Client's Shoes

As a practitioner, it is very important to appreciate the effect that an orthosis will have on your client's daily occupations. The orthosis will most likely interfere with many, if not all, of your client's daily activities. You should experience how it feels to wear an orthosis for an extended period of time. This experience will enable you to be client centered when using orthoses as an intervention strategy in your practice. You must consider how to instruct your client on the importance of the wearing schedule and the benefits of compliance for maximum benefits.

Suggested Reading

Amini, D. (2011). Occupational therapy interventions for work-related injuries and conditions of the forearm, wrist, and hand: A systematic review. *American Journal of Occupational Therapy, 65*(1), 29-36.

Bani, M. A., Arazpour, M., & Kashani, R. V. (2013). Comparison of custom-made and prefabricated neoprene splinting in patients with the first carpometacarpal joint osteoarthritis. *Disability and Rehabilitation: Assistive Technology, 8*(3), 232-237.

Beasley, J. (2012). Osteoarthritis and rheumatoid arthritis: Conservative therapeutic management. *Journal of Hand Therapy, 25*(2), 163-172.

Cantero-Téllez, R., Valdes, K., Schwartz, D. A., Medina-Porqueres, I., Arias, J. C., & Villafañe, J. H. (2018). Necessity of immobilizing the metacarpophalangeal joint in carpometacarpal osteoarthritis: Short-term effect. *Hand (N Y), 13*(4), 412-417 .

Carlsen, B. T., & Moran, S. L. (2009). Thumb trauma: Bennett fractures, Rolando fractures, and ulnar collateral ligament injuries. *Journal of Hand Surgery, 34*(5), 945-952.

Cavaleri, R., Schabrun, S. M., Te, M., & Chipchase, L. S. (2016). Hand therapy versus corticosteroid injections in the treatment of de Quervain's disease: A systematic review and meta-analysis. *Journal of Hand Therapy, 29*(1), 3-11.

Chan, R. K. (2002). Splinting for peripheral nerve injury in upper limb. *Hand Surgery, 7*(2), 251-259.

Coldham, F. (2006). The use of splinting in the non-surgical treatment of de Quervain's disease: A review of the literature. *British Journal of Hand Therapy, 11*(2), 48-55.

Dell, P. C., Dell, R. B., & Griggs, R. (2011). Management of carpal fractures and dislocations. In T. Skirven, A. Osterman, J. Fedorczyk, & P. Amadio (Eds.), *Rehabilitation of the hand and upper extremity* (6th ed., pp. 988-1001). Philadelphia, PA: Mosby.

Doornberg, J. N., Buijze, G. A., Ham, S. J., Ring, D., Bhandari, M., & Poolman, R. W. (2011). Nonoperative treatment for acute scaphoid fractures: A systematic review and meta-analysis of randomized controlled trials. *Journal of Trauma and Acute Care Surgery, 71*(4), 1073-1081.

Hart, R. G., Kleinert, H. E., & Lyons, K. (2005). A modified thumb spica for thumb injuries in the emergency department. *American Journal of Emergency Medicine, 23*(6), 777-781.

Huisstede, B. M., Coert, J. H., Fridén, J., & Hoogvliet, P. (2014). Consensus on multidisciplinary treatment guidelines for de Quervain disease: Results from the European HANDGUIDE study. *Physical Therapy, 94*(8), 1095-1190.

Lawton, J. N., Nicholls, M. A., & Charoglu, C. P. (2007). Immobilization for scaphoid fracture: Forearm rotation in long arm thumb-spica versus Munster thumb-spica casts. *Orthopedics, 30*(8), 612-614.

Leggett, J., & Meko, C. (2006). Acute finger injuries: Part II. Fractures, dislocations, and thumb injuries. *American Family Physician, 73*(5), 827-834.

Mallee, W. H., Doornberg, J. N., Ring, D., Maas, M., Muhl, M., van Dijk, C. N., & Goslings, J. C. (2014). Computed tomography for suspected scaphoid fractures: comparison of reformations in the plane of the wrist versus the long axis of the scaphoid. *Hand, 9*(1), 117-121.

Menendez, M. E., Thornton, E., Kent, S., Kalajian, T., & Ring, D. (2015). A prospective randomized clinical trial of prescription of full-time versus as-desired splint wear for de Quervain tendinopathy. *International Orthopaedics, 39*(8), 1563-1569.

Michaud, E. J., Flinn, S., & Seitz, W. H., Jr. (2010). Treatment of grade III thumb metacarpophalangeal ulnar collateral ligament injuries with early controlled motion using a hinged splint. *Journal of Hand Therapy, 23*(1), 77-82.

Mulligan, J., & Amblum, J. (2014). Diagnosis and treatment of scaphoid fracture. *Emergency Nurse, 22*(3), 18-23.

Sillem, H., Backman, C. L., Miller, W. C., Li, L. C. (2011). Comparison of two carpometacarpal stabilizing splints for individuals with thumb osteoarthritis. *Journal of Hand Therapy, 24*(3), 216-225.

Smith, M. (2009). Literature review: Splinting and education in the treatment of de Quervain's disease: Effect and practability. *Irish Journal of Occupational Therapy, 37*(1), 38-46.

Ten Berge, S. R., Boonstra, A. M., Dijkstra, P. U., Hadders-Algra, M., Haga, N., & Maathuis, C. G. (2012). A systematic evaluation of the effect of thumb opponens splints on hand function in children with unilateral spastic cerebral palsy. *Clinical Rehabilitation, 26*(4), 362-371.

Valdes, K., & Marik, T. (2010). A systematic review of conservative interventions for osteoarthritis of the hand. *Journal of Hand Therapy, 23*, 334-351.

Willey, M. (2004). Modification to a pediatric thumb splint. *Journal of Hand Therapy, 17*(3), 379-380.

Test Your Knowledge

SHORT ANSWER

1. Identify the anatomical landmarks associated with a hand-based thumb orthosis

2. Describe the biomechanical principles that apply to a hand-based thumb orthosis.

3. Identify the recommended thumb position and discuss the rationale behind it.

4. List the movements that a client should be able to perform without difficulty when wearing a hand-based thumb orthosis.

5. Describe the three different hand-based thumb designs and discuss the rationale for each.

6. List the appropriate orthotic design and thermoplastic material suitable for the following:

   ○ A 45-year-old woman with OA of the CMC joint where the orthosis is worn at night only

   ○ A 6-year-old boy with a cerebral palsy and an adducted thumb

   ○ A 35-year-old man with an ulnar collateral ligament injury

   ○ An 80-year-old woman with RA

7. Identify the anatomical landmarks associated with a forearm-based thumb orthosis.

8. Describe the biomechanical principles that apply to a forearm-based thumb orthosis.

9. Identify the recommended wrist position and the recommended thumb position and discuss the rationale behind these positions.

10. List the movements that a client should be able to perform without difficulty when wearing a forearm-based thumb orthosis.

11. Describe the three different forearm-based thumb designs and discuss the rationale for each.

12. List the appropriate orthotic design and thermoplastic material suitable for the following:
    ◦ A 45-year-old woman with OA of the wrist and CMC joint where the orthosis is worn at night only
    ◦ An 11-year-old boy with a scaphoid fracture
    ◦ A 35-year-old man with a de Quervain's syndrome from a work injury
    ◦ An 80-year-old woman with radial nerve palsy undergoing tendon transfers

MULTIPLE CHOICE

13. What type of lever system does a hand-based thumb orthosis represent?
    a. Third class
    b. First class
    c. Second class
    d. Fourth class

14. What will occur if the lever system represented by a hand-based thumb orthosis is not balanced?
    a. The wrist will not be sufficiently supported in the orthosis.
    b. The fingers will not be able to move fully.
    c. The elbow will not be able to flex fully.
    d. The thumb will not be supported properly.

15. Which of the following landmarks do not apply to a hand-based thumb orthosis?
    a. The olecranon
    b. The pisiform
    c. The CMC joint
    d. The MCP joint

16. What is the recommended method of preventing pressure on a bony prominence when fabricating a hand-based thumb orthosis?
    a. Pad the area after molding the orthosis.
    b. Flare the LTTM away from the area after molding the orthosis.
    c. Pad the area prior to molding the orthosis.
    d. Make the forearm component of the orthosis as long as possible.

17. What functional movement should the client be able to do while wearing a hand-based thumb orthosis?
    a. Thumb opposition to each fingertip
    b. Lateral pinch
    c. Power grasp
    d. Tenodesis grasp

18. What will the client experience if the thumb is not properly positioned in his or her orthosis?
    a. The client will be unable to move his or her thumb fully.
    b. The client will be unable to flex the CMC joint.
    c. The client will be unable to fully flex or extend his or her fingers.
    d. The client will have difficulty getting the orthosis on and off.

19. Why is it important to clear the wrist crease completely when fabricating a hand-based thumb orthosis?
    a. This allows for full thumb mobility in the orthosis.
    b. This allows for full PIP and DIP joint mobility in the orthosis.
    c. This allows for full wrist mobility in the orthosis.
    d. This allows for full flexion and gripping in the orthosis.

20. What is the primary advantage of the dorsal hand-based thumb orthosis design?
    a. It allows for more sensory input in the palm.
    b. It allows for more digit mobility.
    c. It allows for more thumb mobility.
    d. It is easier to fabricate than the volar designs.

21. Why might a practitioner choose a simple cone thumb design over a volar or dorsal design?
    a. When a client needs more rigid support.
    b. When a client has difficulty putting the orthosis on.
    c. When a client needs light support for function.
    d. When a client needs to wear the orthosis only at night.

CASE STUDIES

Case Study 1

Jeanne is a 67-year-old, right-hand-dominant woman who describes intense pain at the base of her thumbs while doing everyday household chores that also affects her hobbies of knitting and gardening. She was seen by her family doctor, who felt she might have some OA in her thumb joints and sent her to a specialist for further evaluation. He also recommended a visit to therapy for custom-fitted orthoses. Jeanne says her right thumb aches more than the left one at this time.

She presents for therapy with a prescription that reads:

Thumb pain, right and left hands:

1. *Evaluate and treat.*

2. *Provide right thumb orthosis.*

3. *Joint protection tips.*

Your assessment:

Jeanne presents to therapy for an evaluation and custom thumb orthosis on the right thumb. The right thumb CMC joint displays mild erythema and swelling. Active ROM is within normal limits. Grip and pinch strength are also within functional range, but the client has pain with key, lateral, and 3-point pinch on the right side. Pain was evaluated using the visual analog scale and rated as 6/10 with activity on the right and 3/10 at rest. Jeanne states that the pain and aching in her right thumb worsen at night. She lives with her husband and is quite active with volunteer work and leisure activities.

Using different clinical reasoning approaches, answer the following questions about this client and the prescribed orthosis:

Procedural Reasoning

1. What client factors are important to consider when determining the most suitable orthotic design for this client?

2. Which hand-based thumb orthotic design would be most appropriate for this client? Why?

3. What LTTM properties are important to consider?

4. Describe the instructions you would give this client on:
   ○ How to care for the orthosis
   ○ Wearing schedule
   ○ Precautions
   ○ Exercises/activities

Pragmatic Reasoning

5. What resources are available to fabricate this orthosis (time, materials, expertise)?

6. Are you able to clearly document the need for this orthosis?

7. Does evidence-based practice support the use of this orthosis for this client's diagnosis?

Interactive Reasoning

8. What are the client's goals and valued occupations?

9. What impact will the client's injury and use of the orthosis have on her ADL?

Conditional Reasoning

10. What factors will influence this client's compliance to the wearing schedule of this orthosis?

Narrative Reasoning

11. How does this condition and, more specifically, this orthotic intervention affect this client's valued occupations?

12. What activities is this client most concerned about?

Ethical Reasoning

13. Does the client understand the need for the orthosis?

14. Does the client have the resources to be able to pay for the orthosis (as applicable)?

15. What other options are available to this client if she lacks the resources necessary to pay for the orthosis?

16. Write one short-term goal (1 to 2 weeks) and one long-term goal (6 to 8 weeks) for this client.

Case Study 2

Steven is a 34-year-old, right-hand-dominant high school teacher who injured his right thumb while playing basketball in the neighborhood. Steven states that he fell quite hard and landed with his thumb widely abducted. He was seen by an orthopedic surgeon, who diagnosed him with a right ulnar collateral ligament injury. He now presents for therapy with a prescription that reads:

Right thumb ulnar collateral ligament sprain:

1. *Evaluate and treat.*

2. *Provide thumb orthosis.*

3. *Active ROM exercises.*

Your assessment:

Steven's right thumb MCP joint is red and swollen in comparison to the left. Base of thumb circumference is measured as 6.4 cm on the left and 7.0 cm on the right. The MCP joint is tender to palpation, and the client reports pain on the ulnar aspect of the thumb MCP joint. Active thumb abduction and opposition is limited and painful on the right as compared with the left. IP flexion and extension are within normal limits. Pain was evaluated using the visual analog scale and rated as 8/10 with thumb movement and 5/10 at rest. Steven denies any numbness, tingling, or other sensory symptoms in his right thumb.

Steven is newly married. He is having difficulties with all ADL, including dressing, helping with chores around the house, and doing some work activities. He is eager to regain full motion and function in his injured thumb and return to his valued leisure occupation of playing basketball with his friends.

Using different clinical reasoning approaches, consider the following questions about this client and the prescribed orthosis. Some questions may be directed more toward the client, and some questions may be directed more toward you as the practitioner for reflection:

Procedural Reasoning

1. What client factors are important to consider when determining the most suitable orthotic design for this client?

2. Which hand-based thumb orthotic design would be most appropriate for this client? Why?

3. What LTTM properties are important to consider?

4. Describe the instructions you would give this client on:
   - How to care for the orthosis
   - Wearing schedule
   - Precautions
   - Exercises/activities

Pragmatic Reasoning

5. What resources are available to fabricate this orthosis (time, materials, expertise)?

6. Are you able to clearly document the need for this orthosis?

7. Does evidence-based practice support the use of this orthosis for this client's diagnosis?

Interactive Reasoning

8. What are the client's goals and valued occupations?

9. What effect will the client's injury and use of the orthosis have on his ADL?

Conditional Reasoning

10. What factors will influence this client's compliance to the wearing schedule of this orthosis?

Narrative Reasoning

11. How does this injury and, more specifically, this orthotic intervention affect this client's valued occupations?

12. What activities is this client most concerned about?

Ethical Reasoning

13. Does the client understand the need for the orthosis?

14. Does the client have the resources to be able to pay for the orthosis (as applicable)?

15. What other options are available to this client if he lacks the resources necessary to pay for the orthosis?

16. Write one short-term goal (1 to 2 weeks) and one long-term goal (6 to 8 weeks) for this client.

Appendix

STUDENT ASSIGNMENTS

1. Define all the key terms used in this chapter.

2. As an occupational therapy practitioner, you must provide your client with detailed instructions for wearing and caring for his or her orthosis. This document must be required for the client's official records and insurance payments. Select one of the thumb orthotic designs from this chapter and prepare a client-centered handout for wearing this orthosis. Base your client description on one of the two case studies in this chapter. Include the following in the handout:
   - A description/name of the orthosis
   - An outline of the wearing schedule (remember this will vary depending on the client's condition)
   - A description of how to clean and care for the orthosis
   - Instructions on what the client should be aware of when wearing the orthosis (red areas on skin, pain, increased swelling, etc.)
   - Contact information and follow-up instructions

3. Prepare a case study of a client requiring a thumb orthosis. Use one of the evidence-based resources cited in the chapter to support your orthotic intervention. Summarize the research and explain the outcomes of the study.

4. As an occupational therapy practitioner, it will be interesting and informative for you to spend an extended period wearing an orthosis to appreciate the effect that an orthosis will have on your client's daily occupations. Wear a thumb orthosis designed by your lab partner for a 24-hour period. Take note of how it feels to have one body part immobilized. Elaborate in paragraphs on the following:
   - Describe the orthosis, material used, positioning, and typical diagnosis for this particular orthosis. (Which arm was splinted, when did you wear it, what did you do with it on?)
   - Comfort and ease of use: Is it easy to take on and off? Does the orthosis fit under clothing? Are there any pressure areas? What needs to be modified and how?

- ○ Personal and public image: Does the orthosis attract attention in public? Does the orthosis attract attention in your family? How did this make you feel, even as a class assignment?

- ○ Functionality: How were you able to function with the orthosis? Was the position helpful or harmful? What would the typical wearing schedule be for a client with the typical need for this orthosis? What instructions should be given to the typical client with the need for this orthosis?

- ○ How does this change your appreciation of what your clients are experiencing with their orthoses?

5. Complete the check-out form on the next page.

Multiple Choice Answer Key

13. 6
14. d
15. a
16. c
17. b
18. c
19. c
20. a
21. c

Thumb Orthosis Check-Out Form

*(This can be used for faculty to evaluate students' completed orthoses,
as well as for students to reference when evaluating their own completed orthosis.)*

Fabricate one of the orthotic designs for a thumb orthosis on your classmate and complete the following check-out form:

Name of Orthosis:

Purpose of Orthosis:

Design/Function

_____ The thumb is in the correct position (allows for lateral pinch).

_____ Uninvolved joints can move freely: thumb IP, fingers, and wrist for hand-based designs.

_____ The orthosis is two-thirds the length of the forearm (for forearm-based designs).

_____ The orthosis is one-half the width of the forearm (for forearm-based designs).

Straps/Orthosis Appearance

_____ The straps are in the correct position.

_____ The Velcro hook is secure and covered completely.

_____ The orthosis edges are smooth with rounded corners.

_____ The proximal edge is flared.

_____ The orthosis does not cause impingement or pressure areas.

_____ The orthosis is free of fingerprints, pen marks, or indentations.

Elbow, Wrist, and Hand Immobilization Orthoses

Key Terms

Complex forearm fractures

Constraint induced movement therapy (CIMT)

Cubital tunnel syndrome

Distal humerus

Distal radioulnar joint

Dysesthesias

Extra-articular fractures

Fall on an outstretched hand (FOOSH)

Interosseous membrane

Intra-articular fractures

Joint dislocation

Open reduction internal fixation (ORIF)

Paresthesia

Proximal radioulnar joint

Radial head

Radial neck

Supracondylar

Ulnar claw hand

Learning Outcomes

Upon completion of this chapter, you will be able to:

1. Describe the clinical conditions and goals for prescribing an elbow, wrist, and hand immobilization orthosis.

2. Identify pertinent anatomical structures and biomechanical principles involved in an elbow, wrist, and hand immobilization orthosis and apply these concepts to orthotic design and fabrication.

3. Identify the most commonly selected orthotic designs and describe the rationale for choosing one design over another.

4. Design suitable patterns for the two common types of elbow, wrist, and hand immobilization orthoses and one forearm-based orthosis and identify the pertinent anatomical landmarks.

5. After reviewing the instructional videos:

   a. Outline the steps involved in the fabrication of an elbow, wrist, and hand immobilization orthosis.

   b. Complete the molding and finishing of an elbow, wrist, and hand immobilization orthosis.

   c. Evaluate the fit and function of a completed elbow, wrist, and hand immobilization orthosis and identify and address all areas needing adjustment.

Schofield, K., & Schwartz, D. *Orthotic Design and Fabrication
for the Upper Extremity: A Practical Guide* (pp 125-142).
© 2019 Taylor & Francis Group.

Box 7-1. Common Goals of Elbow, Wrist, and Hand Immobilization Orthoses

PROTECTION

- Support and protect the humerus, radius, and/or ulna following fracture.
- Support and protect the humerus, radius, and/or ulna following surgical repair of structures.
- Offer pain relief and joint protection from a painful tendinitis or arthritis or other inflammatory conditions.
- Support and protect unstable joints (from arthritis or other similar diagnoses).
- Prevent self-biting or other harmful behaviors.

POSITIONING

- Position the elbow to prevent development of joint or soft tissue contracture following injury.
- Position the elbow to limit motion and rest the ulnar nerve.

IMPROVE FUNCTION

- Provide stability to the upper arm for improved reach, grasp, and finger manipulation.
- Provide a static controlled stretch toward increased elbow extension or flexion.
- Use as a base for outrigger attachments to create mobilization orthoses to provide a controlled stretch toward increased elbow extension or flexion.

6. Identify elements of a client education program following provision of an elbow, wrist, and hand immobilization orthosis.

7. Describe special considerations of an elbow, wrist, and hand immobilization orthotic design and fabrication for pediatric and geriatric clients.

Introduction

Clients with a variety of different clinical conditions may benefit from an elbow, wrist, and hand immobilization orthosis. These orthoses are commonly prescribed following traumatic injury to the **distal humerus**, radius, and ulna and supporting ligaments, muscles, and other soft tissues surrounding the elbow, wrist, and hand. Other indications include supporting unstable or painful joints (osteoarthritis [OA] or rheumatoid arthritis [RA]), restricting movement

to protect and rest structures (the ulnar nerve in the cubital tunnel), and providing controlled stress to contracted tissues to improve joint motion (joint stiffness following trauma). Elbow, wrist, and hand orthoses might also be use in **constraint-induced movement therapy (CIMT)**, a treatment intervention that restricts motion in the unaffected limb and encourages or promotes active movement of an involved limb in patients following stroke or other neurological disorders. CIMT is a treatment strategy often also used with children with cerebral palsy. Sometimes elbow, wrist, and hand orthoses are used to prevent clients from hurting themselves with harmful or disruptive habits such as biting themselves or mouthing their hands. The choice of orthotic type and design depends on the clinical condition and physician preference, therapist experience, and needs of the client. A thorough assessment of the client's current functional status must always be done in conjunction with orthotic provision to ensure that the orthotic design chosen meets the needs of the client.

Goals for Use of an Elbow, Wrist, and Hand Immobilization Orthosis

The goals of an elbow, wrist, and hand immobilization orthosis are outlined in Box 7-1.

Clinical Conditions and Wearing Schedules

This section describes common clinical conditions where an elbow, wrist, and hand immobilization orthosis is typically prescribed; recommended wearing schedules; and the current evidence supporting this type of orthosis as an appropriate intervention strategy. Readers are encouraged to review the references provided for additional details regarding each clinical condition and search current research databases for updated evidence as it becomes available.

ELBOW FRACTURES AND JOINT DISLOCATION

Fractures of the elbow can involve the distal humerus, proximal radius, proximal ulna, and/or the **radial head**. Fractures may be nondisplaced, where the bony alignment is maintained even with partial or full break of the involved bone, or displaced, where movement of the bone segments has occurred. Concurrent injury to soft tissue structures, such as the muscles, nerves, blood vessels, and ligaments, can occur with these injuries and may complicate recovery. **Joint dislocation**, where the articulating surfaces of a joint

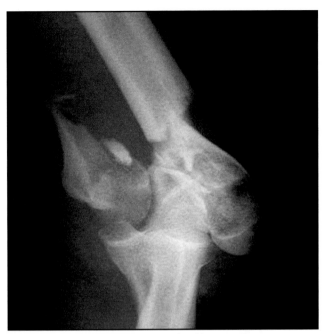

Figure 7-1. This X-ray demonstrates a distal humerus fracture.

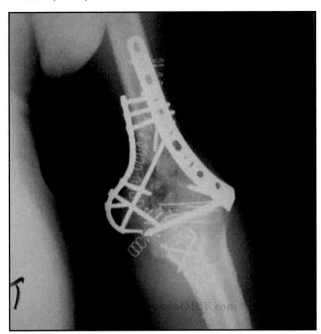

Figure 7-2. The typical treatment of a distal humeral fracture is ORIF of the distal humerus, shown in this X-ray.

are no longer in contact with each other, can also occur with or without associated fractures and is often associated with injuries to the joint capsule and ligaments.

DISTAL HUMERUS FRACTURES

Fractures of the distal humerus account for approximately one-third of all elbow fractures. They occur commonly as a result of a **fall on an outstretched hand (FOOSH)** or a direct blow or hit to the elbow. **Extra-articular fractures**, indicating fractures that do not involve the articulating surface of the distal humerus, typically occur above the condyles (**supracondylar**) and are treated conservatively or with surgical intervention (Figure 7-1).

Intra-articular fractures, indicating fractures that do involve the articulating surface, are usually treated surgically with **open reduction internal fixation (ORIF)** (Figure 7-2).

A posterior elbow, forearm, and wrist immobilization orthosis may be used instead of a cast to protect the injured structures to promote healing. The advantages of an orthosis over a cast is that the orthosis can be removed for periodic wound care and skin checks. It is also is critical for initiating early range of motion (ROM) exercises to avoid stiffness of the elbow joint. The elbow is typically positioned at 90 degrees of flexion, with the forearm in neutral and wrist at 0 degrees (Figure 7-3).

Wearing Schedule

The wearing schedule for this orthosis will depend in part on the healing time of the involved structures, the health of the client, and the severity of the injury. The

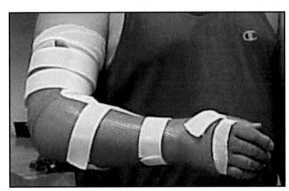

Figure 7-3. A posterior-placed elbow immobilization orthosis protects the fracture during healing.

practitioner must collaborate with the referring physician to determine the appropriate wearing schedule, but typically, a period of 4 to 6 weeks is recommended. Protected movement of the elbow and forearm is strongly encouraged as soon as possible to minimize the risk of joint and soft tissue stiffness that is commonly encountered following elbow trauma.

Evidence

Level V

- Casmus, R. J. (2010). Traumatic distal-third humeral fracture in a collegiate football player: A case review. *Athletic Training and Sports Health Care, 2*(1), 39-42.

  ○ The author describes a case study in which a collegiate football player sustained a traumatic distal-third humeral fracture while tackling an opponent, a high-impact activity. Fractures of the humerus are commonly due to blunt trauma, high-speed collisions, motor vehicle accidents, or falls from heights. Because of the location of the fracture and the degree of angulation, the decision was made to perform distal humerus ORIF. The surgical procedure was performed 48 hours post-injury. Postoperatively, the athlete wore a posterior splint and sling for 2 weeks, followed by a humeral brace for 6 weeks. Due to an intense postoperative therapy regimen, full active ROM of the elbow for flexion and extension was achieved 10 weeks postoperatively. Active ROM for supination and pronation was equal bilaterally at 12 weeks.

PROXIMAL RADIUS FRACTURES

Fractures of the proximal radius are the most common fractures that occur at the elbow and are often a result of FOOSH with the forearm positioned in pronation and the elbow in slight flexion. Most fractures occur at the radial head and/or **radial neck**. Simple, stable fractures are often treated with a posterior elbow, wrist, and hand immobilization orthosis with early active mobilization out of the orthosis. Comminuted or displaced fractures may be treated with ORIF or prosthetic replacement of the radial head if the fracture cannot be repaired. These fractures can also be managed with an elbow, wrist, and hand immobilization orthosis with graded mobilization out of the orthosis. The practitioner must collaborate with the referring physician to determine the ROM that is safe for the client to perform without risk of further injury or disruption of the injury site or surgical repair.

Wearing Schedule

The orthosis wearing schedule will depend in part on the healing time of the involved structures, the health of the client, and the severity of the injury. The practitioner must collaborate with the referring physician to determine the appropriate wearing schedule. For stable, simple fractures, typically a period of 1 to 3 weeks is recommended. Protected movement of the elbow and forearm is strongly encouraged as soon as possible to minimize the risk of joint and soft tissue stiffness that is commonly encountered following elbow trauma.

PROXIMAL ULNA FRACTURES

The majority of proximal ulna fractures occur at the olecranon or at the coronoid process of the ulna. These fractures can be associated with concurrent injury to the triceps insertion. Most are treated with ORIF and immobilized in an elbow, wrist, and hand orthosis with the elbow at 30 to 40 degrees of flexion to avoid stress on the triceps tendon. Fractures of the coronoid process are often associated with significant joint instability and are typically treated with cast immobilization or surgical intervention.

Wearing Schedule

The orthosis wearing schedule will depend in part on the healing time of the involved structures, the health of the client, and the severity of the injury. The practitioner must collaborate with the referring physician to determine the appropriate wearing schedule. For stable fractures, typically a period of 4 to 6 weeks is recommended. As with other fractures involving the elbow, protected movement of the elbow and forearm is strongly encouraged as soon as possible to minimize the risk of joint and soft tissue stiffness that is commonly encountered following elbow trauma.

COMPLEX FOREARM FRACTURES

Complex forearm fractures are those that involve both the radius and ulna and may also include injury to the **proximal radioulnar** and/or **distal radioulnar joints**. The **interosseous membrane**, a fibrous membrane that unites the radius and ulna together, is also susceptible to injury. The following are three such fractures:

- Galeazzi: Fracture of the middle shaft of the radius with distal radioulnar joint disruption

- Monteggia: Ulna fracture with anterior dislocation of the radial head

- Essex-Lopresti: Radial head fracture with interosseous membrane disruption and distal radioulnar joint dislocation

Managing these injuries involves controlling the amount of available forearm, elbow, and wrist motion during the healing process with the use of appropriate orthoses. Clinicians can use one of two different orthoses to limit forearm rotation to allow for adequate healing of structures: a sugar tong orthosis design or a Muenster design. Both of these designs limit full forearm rotation while allowing elbow flexion and extension during the healing process (Figure 7-4).

Wearing Schedule

The orthosis wearing schedule will depend in part on the healing time of the involved structures, the health of the client, and the severity of the injury. The practitioner must collaborate with the referring physician to determine the appropriate wearing schedule. For stable fractures, typically a period of 4 to 6 weeks is recommended. As with other fractures involving the elbow, protected movement of the elbow and forearm is strongly encouraged as soon as possible to minimize the risk of joint and soft tissue stiffness that is commonly encountered following elbow trauma.

Evidence

Level II

- Levy, J., Ernat, J., Song, D., Cook, J. B., Judd, D., & Shaha, S. (2015). Outcomes of long-arm casting versus double-sugar-tong splinting of acute pediatric distal

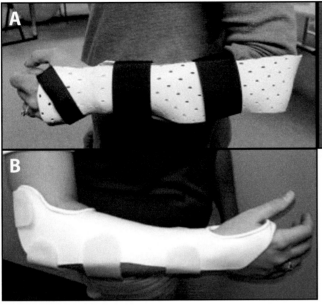

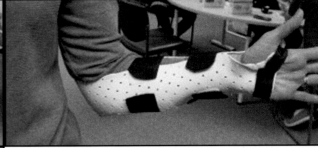

Figure 7-4. Orthoses that limit forearm rotation. (A) Sugar tong orthosis. (Reprinted with permission from Orfit Industries.) (B) Muenster orthosis. (Reprinted with permission from Chad Royer.)

forearm fractures. *Journal of Pediatric Orthopedics, 35*(1), 11-17.

○ This prospective comparative study examined the effectiveness of a double sugar tong orthosis versus a long arm cast in maintaining distal radius or double forearm bone fractures in a pediatric population. Seventy-one subjects participated in the study; 37 with a long arm cast and 34 in a double sugar tong orthosis after fracture reduction. The double sugar tong orthosis was described as a sugar tong orthosis fabricated from plaster and bivalved that was then converted into a long arm cast after the initial swelling had decreased. The long arm cast group had significant risk of loss of reduction throughout the study, but no difference between groups was apparent following cast removal. The authors concluded that both the long arm cast and double sugar tong orthoses are comparable and effective methods of immobilization for this population.

- Kim, J. K., Kook, S. H., & Kim, Y. K. (2012). Comparison of forearm rotation allowed by different types of upper extremity immobilization. *Journal of Bone and Joint Surgery, 94*, 455-60.

○ This prospective comparative study examined the degree of allowable forearm rotation of five elbow, wrist, and forearm immobilization devices: short arm splint, short arm cast, sugar tong splint, long arm splint, and long arm cast. Forty healthy subjects participated in the study, 20 men and 20 women. Active forearm pronation and supination with and without each of the five immobilization orthoses was measured with a custom goniometer, and results were compared between each orthosis, as well as between men and women. The long arm cast was the most effective at limiting forearm rotation

(less than 10% of allowable motion); no significant differences were found between the sugar tong, short arm splint, long arm splint, and short arm cast in the degree of allowable forearm rotation (each averaging approximately 30% to 40% of allowable motion). The authors recommend use of a long arm cast if complete forearm immobilization is required.

Level IV

- Slaughter, A., Miles, L., Fleming, J., & McPhail, S. (2010). A comparative study of splint effectiveness in limiting forearm rotation. *Journal of Hand Therapy, 23*, 241-248.

○ This case series study compared the effectiveness of four orthoses that are designed to limit forearm rotation: Muenster, sugar tong, wrist immobilization, and anti-pronation. Five healthy, uninjured subjects participated in the study. All four orthoses were fabricated for each participant with the forearm in neutral rotation. Outcome measures included the degree of active forearm rotation to the point of sensory feedback and forearm supination and pronation to the point of maximum force for each of the four orthoses. Results indicated statistically significant differences in active ROM for all four orthoses. The sugar tong design was more restrictive than the Muenster orthosis for forearm pronation, and the anti-pronation orthosis was more restrictive in pronation compared with the wrist orthosis. None of the orthoses immobilized the forearm completely. The authors recommend the sugar tong design to restrict forearm pronation and note that further study is warranted to assess orthoses effectiveness when the forearm is positioned in supination (to limit pronation) and pronation (to limit supination).

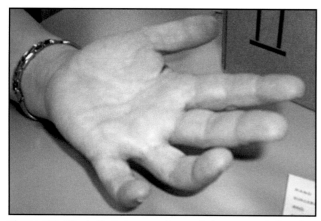

Figure 7-5. Client displaying symptoms of ulnar nerve dysfunction: clawing of the ulnar digits.

DISTAL BICEPS AND TRICEPS INJURIES

Injuries to the distal biceps and or triceps tendons are typically avulsion injuries and may be treated conservatively or surgically. Clients may include workers, weight lifters, and professional athletes, and these injuries occur most commonly in males aged 40 to 60 years. Typically, the mechanism of acute injury involves an eccentric load placed across a contracting muscle belly. Both the triceps and biceps muscles span two joints, and they can be particularly at risk when placed in an unfavorable loading condition such as lowering a very heavy object.

Both operative and nonoperative treatments have been reported, but recommendations for surgical repair are supported in the literature. Nonoperative treatment typically includes splinting the elbow at 90 degrees for several weeks and, if needed, using physical agents for pain relief.

Biceps repairs are immobilized initially in a long arm splint positioning the elbow in 90 degrees of flexion, the forearm in neutral rotation, and the wrist supported. Following triceps repairs, the elbow is typically immobilized in a long arm splint, initially positioning the elbow in 30 to 45 degrees of elbow flexion, the forearm in neutral, and the wrist often supported.

Evidence

Level V

- Blackmore, S. M., Jander, R. M., & Culp, R. W. (2006). Management of distal biceps and triceps ruptures. *Journal of Hand Therapy, 19*(2), 154-169.

    ○ The authors outline the management of distal biceps and triceps ruptures and describe in detail the clinical presentation, evaluation, surgical management, and nonoperative management protocols. They describe therapeutic interventions and orthotic options for these injuries. Although they highlight the numerous surgical procedures and techniques used by surgeons to repair tears and list the postsurgical complications, the more interesting

components to this article for therapists are the postoperative time tables for rehabilitation procedures and orthotic design options for both immobilization and mobilization orthoses.

CUBITAL TUNNEL SYNDROME

Cubital tunnel syndrome, the second most common compressive nerve syndrome in the upper extremity (UE) after carpal tunnel syndrome, is defined as compression of the ulnar nerve at the elbow as it courses through the cubital tunnel, a bony canal formed by the medial epicondyle and olecranon. Tension on the ulnar nerve in this area can occur secondary to compression, friction, or elongation. Some examples include resting the elbow on a hard surface such as a desk or car door, holding the elbow in a fully flexed position for a prolonged period, or moving the elbow in a repetitive manner, such as seen with individuals who use a manual wheelchair for mobility. Elbow flexion in particular narrows the space within the cubital tunnel. Clients with this condition often present with symptoms of pain, **dysesthesias** (reports of pain from normally nonpainful touch), and **paresthesias** (numbness/tingling) on the volar and dorsal aspects of the ulnar half of the ring finger and entire small finger, along with impaired grip and pinch strength. In more advanced cases, clawing of the ring and small fingers may be observed due to weakened fourth and fifth digit lumbricals and volar and dorsal interossei and loss of balance between the extrinsic flexor and extensor muscles of the fingers. This position is characterized by hyperextension of the metacarpophalangeal (MCP) joints of the ring and small fingers, with concurrent flexion of the proximal interphalangeal and distal interphalangeal joints, and is commonly referred to as **ulnar claw hand** (Figure 7-5).

An elbow immobilization orthosis is commonly prescribed for clients with cubital tunnel syndrome to reduce tension and rest the ulnar nerve at the cubital tunnel. The elbow is positioned between 30 and 45 degrees of flexion, and the orthosis is typically worn at night to prevent full elbow flexion while sleeping. An elbow pad may also be prescribed for use during the day to protect and pad the ulnar nerve (Figure 7-6).

Wearing Schedule

When an orthosis is used as part of conservative treatment of cubital tunnel syndrome, a minimum of 3 months of consistent use of the orthosis at night is recommended, along with avoiding provocative activities during the day such as repetitive elbow flexion and direct pressure on the ulnar nerve/medial epicondyle during daily tasks.

Evidence

Level III

- Shah, C. M., Calfee, R. P., Gelberman, R. H., & Goldfarb, C. A. (2013). Outcomes of rigid night splinting and

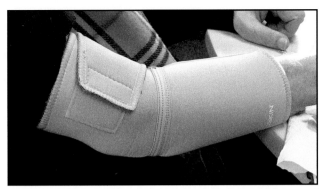

Figure 7-6. Elbow pad for use during the day to treat cubital tunnel syndrome. (Reprinted with permission from Michelle Blumenstyk.)

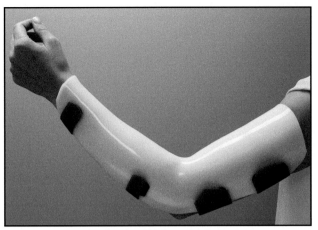

Figure 7-7. Anterior elbow immobilization orthosis.

activity modification in the treatment of cubital tunnel syndrome. *Journal of Hand Surgery, 38*, 1125-1130.

○ This prospective quasi-experimental study analyzed the effectiveness of a 3-month course of night splinting and activity modification for cubital tunnel syndrome. Nineteen subjects (25 extremities) participated in the study with a diagnosis of idiopathic cubital tunnel syndrome; 85% of the participants had positive nerve conduction studies. Treatment consisted of a 3-month course of education on activity modification to reduce "daytime aggravation of the ulnar nerve" and rigid night time splinting with the elbow at 45 degrees of flexion. Outcome measures included the Disabilities of the Arm, Shoulder and Hand score, self-report of splint compliance, the Short Form 12, grip strength, and ulnar nerve provocative testing. All were measured at baseline, 6 weeks, 3 months, and 1 and 2 years. A total of 24 of the 25 extremities were available at final follow-up; 21 of the 24 extremities demonstrated significant improvement in all outcomes measured. The authors conclude that rigid splinting, along with activity modification, is an effective intervention for clients with mild to moderate cubital tunnel syndrome.

ELBOW STIFFNESS/ELBOW FLEXION CONTRACTURE

Elbow stiffness and elbow flexion contractures are a common occurrence after trauma or injury to elbow structures. Anteriorly placed elbow, wrist, and hand orthoses are often used to treat elbow flexion contractures and elbow stiffness when clients have difficulty maintaining elbow extension. An orthosis can be fabricated on the anterior arm and molded to hold the limb in maximum extension (Figure 7-7). This orthosis should be worn at a minimum every night for maximum benefit. Over time, the orthosis can be remolded to accommodate changes and gains in

joint position. This is known as *serial splinting*, or periodic changes to the molded orthosis to achieve gains in passive joint ROM.

Biomechanical Concepts of Elbow, Wrist, and Hand Immobilization Orthoses

Orthoses that are designed to immobilize the elbow and wrist are first-class lever systems. As discussed in Chapter 1, a first-class lever system has three components:

1. A fulcrum, which is typically the target joint that the orthosis is acting on

2. An effort force, the component of the orthosis applying the effort force

3. A resistance force, the component of the orthosis resisting the effort force

Specific to an elbow immobilization orthosis, the elbow is the fulcrum, the orthosis proximal to the elbow along the humerus is the effort force, and the orthosis segment distal to the elbow the resistance force (Figure 7-8).

The practitioner should follow some basic biomechanical principles when designing an elbow, wrist, and hand immobilization orthosis to optimize effectiveness and comfort:

• Less force is needed to stabilize/immobilize the elbow when the resistance force is as long as possible.

• The orthosis will be more balanced if the effort force is also as long as possible.

• Make the orthosis as wide as possible to distribute the forces over a large area. This will lessen the compressive and shear forces on the tissues/structures that the orthosis influences.

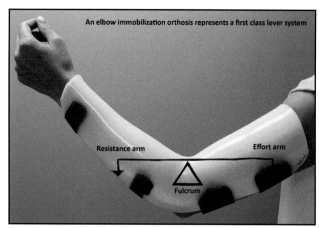
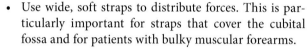

Figure 7-8. Elbow immobilization orthosis with components of first-class lever system outlined.

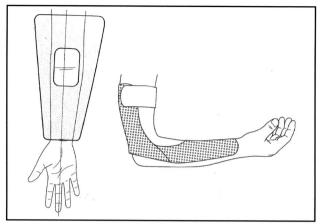

Figure 7-9. Elbow extension orthosis with cut out. (Reprinted with permission from Orfit Industries.)

- Use wide, soft straps to distribute forces. This is particularly important for straps that cover the cubital fossa and for patients with bulky muscular forearms.

- Pay attention to the bony prominences: the lateral and medial epicondyles, the olecranon, and the radial styloid and ulnar head. Either pad these areas before applying the low-temperature thermoplastic material (LTTM) or bump them out afterward. You can also select a highly conforming material or use an elastic based material with stretch. This is particularly important for orthoses that are on the posterior aspect of the elbow.

- Consider including the wrist because this will lengthen the resistance force and lessen the force needed to stabilize the elbow.

- Use highly conforming LTTM to lessen the likelihood of compressive and shear forces over bony prominences and other tissues.

Elbow, Wrist, and Hand Immobilization Orthotic Designs

Two common designs for orthoses that immobilize the elbow, forearm, and wrist are the posterior and anterior elbow, wrist, and hand immobilization orthoses (see Figures 7-3 and 7-7). Other designs, such as the previously mentioned Muenster orthosis and the sugar tong orthosis, are designed to limit forearm rotation while allowing for elbow motion. The specific design will depend on the individual client's clinical condition, current functional needs, specific indications requested by the referring physician, and practitioner preference. The practitioner must consider the anatomy of the elbow, forearm, and wrist and how the

orthosis will influence these structures when determining the most appropriate orthosis design.

POSTERIOR ELBOW IMMOBILIZATION ORTHOSIS

The posterior elbow immobilization orthosis design immobilizes the elbow, wrist, and hand and may include the wrist depending on the client's condition. It sits on the posterior aspect of the humerus, elbow, and forearm, and the typical position in the orthosis is 90 degrees of elbow flexion and neutral forearm rotation. If included in the orthosis, the wrist should be positioned at 0 to 20 degrees of extension to prevent stiffness and shortening of structures. The practitioner may vary the position of the elbow and forearm based on the client's particular injury/surgery and physician preference. Care must be taken to protect the ulnar nerve at the cubital tunnel, the medial and lateral epicondyles, and the olecranon with this design because the LTTM covers these structures. Measures to do this include judicious use of padding prior to molding; use of highly conforming LTTM; and wide, soft straps

ANTERIOR ELBOW IMMOBILIZATION ORTHOSIS

The anterior elbow immobilization orthosis design also immobilizes the elbow, forearm, and wrist. It covers the anterior aspect of the humerus, cubital fossa, forearm, and palm. This design is well-suited for conditions where limited elbow flexion is desired, such as cubital tunnel syndrome; to apply gentle, controlled force to a stiff, contracted elbow in the direction of extension; or if there is a wound on the posterior aspect of the elbow/arm.

For clients who present with elbow flexion contractures, a small opening can be created at the level of the cubital fossa, and the proximal material slipped over the posterior aspect of the upper arm, while the distal material is placed over the anterior forearm, to provide a gentle stretching force into elbow extension (Figure 7-9).

SUGAR TONG AND MUENSTER ORTHOSES

The goal of sugar tong and Muenster orthoses is to limit or minimize forearm rotation but still allow for elbow movement, in conditions such as mid-shaft radius fractures, ulna fractures, distal radius fractures, injury or instability of the distal radioulnar joint, or injury/inflammation of the extensor carpi ulnaris tendon at the wrist. These orthotic designs limit rotation of the radius on the ulna that occurs with forearm pronation and supination by immobilizing the distal radioulnar joint and prevent the extensor carpi ulnaris from rotating over the ulnar head with forearm pronation. The Muenster orthosis can be fabricated to rest on the anterior or posterior aspect of the forearm and wrist, with LTTM extending proximally to cover the medial and lateral epicondyles above the olecranon. A strap can be used to join the proximal ends on the posterior aspect of the distal humerus or the material can be joined together. The sugar tong orthosis design is similar, with the LTTM covering both the anterior and posterior aspects of the forearm with the medial and lateral aspects of the forearm free of LTTM. This design may be better suited for clients who present with significant edema.

Orthotic Fabrication Steps

Orthotic fabrication begins after the practitioner has determined which design is most suited to the client's condition, specific needs, and physician referral specifications. The process begins with designing the pattern, followed by selecting the LTTM, positioning the client, molding the LTTM to the client, fitting and adjusting the orthosis, applying straps, and ending with evaluating the orthosis for fit and comfort. The final step in this process is educating the client on the purpose, wearing schedule, and care of the orthosis.

Refer to the instructional video for detailed step-by-step instructions.

PATTERN MAKING

Designing a pattern for an elbow immobilization orthosis differs from wrist and hand orthoses patterns. Because these orthoses are larger in size, measurements are taken with a tape measure and transferred to paper toweling, paper, or directly onto the LTTM.

Posterior Elbow Design

1. Measure the following on the client's UE:
   - The length of the UE from the distal palmar crease to approximately 2 inches distal to the axilla. (If the wrist is not included in the orthosis, use the wrist crease instead of the distal palmar crease.)
   - The width of the proximal arm

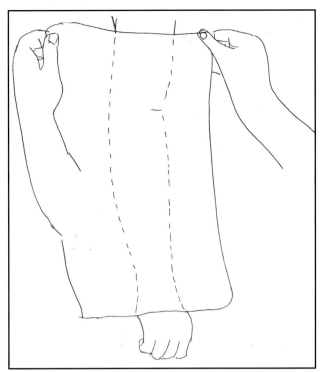

Figure 7-10. Placement of material on arm for anterior or posterior elbow immobilization orthosis.

   - The width of the elbow from the lateral epicondyle to the medial epicondyle (measured on posterior elbow)
   - The width of the mid-forearm
   - The width of the hand (approximately two-thirds the circumference of the hand from the long finger MCP head volarly to the same landmark dorsally). (If the wrist is not included in the orthosis, measure two-thirds the circumference of the wrist.)

2. Transfer the measurements to a paper towel or directly onto a piece of LTTM. Hint: When preparing the material, use up to one-third less than the measurements that you took in order to stretch the LTTM around the proximal arm and distal forearm for improved conformity.

3. Mark the medial and lateral epicondyles for reference (Figure 7-10).

Anterior Elbow Design

1. Measure the following on the client's UE:
   - The length of the UE from the distal palmar crease to approximately 2 inches distal to the axilla (If the wrist is not included in the orthosis, use the wrist crease instead of the distal palmar crease.)
   - The width of the proximal arm at the proximal border of the biceps brachii muscle belly

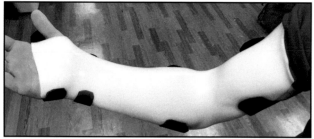

Figure 7-11. Long arm anterior elbow orthosis with wrist included.

- The width of the elbow from the lateral epicondyle to the medial epicondyle (measured on the anterior elbow across the cubital fossa)

- The width of the mid forearm (approximately two-thirds the circumference of the forearm)

- The width of the hand (approximately two-thirds the circumference of the hand from the long finger MCP head volarly to the same landmark dorsally). (If the wrist is not included in the orthosis, measure two-thirds the circumference of the wrist.)

2. Transfer the measurements to a paper towel or directly onto a piece of LTTM. Mark the medial and lateral epicondyles for reference and a small circle (for the thumb to pass through) approximately 1 inch from the distal border in the center (if the wrist is included in the orthosis; Figure 7-11). When preparing the material, be sure to use up to one-third less than the measurements that you took to stretch the LTTM around the proximal arm and distal forearm for improved conformity. Use the pinch method to secure the LTTM in place. When cooled and hardened, open the pinch marks.

Muenster Design

A pattern for the Muenster orthosis is outlined in Figure 7-12.

MATERIAL SELECTION

A variety of factors are important to consider when selecting an appropriate LTTM for elbow immobilization orthoses. These factors include the following:

- Thickness: 1/8 inch/2.4 mm for most designs. A thinner material may be suitable for pediatric clients or for those who do not require rigid support.

- High degree of conformability, drape, and stretch to conform well over the elbow bony prominences.

- Memory for conditions requiring frequent adjustments or if edema is present.

- Material with coating to allow the practitioner to use the **pinch method** during molding: The practitioner pinches the edges of the LTTM together at the

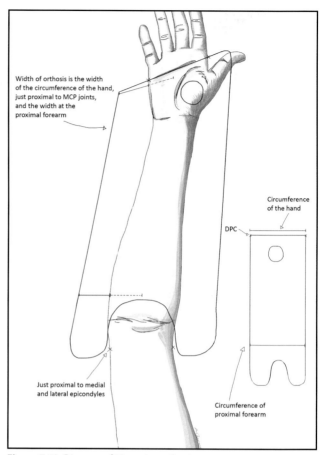

Width of orthosis is the width of the circumference of the hand, just proximal to MCP joints, and the width at the proximal forearm

Circumference of the hand

DPC

Just proximal to medial and lateral epicondyles

Circumference of proximal forearm

Figure 7-12. Diagram of Muenster orthosis pattern.

proximal edge, middle around the elbow, mid-forearm, and wrist. This allows the material to stretch and conform perfectly over the client's joints and soft tissues. The material can then be pulled apart when cool and cut off. This creates a nice smooth edge with no seams or overlapping material (Figure 7-13).

- Choose colored material for client preference to optimize compliance.

Client Positioning

Watch the video demonstration to see how to position the client in standing to accommodate an anterior- or posterior-placed elbow orthosis. Figure 7-14 highlights the positioning of a client in standing to be fitted with a posterior elbow orthosis.

Molding Techniques

Watch the video demonstration to see how the stretch and pinch method is used to create a circumferential orthosis. Pinch the warm material together, and it stays in place. When cooled and hardened, the pinches can be opened and trimmed away, leaving an opening along the anterior or posterior arm for ease of putting the orthosis on or taking it off.

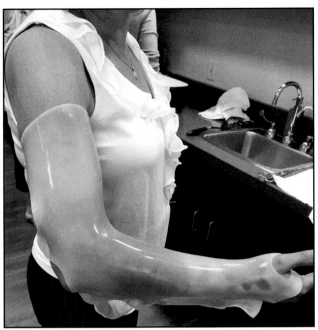

Figure 7-13. The pinch method used when molding an elbow immobilization orthosis.

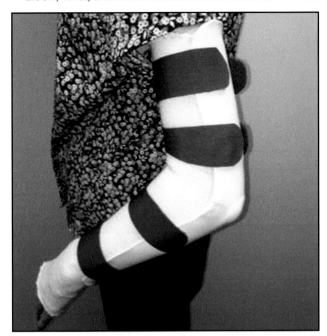

Figure 7-14. Posterior elbow immobilization orthosis. (Reprinted with permission from Chad Royer.)

Finishing Techniques: Edges and Strapping

Watch the video demonstration for finishing techniques, including strapping, finishing of the edges, and addressing bony landmarks.

Orthosis Check-Out

- Can the client fully flex and extend his or her fingers?

  If no, adjust the distal edge of the orthosis so it clears the distal palmar crease.

- For Muenster/sugar tong orthoses, can the client flex his or her elbow fully without the orthosis interfering with this motion?

  If no, the proximal edge may not flared adequately, or the cubital fossa is not cleared enough.

- For Muenster/sugar tong orthoses, does the client complain of discomfort when moving his or her hand or elbow in the orthosis?

  If yes, locate the area(s) of discomfort. Some possible solutions:

  ◦ *Flare the distal edge and be sure it clears the distal palmar crease.*

  ◦ *Smooth and round all rough edges.*

  ◦ *Be sure the area around the ulnar head is clear or flared well.*

- For anterior/posterior elbow orthoses, are the bony prominences protected?

  If no, flare the LTTM away from the prominence(s) and add padding for comfort.

- Are the corners of the orthosis rounded and smooth?

  If no, round and smooth all corners of the orthosis.

- Are the straps secure and edges rounded?

  If no, adjust the straps: the wrist and mid-forearm straps should go in a circumferential fashion around the wrist and mid forearm; the ends should meet together. No Velcro (Velcro BVBA) should be exposed. The strap over the metacarpals should secure the orthosis on the hand. For anterior and posterior elbow orthoses, the elbow may be more secure in the orthosis if the straps are crisscrossed in front or behind the elbow. Soft Velfoam (Velcro BVBA)-type straps may also be more comfortable.

- Are all indentations and pattern marks removed?

  If no, use a heat gun to smooth the LTTM. Rubbing alcohol can be used to remove wax pencil marks. Ink cannot be removed, so refrain from using this when drawing your pattern on the LTTM.

- Remove the orthosis after 5 to 10 minutes and observe the skin. Are there any reddened areas?

  If yes, adjust the orthosis by flaring and smoothing edges and/or flaring material away from bony prominences.

- Review the purpose and care of the elbow immobilization orthosis with the client. Does he or she understand why he or she is wearing it? When he or she should wear it? How to take care of it?

  If no, discuss the wearing schedule and care of the orthosis with the client before he or she leaves the clinic and provide clear written instructions to take home with him or her (refer to the Appendix at the end of the chapter).

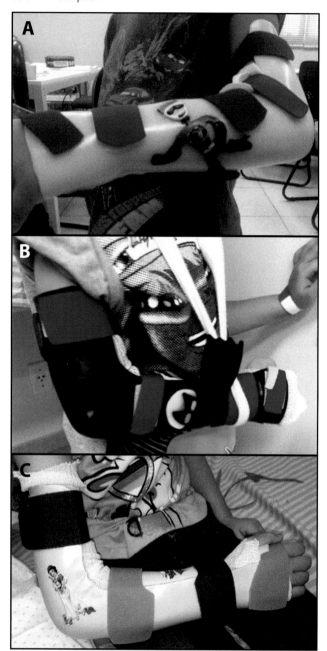

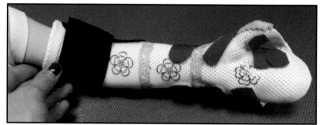

Figure 7-16. Special client touches on an elbow, wrist, and hand immobilization orthosis. (Reprinted with permission from Anna Ovsyannikova.)

Coban wrap (3M), or other cohesive bandaging on top of the LTTM to secure the orthosis on the arm until the material has set and hardened during the fabrication process. This approach may be helpful in preventing children from removing their orthoses. The practitioner may also consider covering the orthosis with a sleeve or a long stockinette to prevent a young client from taking the orthosis off (Figures 7-15 and 7-16).

Geriatric Clients

- Consider using contrasting-colored materials and straps for visually impaired clients.

- Straps can be attached directly to the LTTM by the use of dry heat or metal rivets so that elderly clients do not lose the straps at night.

- Clients with fragile skin may require additional skin protection through the use of padding, extra layers of stockinette, lightweight LTTM, and special soft straps (Box 7-2).

Summary

- Knowledge of the key anatomical structures affected by an elbow, wrist, and hand immobilization orthosis will help the practitioner understand how the orthosis will influence these structures and assist them in determining the most appropriate orthotic design and wearing schedule.

- The goals of an elbow, wrist, and hand immobilization orthosis and the specifics of each individual wearing schedule will vary depending on the client's needs and the diagnosis.

- An elbow, wrist, and hand immobilization orthosis represents a first-class lever system.

- Elbow, wrist, and hand immobilization orthoses can be fabricated using an anterior or posterior design. The design chosen depends on the client's clinical condition, current functional needs, specific indications requested by the referring physician, and practitioner preference.

Figure 7-15. Three pediatric clients with decorated elbow orthoses. (Reprinted with permission from Maria Candida Miranda Luzo.)

SPECIAL CONSIDERATIONS

Pediatric Clients

- Consider using colored LTTM and colored straps to appeal to younger clients. Allow them to choose decorations like stickers or add thermoplastic designs to their orthoses to help them to feel that they are part of the process.

- Consider wrapping the orthosis in place using an Ace bandage (3M), TheraBand (Performance Health),

Box 7-2. Helpful Hints

- Each client is an individual, and the selected orthosis must match the individual's needs, size, and functional demands.

- Perforated materials are appropriate for warmer climates, clients with open wounds, or clients who need more ventilation. However, be mindful when stretching the material around the elbow/bony prominences because the individual perforations may stretch too much.

- LTTM with memory is important when frequent readjustments of the orthosis are required (e.g., clients with edema or tendon injury). This makes remolding the orthosis easier and is cost efficient.

- It is very important to make the initial pattern large enough, especially when using the pinch method during the molding process. Material that is stretched excessively during the molding process will return to its original shape when reheated and may be too small as a result.

- LTTM with a nonstick coating is preferable when using the pinch method during molding. This allows the practitioner to pull the material apart after it has cooled and remove it from the client's arm easily.

- Consider including the wrist in the orthosis to increase the mechanical advantage and lessen the force needed to position the elbow comfortably in the orthosis.

- Consider using soft straps such as Velfoam around the cubital fossa and posterior elbow to optimize comfort.

- Positioning the client in supine during the molding process allows gravity to assist while conforming the LTTM around the arm.

- Muenster and sugar tong orthoses are specifically designed to limit forearm rotation but allow clients to move their elbows while in the orthosis.

- Special populations such as pediatric and/or geriatric clients may require specific orthotic designs or adaptations to achieve the best outcomes.

- Each orthosis must be molded to the individual anatomy for the best fit. Post-fabrication critique and check out help identify areas for modification and optimize client comfort.

In Your Client's Shoes

As a practitioner, it is very important to appreciate the impact that an elbow orthosis will have on your client's daily occupations. These orthoses, especially those designed to immobilize the elbow, significantly limit the client's ability to use his or her affected extremity in activities of daily living (ADL) tasks. You should experience how it feels to wear an orthosis for an extended period of time. This experience will enable you to be client centered when using orthoses as an intervention strategy in your practice. You must consider how to instruct your client on the importance of the wearing schedule and the benefits of compliance for maximum benefits.

Suggested Reading

Blackmore, S. M., Jander, R. M., & Culp, R. W. (2006). Management of distal biceps and triceps ruptures. *Journal of Hand Therapy, 19*(2), 154-169.

Casmus, R. J. (2010). Traumatic distal-third humeral fracture in a collegiate football player: A case review. *Athletic Training and Sports Health Care, 2*(1), 39-42.

Coppard, B. M., & Lohman, H. (2014). *Introduction to orthotics: A clinical reasoning and problem-solving approach* (4th ed.). St. Louis, MO: Elsevier Mosby.

Humans, J. M., Postema, K., & Geertzen, J. H. B. (2004). Elbow orthoses: A review of literature. *Prosthetics and Orthotics International, 28*(3), 263-272.

Jacobs, M. A., & Austin, N. M. (2014). *Orthotic intervention for the hand and upper extremity* (2nd ed.). Baltimore, MD: Lippincott Williams & Wilkins.

Kim, J. K., Kook, S. H., & Kim, Y. K. (2012). Comparison of forearm rotation allowed by different types of upper extremity immobilization. *Journal of Bone and Joint Surgery, 94,* 455-460.

Levy, J., Ernat, J., Song, D., Cook, J. B., Judd, D., & Shaha, S. (2015). Outcomes of long-arm casting versus double-sugar-tong splinting of acute pediatric distal forearm fractures. *Journal of Pediatric Orthopedics, 35*(1), 11-17.

Muller, A. M., Sadoghi, P., Lucas, R., Audige, L., Delaney, R., Klein, M., … Vavken, P. (2013). Effectiveness of bracing in the treatment of nonosseous restriction of elbow mobility: A systematic review and meta-analysis of 13 studies. *Journal of Shoulder and Elbow Surgery, 22,* 1146-1152.

Palmar, B. A., & Hughes, T. B. (2010). Cubital tunnel syndrome. *Journal of Hand Surgery, 35,* 153-163.

Rinkel, W. D., Schreuders, T. A., Koes, B. W., & Huisstede, B. M. (2013). Current evidence for effectiveness of interventions for cubital tunnel syndrome, radial tunnel syndrome, instability, or bursitis of the elbow: A systematic review. *Clinical Journal of Pain, 29*(12), 1087-1096.

Shah, C. M., Calfee, R. P., Gelberman, R. H., & Goldfarb, C. A. (2013). Outcomes of rigid night splinting and activity modification in the treatment of cubital tunnel syndrome. *Journal of Hand Surgery, 38*, 1125-1130.

Slaughter, A., Miles, L., Fleming, J., & McPhail, S. (2010). A comparative study of splint effectiveness in limiting forearm rotation. *Journal of Hand Therapy, 23*, 241-248.

Szabo, R. M., & Kwak, C. (2007). Natural history and conservative management of cubital tunnel syndrome. *Hand Clinics, 23*, 311-318.

Test Your Knowledge

SHORT ANSWER

1. Identify the anatomical landmarks associated with an elbow, wrist, and hand immobilization orthosis.

2. Describe the biomechanical principles that apply to an elbow, wrist, and hand immobilization orthosis.

3. Identify the recommended elbow, wrist, and hand position in an elbow, wrist, and hand immobilization orthosis and discuss the rationale behind it.

4. List the movements that a client should be able to perform without difficulty when wearing a sugar tong or Muenster immobilization orthosis.

5. Describe the three different elbow, wrist, and hand immobilization designs and discuss the rationale for each.

6. List the appropriate orthotic design and LTTM suitable for the following:
   ◦ A 30-year-old man with a distal humerus fracture
   ◦ A 6-year-old boy with cerebral palsy who presents with moderate spasticity in his elbow flexor muscles
   ◦ An 80-year-old woman with RA who presents with a painful, swollen elbow

MULTIPLE CHOICE

7. How can you lessen the force needed to immobilize the elbow when fabricating an elbow immobilization orthosis?
   a. Make the resistance force as short as possible.
   b. Make the resistance force as long as possible.
   c. Make the effort force as short as possible.
   d. Use extra padding around the elbow.

8. Which of the following landmarks do not apply to an elbow, wrist, and hand immobilization orthosis?
   a. The olecranon
   b. The lateral epicondyle
   c. The elbow crease
   d. The MCP joint

9. What is the recommended method of preventing pressure on a bony prominence when fabricating an elbow, wrist, and hand immobilization orthosis?
   a. Pad the area after molding the orthosis.
   b. Flare the thermoplastic material away from the area after molding the orthosis.
   c. Pad the area prior to molding the orthosis.
   d. Make the forearm component of the orthosis as long as possible.

10. What functional movement should the client be able to do while wearing a Muenster or sugar tong immobilization orthosis?
    a. Forearm supination
    b. Elbow flexion
    c. Forearm pronation
    d. Wrist extension/power grasp

11. Which orthosis design is well-suited for a client with cubital tunnel syndrome?
    a. Sugar tong orthosis
    b. Muenster orthosis
    c. Anterior elbow immobilization orthosis
    d. Posterior elbow immobilization orthosis

12. Why is it important to clear the cubital fossa completely when fabricating a Muenster immobilization orthosis?
    a. This allows for full wrist mobility in the orthosis.
    b. This allows for unrestricted forearm rotation in the orthosis.
    c. This allows for full elbow mobility in the orthosis.
    d. This allows for full flexion and gripping in the orthosis.

13. What is the primary advantage of the anterior elbow, wrist, and hand immobilization orthosis design?
    a. It allows for more sensory input in the palm.
    b. It allows for more digit mobility.
    c. It minimizes pressure on the bony prominences around the elbow.
    d. It is easier to fabricate than the posterior design.

14. When might a practitioner choose a prefabricated elbow pad over a custom elbow, wrist, and hand immobilization orthosis for a client?
    a. When a client needs more rigid support.
    b. When a client has difficulty putting the orthosis on.
    c. When a client is unable to tolerate a rigid orthosis at night.
    d. When a client needs to wear the orthosis during the day only.

CASE STUDIES

Case Study 1

Joy is a 28-year-old, right-hand–dominant woman who presents with complaints of aching, constant tingling in her right ring and small fingers, and a sense of clumsiness/weakness in her hand. She reports that her symptoms started about 1 month ago, and they appear to be getting worse, particularly at night. She is currently in her second year in a master's degree program in occupational therapy and is concerned that her symptoms will interfere with school.

She presents for therapy with a prescription that reads:

Right cubital tunnel syndrome:

1. *Evaluate and treat.*

2. *Provide right elbow, wrist, and hand immobilization orthosis for night use.*

3. *Provide instructions on activity modification.*

Your assessment:

Joy presents to therapy for her an evaluation and custom elbow orthosis for her right UE. Your evaluation reveals the following:

- Positive Tinel's at the cubital tunnel
- Impaired light touch sensation in her ring and small fingers
- Mild weakness in her abductor digiti minimi muscle (grade 4/5) on the right
- Reports of pain at 7/10 on a 0 to 10 visual analog scale
- Mild impairment in grip and pinch strength on the right side
- Full ROM right UE

Using different clinical reasoning approaches, answer the following questions about this client and the prescribed orthosis:

Procedural Reasoning

1. What client factors are important to consider when determining the most suitable orthotic design for this client?

2. Which immobilization orthotic design would be most appropriate for this client? Why?

3. What LTTM properties are important to consider?

4. Describe the instructions you would give this client on:
   - How to care for the orthosis
   - Wearing schedule
   - Precautions
   - Exercises/activities

Pragmatic Reasoning

5. What resources are available to fabricate this orthosis (time, materials, expertise)?

6. Are you able to clearly document the need for this orthosis?

7. Does evidence-based practice support the use of this orthosis for this client's diagnosis?

Interactive Reasoning

8. What are the client's goals and valued occupations?

9. What effect will the client's injury and use of the orthosis have on her ADL?

Conditional Reasoning

10. What factors will influence this client's compliance to the wearing schedule of this orthosis?

Narrative Reasoning

11. How does this condition and, more specifically, this orthotic intervention affect this client's valued occupations?

12. What activities is this client the most concerned about?

Ethical Reasoning

13. Does the client understand the need for the orthosis?

14. Does the client have the resources to be able to pay for the orthosis (as applicable)?

15. What other options are available to this client if she lacks the resources necessary to pay for the orthosis?

16. Write one short-term goal (1 to 2 weeks) and one long-term goal (6 to 8 weeks) for this client.

Case Study 2

Cole is an active 14-year-old boy who fell from the rings while doing gymnastics during his physical education class at school. He fractured his radius and ulna mid-shaft and underwent surgery (ORIF) of both fractures 3 days ago. He has been referred to occupational therapy for provision of a custom orthosis to protect the fracture. His referral reads:

Right mid-shaft radius and ulna fracture:

1. *Provide custom orthosis to limit right forearm rotation but allow for some elbow flexion and extension (a Muenster or sugar tong orthosis).*

Your assessment:

Cole presents in therapy with a postoperative dressing and plaster slab in place with his elbow immobilized at 90 degrees of flexion and his forearm in neutral rotation. He is wearing a sling. He is doing surprisingly well and complains of moderate pain in his forearm and swelling in his hand and fingers in the cast/splint. He denies any numbness or tingling in his fingers. His mother reports that he is anxious to get the splint and dressing off and is nervous about what his arm will look like. He wants to get back to school as quickly as possible but is worried about not being able to use his computer or play video games at home.

Using different clinical reasoning approaches, consider the following questions about this client and the prescribed orthosis. Some questions may be directed more toward the client, and some questions may be directed more toward you as the practitioner for reflection.

Procedural Reasoning

1. What client factors are important to consider when determining the most suitable orthotic design for this client?

2. Which immobilization orthotic design would be most appropriate for this client? Why?

3. What LTTM properties are important to consider?

4. Describe the instructions you would give this client on:
   ◦ How to care for the orthosis
   ◦ Wearing schedule
   ◦ Precautions
   ◦ Exercises/activities

Pragmatic Reasoning

5. What resources are available to fabricate this orthosis (time, materials, expertise)?

6. Are you able to clearly document the need for this orthosis?

7. Does evidence-based practice support the use of this orthosis for this client's diagnosis?

Interactive Reasoning

8. What are the client's goals and valued occupations?

9. What effect will the client's injury and use of the orthosis have on his ADL?

Conditional Reasoning

10. What factors will influence this client's compliance to the wearing schedule of this orthosis?

Narrative Reasoning

11. How does this injury and, more specifically, this orthotic intervention affect this client's valued occupations?

12. What activities is this client the most concerned about?

Ethical Reasoning

13. Does the client understand the need for the orthosis?

14. Does the client have the resources to be able to pay for the orthosis (as applicable)?

15. What other options are available to this client if he lacks the resources necessary to pay for the orthosis?

16. Write one short-term goal (1 to 2 weeks) and one long-term goal (6 to 8 weeks) for this client.

Appendix

1. Define all the key terms used in this chapter.

2. As an occupational therapy practitioner, you must provide your client with detailed instructions for wearing and caring for his or her orthosis. This document must be required for the client's official records and insurance payments. Select one of the elbow, wrist, and hand immobilization orthotic designs from this chapter and prepare a client-centered handout for wearing this orthosis. Base your client description on one of the two case studies in this chapter. Include the following in the handout:
   ◦ A description/name of the orthosis
   ◦ An outline of the wearing schedule (remember this will vary depending on the client's condition)
   ◦ A description of how to clean and care for the orthosis
   ◦ Instructions on what the client should be aware of when wearing the orthosis (red areas on skin, pain, increased swelling, etc.)
   ◦ Contact information and follow-up instructions

3. Prepare a case study of a client requiring an elbow, wrist, and hand immobilization orthosis. Use one of the evidence-based resources cited in the chapter to support your orthotic intervention. Summarize the research and explain the outcomes of the study.

4. As an occupational therapy practitioner, it will be interesting and informative for you to spend an extended period wearing an orthosis to appreciate the effect that an orthosis will have on your client's daily occupations. Wear an elbow immobilization orthosis designed by your lab partner for a 24-hour period. Take note of how it feels to have one body part immobilized. Elaborate in paragraphs on the following:
   ◦ Describe the orthosis, material used, positioning, and typical diagnosis for this particular orthosis. (Which arm was splinted, when did you wear it, what did you do with it on?)
   ◦ Comfort and ease of use: Is it easy to take on and off? Does the orthosis fit under clothing? Are there any pressure areas? What needs to be modified and how?

- Personal and public image: Does the orthosis attract attention in public? Does the orthosis attract attention in your family? How did this make you feel, even as a class assignment?

- Functionality: How were you able to function with the orthosis? Was the position helpful or harmful? What would the typical wearing schedule be for a client with the typical need for this orthosis? What instructions should be given to the typical client with the need for this orthosis?

- How does this change your appreciation of what your clients are experiencing with their orthoses?

5. Complete the check-out form on the next page.

Multiple Choice Answer Key

7. b
8. d
9. c
10. b
11. c
12. c
13. c
14. c

Elbow Orthosis Check-Out Form

*(This can be used for faculty to evaluate students' completed orthoses,
as well as for students to reference when evaluating their own completed orthosis.)*

Fabricate one of the orthotic designs for an elbow immobilization orthosis on your classmate and complete the following check-out form:

Name of Orthosis:

Purpose of Orthosis:

Design/Function

_____ The elbow and/or forearm is positioned correctly for the condition.

_____ The thenar area is cleared adequately to allow for full thumb motion.

_____ The distal palmar crease is clear/full MCP joint motion is observed to allow for full finger motion.

_____ The orthosis effectively immobilizes the elbow (as applicable).

_____ The orthosis limits forearm rotation (as applicable).

_____ The orthosis allows for elbow flexion and extension (as applicable).

_____ The hand arches are supported: distal and proximal transverse arches, longitudinal arch.

_____ The orthosis does not cause impingement or pressure areas.

_____ The orthosis clears all bony prominences.

Straps/Orthosis Appearance

_____ The straps are in the correct position: elbow, wrist, forearm, and hand.

_____ The straps are secure and corners rounded.

_____ The orthosis edges are smooth and corners rounded.

_____ The proximal edge is flared.

_____ The orthosis is free of fingerprints, pattern marks, or indentations.

CHAPTER 8

Hand-Based Orthoses

Key Terms

Angulation	Dupuytren's contracture	Needle fasciotomy
Boxer's fracture	Extension lag	Three-point fixation
Buddy strapping or taping	Metacarpophalangeal (MCP) ulnar drift	Trigger finger
Collagenase injection		

Learning Outcomes

Upon completion of this chapter, you will be able to:

1. Describe the clinical conditions and goals for prescribing a hand-based orthosis.

2. Identify pertinent anatomical structures and biomechanical principles involved in a hand-based orthosis and apply these concepts to orthotic design and fabrication.

3. Identify the most commonly selected orthotic designs and describe the rationale for choosing one design over another.

4. Design a pattern for two different types of hand-based orthoses.

5. After reviewing the instructional videos:

   a. Outline the steps involved in the fabrication of a hand-based orthosis.

   b. Complete the molding and fabrication steps of a hand-based orthosis.

   c. Evaluate the fit and function of a completed hand-based orthosis and identify and address all areas needing adjustment.

6. Identify elements of a client education program following provision of a hand-based orthosis.

7. Describe special considerations of hand-based orthotic design and fabrication for pediatric and geriatric clients.

Schofield, K., & Schwartz, D. *Orthotic Design and Fabrication*
for the Upper Extremity: A Practical Guide (pp 143-166).
© 2019 Taylor & Francis Group.

Box 8-1. Common Goals of Hand-Based Orthoses

PROTECTION

- Support and protect the metacarpals and proximal and/or middle phalanges of digits II through V following a metacarpal or proximal phalanx fracture.

- Offer pain relief for injured, edematous joints or soft tissues.

- Support and protect unstable joints from arthritis or injury (e.g., sagittal band rupture).

POSITIONING

- Position the digits to prevent development of joint or soft tissue contracture following injury or surgery (e.g., **Dupuytren's contracture** release).

- Position the digit(s) to limit movement of the flexor tendon to enhance healing from **trigger finger**.

- Position the fourth and fifth metacarpophalangeal (MCP) joints in flexion to prevent development of soft tissue and/or joint contractures following injury to the ulnar nerve.

IMPROVE FUNCTION

- Substitute for loss of muscle function and facilitate muscle balance in the affected digit(s) following ulnar nerve injury.

- Improve the alignment of the joints affected by a disease process or injury (e.g., rheumatoid arthritis).

Introduction

Clients with a variety of different clinical conditions may benefit from a hand-based orthosis. These orthoses are commonly prescribed following injury to the bones of the hand (metacarpals and digit phalanges); joints (MCP, proximal interphalangeal [PIP], and distal interphalangeal [DIP]); supporting ligaments, tendons, and muscles; and other soft tissue structures. Other indications include positioning the digits following surgery or injury to prevent development of joint or soft tissue contractures or limiting tendon movement following tendon repair or trigger finger. The choice of orthotic type and design depends on the clinical condition and physician preference, therapist experience, and client needs. A thorough assessment of the client's current functional status must always be done in conjunction with orthotic provision to ensure that the orthotic design chosen meets the clinical and personal needs of the client.

Goals for Use of a Hand-Based Orthosis

The goals of a hand-based orthosis will depend on the condition or diagnosis for which the orthosis is being prescribed, the order from the referring physician, the therapist's experience and clinical judgement, and the client's needs (Box 8-1).

When fabricating hand-based orthoses, the practitioner must consider the specific diagnosis and the purpose of the orthosis and use clinical reasoning to select the most appropriate design. As discussed, the particular design chosen depends on multiple factors. The orthosis can be volar, dorsal, radial, ulnar, or circumferential in design, depending on the involved structures and the client's needs (Figure 8-1).

Practitioners treating clients with hand injuries (fractures, sprains, ligament injuries, or other pathologies) must recognize the benefits that immobilization orthoses can offer their clients. These benefits include relief from pain, provision of stability, prevention or correction of deformity, positioning during healing, and improved functional ability. It is critical to perform an ongoing assessment of a client's current status, particularly in relation to his or her functional ability. A custom-made hand orthosis may require adaptations to meet the client's changing needs. Inflamed or injured swollen joints require rest and immobilization; however, prolonged immobilization may lead to loss of range of motion (ROM) due to joint stiffness. This is especially true for the MCP, PIP, and DIP joints of the digits. The use of orthoses helps prevent the development of soft tissue or joint contractures and improve function, allowing the client to maintain independence.

Clinical Conditions and Wearing Schedules

This section describes common clinical conditions where a hand-based orthosis is typically prescribed, recommended wearing schedules, and the current evidence supporting this orthosis as an appropriate intervention strategy. Readers are encouraged to review the references provided for additional details regarding each clinical condition and search current research databases for updated evidence as it becomes available.

METACARPAL FRACTURES

Hand fractures are the most common fractures of the human skeleton. Metacarpal fractures collectively account for 30% to 50% of all hand fractures, with fractures of the fourth and fifth metacarpal neck occurring most often. These are commonly referred to as **boxer's fractures** when

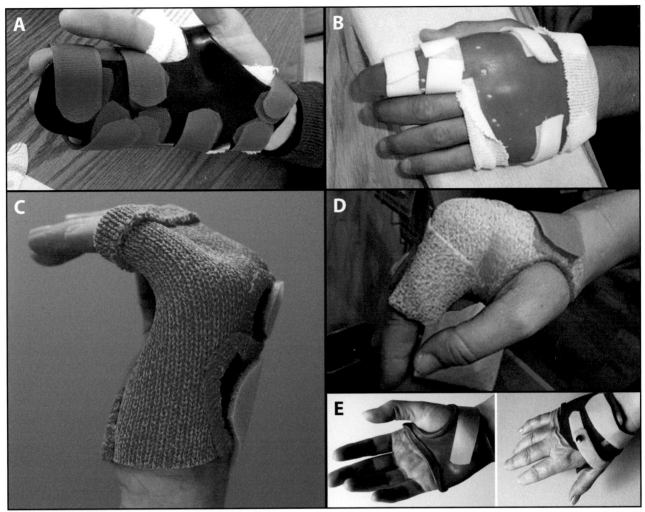

Figure 8-1. The designs for a hand-based orthosis: (A) volar digit-based orthosis, (B) dorsal hand-based orthosis, (C) ulnar gutter orthosis, (D) radial gutter orthosis, (E) circumferential hand-based orthosis.

they involve the fifth metacarpal bone (Figure 8-2). These fractures are extra-articular in nature, meaning the fracture does not involve the articulating surface of the metacarpal head. These fractures frequently occur as a result of direct impact from a hard object on the metacarpal head. The force from the impact is then transferred to the metacarpal neck, causing displacement of the metacarpal head volarly. The majority of these fractures do not require surgery and are treated conservatively with hand-based ulnar gutter design immobilization orthoses. The position of protection for a metacarpal fracture is with the MCP joints positioned in 70 degrees of flexion. Inclusion of the wrist, PIP, or DIP joints depends on fracture stability, presence of edema or pain, and surgeon preference. If included, the PIP and DIP joints should be in full extension to prevent stiffness. Fractures involving the second or third metacarpals are immobilized in the same position, but with a hand-based radial gutter design.

Metacarpal shaft fractures are typically classified as either transverse or oblique and are subject to considerable deforming forces from the interossei muscles, which can result in dorsal **angulation** at the fracture site, where the fracture "ends" move dorsally (Figure 8-3). Treatment of these fractures depends on the degree of angulation and fracture stability. Stable fractures are typically treated with immobilization in a hand-based metacarpal orthosis that employs the **three-point fixation** concept: one pressure point over the fracture site and two pressure points on either side of the fracture (Figure 8-4). The MCP joints are left free to move in this orthosis. **Buddy strapping** of the adjacent uninjured digits may be used in conjunction with this orthosis to prevent rotation at the fracture site (Figure 8-5).

Wearing Schedule

Metacarpal neck and shaft fractures heal rapidly. Immobilization for 3 to 4 weeks is recommended. Active PIP and DIP joint motion, both flexion and full interphalangeal (IP) joint extension, are encouraged within the orthosis. The IP joints can be placed in an extension orthosis at night if an **extension lag** develops (loss of active PIP and/or DIP joint extension).

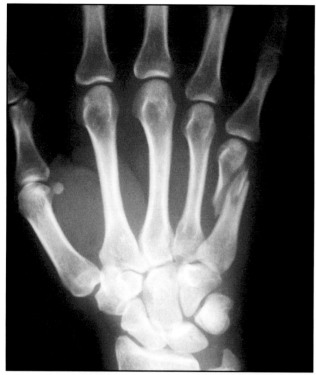

Figure 8-2. X-ray illustrating a boxer's fracture of the fifth metacarpal.

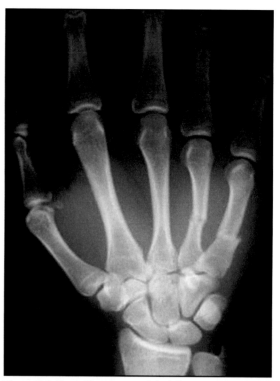

Figure 8-3. X-ray of a metacarpal shaft fracture.

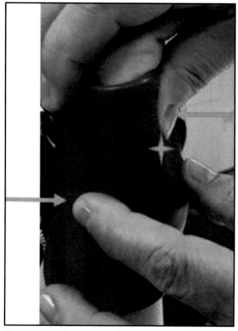

Figure 8-4. Three-point fixation concept for metacarpal fractures.

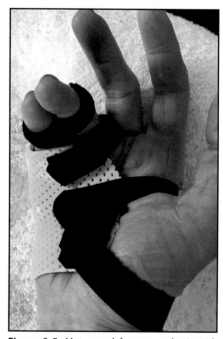

Figure 8-5. Metacarpal fracture orthosis with buddy tapes.

Evidence

Level I

- Harding, I. J., Parry, D., & Barrington, R. (2001). The use of a moulded metacarpal brace versus neighbor strapping for fractures of the little finger metacarpal neck. *Journal of Hand Surgery (British and European Volume), 26*(3), 261-263.

  ○ This prospective, randomized, single-blind study compared the use of a hand-based thermoplastic metacarpal brace with use of neighbor strapping of the fourth and fifth digits for treatment of non-displaced, minimally angulated fifth metacarpal neck fractures. Outcome measures included pain evaluation using a verbal rating scale, active and passive flexion and extension at the fifth MCP joint, and total ROM of the fifth digit. Participants also rated their overall satisfaction during the 3 weeks of immobilization. Participants in the brace group complained of significantly less pain during immobilization and had slightly better digit mobility following healing as compared with the strapping group; the brace group returned to work earlier and reported higher levels of satisfaction. A hand-based custom orthosis is an acceptable treatment option for minimally displaced fifth metacarpal neck fractures.

Level II

- Gülke, J., Leopold, B., Grözinger, D., Drews, B., Paschke, S., & Wachter, N. J. (2018). Postoperative treatment of metacarpal fractures—Classical physical therapy compared with a home exercise program. *Journal of Hand Therapy, 31*(1), 20-28.

  ○ The authors designed a prospective, cohort, randomized, controlled trial to evaluate whether a home exercise program or traditional physical therapy was more effective in the postoperative management of metacarpal fractures. Their study included 60 patients suffering from digital metacarpal fractures. Fractures of the first metacarpal were not included. All patients were prospectively randomized into either the physical therapy group or the home exercise group. Follow-up evaluations occurred at 2, 6, and 12 weeks postoperatively. After 2 weeks, the ROM in both groups was still severely reduced. Twelve weeks after surgery, the total digital flexion ROM of the involved digit improved to 245 degrees (physical therapy group) and 256 degrees (home exercise group). Grip strength after 6 weeks was 68% (physical therapy group) and 71% (home exercise group) when compared with the noninjured hand, improving to 91% (physical therapy group) and 93% (home exercise group) after 12 weeks. The results indicate that both home exercise programs and traditional therapy visits are effective in the postoperative management of metacarpal fractures.

- Gulabi, D., Avci, C., Cecen, G., Bekler, H., Saglam, F., & Merih, E. (2014). A comparison of the functional and radiological results of Paris plaster cast and ulnar gutter splint in the conservative treatment of fractures of the fifth metacarpal. *European Journal of Orthopedic Surgery and Traumatology, 24*, 1167-1173.

  ○ In this retrospective comparative study, the authors compared two methods of immobilization of fifth metacarpal neck and shaft fractures: a short arm of Paris cast and a short arm ulnar gutter splint. Both groups were immobilized for an average of 30 days. Outcome measures included fourth and fifth digit mobility using goniometric measurements, grip strength, and radiographic evaluation. No statistical difference was found in both groups when all three outcome measures were compared. The plaster of Paris treatment group did experience pressure sores and pain during the immobilization period, whereas the ulnar gutter splint group did not. The authors found that immobilization in an ulnar gutter orthosis/splint is an acceptable conservative treatment option for fifth metacarpal neck and shaft fractures.

Level IV

- McNemar, T. B., Howell, J. W., & Chang, E. (2003). Management of metacarpal fractures. *Journal of Hand Therapy, 16*(2), 143-151.

  ○ This comprehensive review article outlines the different fractures that occur at the metacarpals and the conservative and operative treatment options for each. The authors outline the importance of orthoses as part of the management of these fractures. Orthoses include custom-fabricated forearm- and hand-based designs for metacarpal head, neck, and shaft fractures and use of prefabricated varieties for stable shaft fractures. The majority of metacarpal fractures can be treated conservatively, and some degree of angulation following fracture healing is acceptable as long as it does not interfere with hand function. The authors recommend immobilizing the MCPs in 70 to 90 degrees of flexion with the wrist in neutral to slight extension. Also important is a dorsal component that allows for IP joint extension positioning between exercise periods and at night but allows for full IP joint flexion within the orthosis.

PROXIMAL PHALANX FRACTURES

Proximal phalanx fractures, similar to metacarpal fractures, commonly involve the neck or shaft. Due to the close relationship of the anatomical structures on the dorsal and volar surfaces of these bones, proximal phalanx fractures can pose more of a challenge for the practitioner. This type of fracture of the proximal phalanx is more susceptible to adhesions of either the extensor or flexor tendon(s) over the fracture site, which can result in loss of active extension or flexion at the PIP joint of the injured digit. Proximal phalanx fractures and PIP joint injuries are also subject to deforming forces at the time of injury and can result in volar or dorsal angulation due to the pull of the intrinsic muscles across the fracture site (Figure 8-6). A hand-based orthosis is typically used to help protect the fracture and promote protected tendon gliding during healing. The MCP joint is positioned at 60 to 70 degrees of flexion with the PIP and DIP joints in full extension (safe position). For stable fractures, the PIP and DIP joints may be left out of the orthosis to promote active tendon movement across the fracture site during healing, helping to discourage development of adhesions.

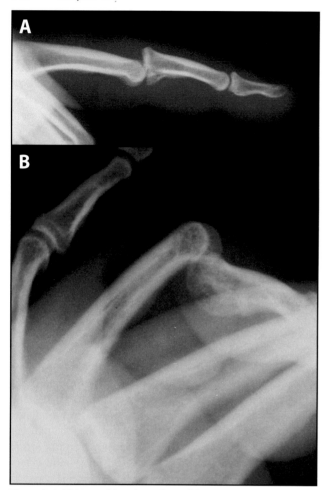

Figure 8-6. (A) X-ray of dorsal angulation following PIP joint fracture. (B) X-ray of volar angulation following PIP joint fracture.

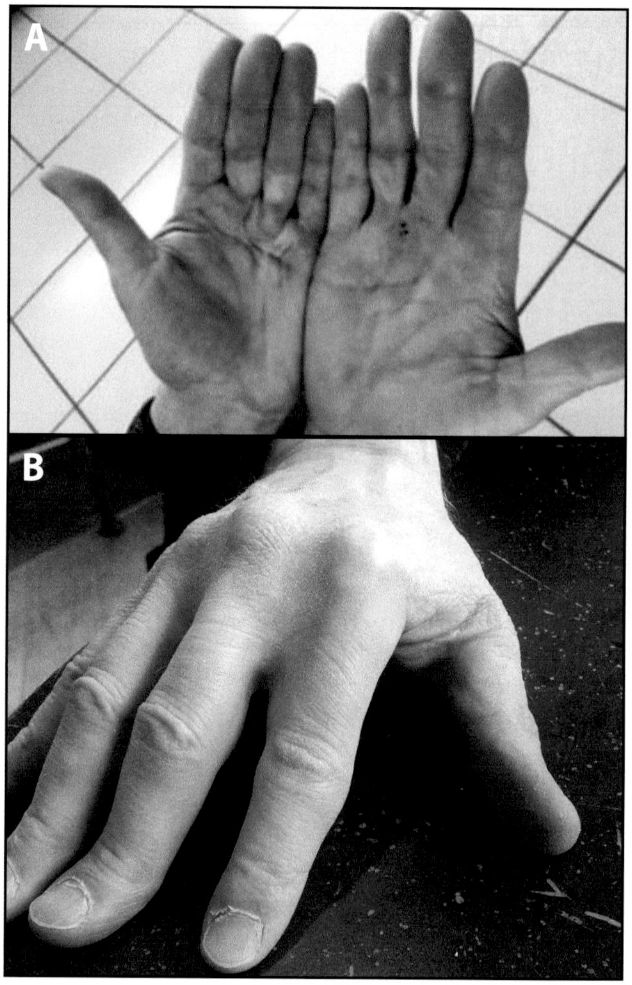

Figure 8-7. (A) Volar view and (B) dorsal view of a client with bilateral Dupuytren's contracture.

Wearing Schedule

The wearing schedule of an orthosis prescribed for a proximal phalanx fracture depends on fracture stability and surgeon preference. Proximal phalanx fractures typically heal quickly. Immobilization for 2 to 4 weeks is recommended, with active PIP and DIP joint motion, both flexion and full IP joint extension, encouraged within the orthosis for stable fractures. As with metacarpal fractures, the PIP joint can be placed in an extension orthosis at night if an extension lag, or loss of active PIP and/or DIP joint extension, develops.

DUPUYTREN'S CONTRACTURE/ DUPUYTREN'S DISEASE

Dupuytren's disease is an irreversible connective tissue disorder that results in progressive fibrosis, or thickening of the palmar fascia that causes development of contractile cords and nodules in the palm of the hand (Figure 8-7). Dupuytren's is characterized by progressive thickening of

the fascia below the skin, which draws the digits in toward the palm. Consequently, the client is unable to place his or her hand flat on a table surface. This condition occurs more frequently in men of European descent and affects up to 20% of men over the age of 65 years. Flexion contractures of the MCP and/or PIP joints of the affected digits is common and can significantly affect an individual's ability to perform daily activities. Surgical intervention with excision of the diseased fascia and release of the contracted joint(s) is the most common treatment. Nonoperative techniques, including **needle fasciotomy** and **collagenase injection** with manipulation, are becoming popular due to decreased complications and faster recovery. In needle fasciotomy, the surgeon uses a needle to repeatedly pierce the skin and diseased cords. The affected digits are then passively extended until the cord is ruptured. With collagenase injection with manipulation, the surgeon injects collagenase into the diseased cord(s) in order to disrupt the collagen bonds and weaken the cord. The client returns the following day to have the affected digit passively extended, rupturing the cord. Researchers are studying the long-term effects of

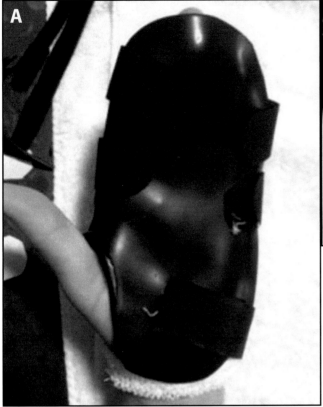

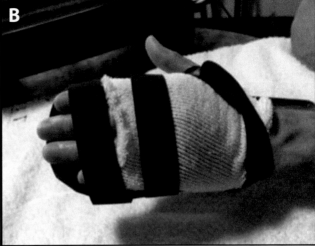

Figure 8-8. Client with a volar hand orthosis with fingers in extension after Dupuytren's release surgery. (A) Volar surface. (B) Dorsum of hand.

these procedures; however, long-term outcomes are currently unknown. Readers are strongly encouraged to seek out current literature as it becomes available.

Hand-based orthoses are commonly used following both surgery and nonoperative procedures to maintain the digit extension achieved and prevent recurrence of flexion contractures. The involved digits are positioned in extension, with care taken to avoid excessive tension on the wound for the first 1 to 2 weeks following surgery (Figure 8-8). Wide variability exists in the frequency in which these orthoses are used, the force and position of the involved digits in the orthosis, and the duration of orthosis use following surgery. The therapeutic effect of orthoses to deliver controlled stress to diseased fascia following surgery is currently unknown, particularly the use of orthoses at night following the initial healing period. The reader is encouraged to refer to current literature as it becomes available.

Wearing Schedule

The wearing schedule of an orthosis following treatment, both surgical and nonoperative, of Dupuytren's disease depends on disease severity, surgeon preference, and degree of preoperative joint contracture. As discussed, the duration of orthosis use for this population remains widely variable. Some surgeons recommend full-time wear until the wounds have healed, with removal on a regular basis for active digit flexion and extension, combined with consistent night wear for 4 to 6 months. Others recommend

orthosis use as needed based on maintenance of digit extension following surgery.

Evidence

Level I

- Jerosh-Herold, C., Shepstone, L., Chojnowsi, A. J., Larson, D., Barrett, E., & Vaughan, S. P. (2011). Nighttime splinting after fasciotomy or dermo-fasciectomy for Dupuytren's contracture: A pragmatic, multi-centre, randomized controlled trial. *BMC Musculoskeletal Disorders, 12*, 136.

  ○ This prospective, randomized, controlled trial evaluated the effectiveness of use of a night digit extension immobilization orthosis following surgery to treat Dupuytren's contracture. Outcome measures included Disabilities of the Arm, Shoulder, and Hand scores, digit ROM, and self-reported patient satisfaction. No statistical differences were noted in all outcome measures at 12 months postsurgery. The authors recommend use of a hand-based digit extension orthosis only if loss of digit extension is observed following surgery and report that routine use of a night orthosis is not necessary.

Level II

- Kemler, M. A., Houpt, P., & van der Horst, C. M. (2012). A pilot study assessing the effectiveness of postoperative splinting after limited fasciectomy for Dupuytren's

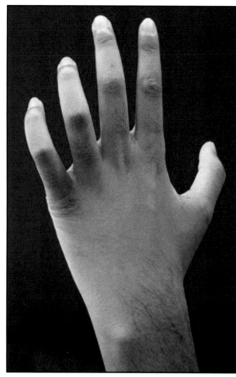

Figure 8-9. Client with a claw hand deformity due to lack of ulnar nerve innervation.

disease. *Journal of Hand Surgery (European Volume), 37*(8), 733-737.

- This study examined the effectiveness of postoperative splinting following surgery for Dupuytren's contracture. All 54 participants had a PIP flexion contracture of at least 30 degrees. PIP extension served as the primary outcome measure; secondary measures included visual analog scale (VAS) for pain, perceived comfort of the splint, and compliance with splint wear. All participants were evaluated at 1 year postsurgery. No statistically significant results were noted in all outcome measures between the two groups. The authors suggest that use of an orthosis following surgery for Dupuytren's disease is not beneficial but note that further study is needed to support their preliminary pilot data.

- Brauns, A., Van Nuffel, M., De Smet, L., & Degreef, I. (2017). A clinical trial of tension and compression orthoses for Dupuytren contractures. *Journal of Hand Therapy, 30*(3), 253-261.

- The authors devised a randomized clinical trial on two patient groups with Dupuytren's disease to evaluate how much improvement two different types of orthoses (tension and compression) can provide to a patient with a Dupuytren's contracture. They wanted to find whether a compression orthosis contributed to better results than a tension orthosis. The trial included 30 patients with measurable flexion contractures of the fingers. Each treatment group consisted of 15 patients. One group received a standard tension orthosis and the other group received a newly designed silicon compression orthosis. Patients were instructed to wear their orthoses 20 hours per day for 3 months. Outcome measures were collected at the initial visit and again after 3 months of orthotic treatment. Primary outcomes were active extension deficit of each joint and total active extension of the digit. Secondary outcomes included patient satisfaction, and a VAS score of function and esthetics (0 to 10 points). The results of this trial showed that, for all patients, the flexion contracture was reduced at least 5 degrees. After 3 months, total active extension was significantly reduced in both groups (both $P < .001$). The mean change in total active extension was 32.36 degrees in the tension orthosis group and 46.47 degrees in the compression orthosis group. Although reduction of total active extension deficit was bigger in the compression group, this difference was not statistically significant ($P = .39$). The VAS score of esthetics and functionality was significantly increased in both treatment groups. The functional VAS after 3 months was 11% higher in the compression group than in the tension group ($P = .03$). A major complication of the tension orthotic was skin ulcers. The authors concluded that both tension and/or compression orthoses can be used as a nonoperative treatment of Dupuytren's disease in both early proliferative untreated hands and aggressive postsurgery recurrence. Although there was no statistically significant difference, compression orthoses appear to be more effective and are better tolerated.

ULNAR NERVE INJURIES

Both high and low injuries to the ulnar nerve can cause significant motor and sensory impairments in the hand. As discussed in Chapter 1, the ulnar nerve innervates the majority of the hand intrinsic muscles, hypothenar muscles, and adductor pollicis. Paralysis or weakness of these muscles causes considerable imbalance of forces across the MCP and IP joints of the fourth and fifth digits, impairment in prehensile function, and sensory impairment on the ulnar aspect of the hand and digits. Ulnar claw hand develops due to the unopposed contraction of the extensor digitorum across the MCP joints and loss of intrinsic muscle power across the IP joints. The ulnar claw hand postures with the fourth and fifth MCP joints in hyperextension and concurrent flexion of the PIP and DIP joints with all attempts at active digit (Figure 8-9). A hand-based orthosis (Figure 8-10) that positions the fourth and fifth MCP joints in flexion helps to transfer the force from the extensor

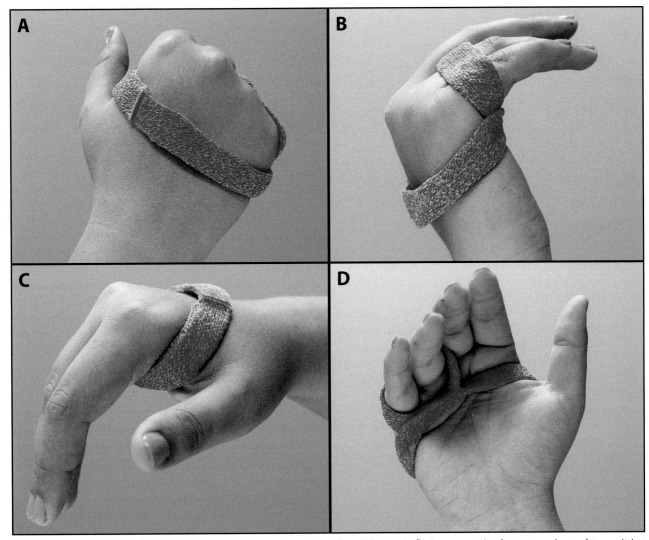

Figure 8-10. An anti-claw orthosis reduces the deformity by positioning the MCP joints in flexion, preventing hyperextension and transmitting force to extend the PIP joints. (A) Dorsal view, (B) ulnar view, (C) radial view, and (D) volar view.

digitorum communis at the MCP joints to the IP joints to prevent MCP hyperextension, as well as prevent development of fixed contractures. For burns or other longstanding injuries with IP flexion contractures, a hand-based orthosis that positions the fourth and fifth MCP joints in flexion with the IP joints in maximum extension is recommended.

Wearing Schedule

The length of orthosis use will depend on the location of the nerve injury/repair, age of the client, and involvement of other structures. Nerve injuries that occur more proximal in the upper extremity will take longer to recover as compared with more distal nerve injuries, hence length of time needed for restoration of muscle function varies considerably. The orthosis should be worn until the interossei and lumbrical muscles are strong enough to prevent MCP hyperextension during active digit extension (typically a minimum of grade 3 muscle strength).

Evidence

Level V

- Dell, P. C., & Sforzo, C. R. (2005). Ulnar intrinsic anatomy and dysfunction. *Journal of Hand Therapy, 18*(2), 198-207.

    ○ The authors provide a detailed description of the ulnar nerve and its course through the palm and provide critical information for clinicians on anatomical considerations that might affect a patient's ability to grasp and release objects. They specifically address disorders that limit active and passive motion, including intrinsic tightness, extrinsic extensor tightness, Landsmeer ligament tightness (tightness of the oblique retinacular ligament), and methods to assess these limitations. Surgical interventions are also described, along with some guidelines for orthotic intervention to improve function.

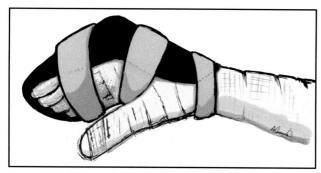

Figure 8-11. Client with a dorsal hand burn wearing a hand-based orthosis.

- Chan, R. K. (2002). Splinting for peripheral nerve injury in upper limb. *Hand Surgery, 7*(2), 251-259.

  ○ The author describes the peripheral nerves and the path of peripheral nerve recovery after trauma. Full recovery of injured nerves will depend greatly on the level of injury, severity of injury, surgical intervention, and postoperative treatment process. Many high-level injuries may take years or months for the affected peripheral nerve to recover. Damage to nerves typically causes imbalance of muscle activity. Prolonged muscle imbalance causes joint contractures and overstretching of denervated muscles. Without proper treatment and attention, hand function recovery may be limited even if the nerve regenerates. During this period of nerve regeneration, orthotic management is one of the most useful modalities to minimize deformities, prevent joint contractures, and substitute lost motor control. Proper splinting encourages early use of the injured hand in daily activities. There are different types of orthotic design for median nerve palsy, ulnar nerve palsy, and radial nerve palsy. Dynamic splinting techniques may also be used to allow early prehension activities.

HAND BURNS

The dorsal aspect of the hand is frequently subject to burn injuries due to the natural response to protect the body and face from injury. Skin on the dorsal hand surface is thin and mobile, with the extensor tendons and blood vessels directly underneath. In contrast, the skin on the palmar surface is thick and immobile and has considerably more subcutaneous tissue to help protect the flexor tendons. Contractures develop more readily on the dorsal aspect of the hand, leading to MCP extension and IP flexion deformities. Therefore, an orthosis that positions the affected digits in a safe position (MCP flexion with full IP joint extension) after injury or surgical intervention is needed to help prevent the onset of contractures (Figure 8-11). The thumb or wrist may be included in the orthosis depending on the location and severity of the burn injury. Burns on

the palmar surface of the hand may require an orthosis that positions the affected digits in extension, including the MCP joints. Following initial healing (typically 2 weeks), compression garments and silicone sheeting may be used under the orthosis for ongoing scar management.

Wearing Schedule

The orthosis wearing schedule for burn management will depend in part on the healing time of the involved structures, the health and age of the client, and the location and severity of the burn injury. The practitioner must collaborate with the referring physician to determine the appropriate wearing schedule. Currently, the optimal amount of time an orthosis should be worn following a burn injury is unknown. In general, the degree of active joint movement following a burn injury/surgery will help dictate the orthosis wearing schedule. If the client can move actively through full joint ROM, then the orthosis should be worn primarily at night to prevent onset of contractures. If limitations in joint ROM, stiffness, or scarring begin to develop, the wearing time should be increased and the client monitored to ensure that contractures do not develop.

Evidence

Level IV

- Fufa, D. T., Chuang, S., & Yang, J. (2014). Prevention and surgical management of postburn contractures of the hand. *Current Review of Musculoskeletal Medicine, 7*, 53-59. doi:10.1007/s12178-013-9192-9

  ○ The authors provide a review of current concepts of acute burn injury management with emphasis on interventions to prevent development of joint and skin contractures, including burn claw hand. Following dorsal hand burn injuries, use of orthoses that position the MCPs in 70 to 90 degrees of flexion and the PIP and DIP joints in full extension is emphasized, along with early supervised controlled ROM. The thumb should also be positioned in full abduction, along with the wrist in extension if these areas are also burned. Although the authors do not directly reference use of a hand-based orthosis, these designs are indicated for burn injuries that do not extend proximally into the wrist and forearm.

SAGITTAL BAND INJURIES

The sagittal bands help to position and maintain the extensor digitorum tendon over the dorsal aspect of the MCP joint during active flexion and extension. Acute rupture or attenuation, stretching of the sagittal bands due to swelling in and around the MCP joint as seen with rheumatoid arthritis (RA), causes the extensor digitorum tendon to sublux ulnarly into the web space of the adjacent digit (Figure 8-12). Conservative treatment of sagittal band dysfunction involves use of a hand-based orthosis

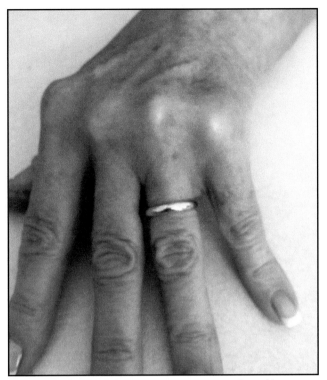

Figure 8-12. Enlarged MCP joints with extensor tendon subluxation in a client with RA.

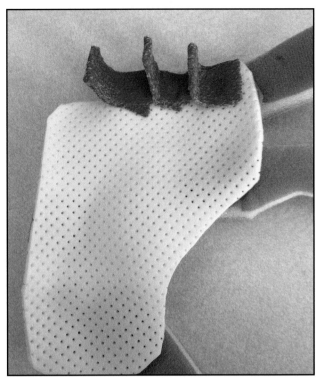

Figure 8-13. Low-temperature thermoplastic material used to separate digits and align them for client with RA in an MCP extension orthosis.

positioning the affected MCP joint in extension, and finger separators may be useful to help align the digits (Figure 8-13). A similar orthosis may be used following surgical repair of the sagittal band for protection and to facilitate optimal healing. A relative motion orthosis may also be used to treat sagittal band injuries. This will be discussed in detail in Chapter 10.

Wearing Schedule

The practitioner must collaborate with the referring physician to determine the appropriate wearing schedule following sagittal band injuries and repairs. A period of 4 weeks of uninterrupted wear is recommended for conservative management of these injuries, followed by buddy taping for an additional 6 weeks. A similar wearing schedule may be indicated following surgical repair.

METACARPOPHALANGEAL JOINT ULNAR DRIFT

MCP ulnar drift is a common deformity seen with RA. Factors that contribute to development of ulnar drift include the following:

- Progressive and longstanding synovitis or inflammation of the synovium inside the joint capsule
- Stretching or attenuation of the MCP joint capsule and radial collateral ligaments with subsequent subluxation of the extensor digitorum and flexor tendons in an ulnar direction

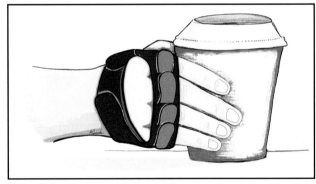

Figure 8-14. Hand-based MCP orthosis to correct ulnar deviation for a client with RA.

- Destruction of the metacarpal head
- Volar dislocation of the proximal phalanx

Additionally, many activities of daily living (ADL), such as gripping a washcloth, and lateral pinching activities place excessive ulnar and volar deviating forces across the MCP joints, thereby increasing the deforming forces (Figure 8-14). MCP anti-ulnar drift orthoses are used to protect the MCP joints and lessen the deforming forces that encourage further MCP ulnar drift during gripping and prehensile tasks. These orthoses position the MCP joints in neutral and help to realign the proximal phalanges. It is important to note that these orthoses cannot correct longstanding deformities such as joint subluxation or dislocation but can gently reposition involved joints to reduce pain and improve functional mobility (Figure 8-15).

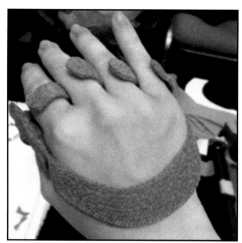

Figure 8-15. A hand-based anti-ulnar drift orthosis is helpful in correcting the ulnar drift deformity.

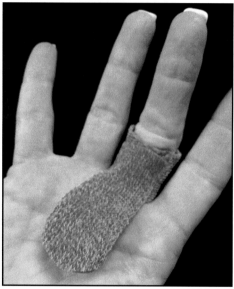

Figure 8-16. An orthosis that prevents full MCP flexion is useful for clients with trigger finger.

Table 8-1

STAGES OF STENOSING TENOSYNOVITIS

STAGE	DESCRIPTION
1	Normal
2	A painful palpable nodule
3	Triggering
4	The PIP joint locks in active flexion and is unlocked with active PIP joint extension.
5	The PIP joint locks in active flexion and is unlocked with passive PIP joint extension.
6	The PIP joint remains locked in a flexed position.

Evidence

Level IV

- Rennie, H. J. (1996). Evaluation of the effectiveness of a metacarpophalangeal ulnar deviation orthosis. *Journal of Hand Therapy, 9,* 371-377.

  ○ This small pilot study investigated the effectiveness of a hand-based ulnar deviation orthosis on grip strength, pain, hand function, and passive correction of MCP ulnar deviation. Outcome measures included the Sollerman assessment of hand grip function, grip and pinch strength, VAS scale for pain, and measurement of MCP ulnar deviation on X-ray with a goniometer. Subjects also completed a post-study questionnaire to obtain their perspectives of the orthosis. Results indicated significant improvement in MCP ulnar deviation angle in all digits except digit II and improved three-point pinch strength with the orthosis on. No statistically significant changes were noted in overall grip strength, pain, or hand function with the orthosis on. Further, no long-term improvements were noted upon orthosis removal with pinch strength of MCP alignment. Collectively, subjects were highly satisfied with the orthosis, and the majority of them reported they would continue to wear the orthosis after the study concluded.

TRIGGER FINGER

Digital stenosing tenosynovitis, commonly referred to as *trigger finger,* is a condition affecting the movement and gliding of the long digit flexor tendons under the A1 pulley. Trigger finger is thought to be caused by inflammation of the flexor tendon sheath, irritation of the tissues, and subsequent narrowing of the space beneath the A1 pulley. Table 8-1 outlines the stages of this condition. Trigger finger is more common in women than in men and typically occurs in the fifth to sixth decades of life. Symptoms include pain, clicking, a catching sensation, and an inability to flex or extend the involved finger. Orthoses are often prescribed to limit the full excursion of the flexor tendon until the inflammation has resolved. Digit-based orthoses that block full MCP motion are commonly fabricated for trigger finger (Figure 8-16).

Wearing Schedule

The appropriate wearing schedule of an orthosis for clients with trigger finger is to wear it as much as possible to reduce the incidence of triggering. Over time, the flexor

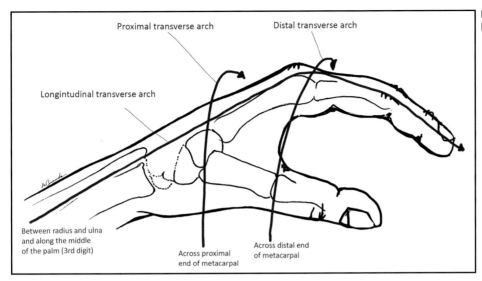

Figure 8-17. Hand arches in resting hand position.

tendon may slide more easily under the A1 pulley and the triggering will resolve. Sometimes the orthosis is offered after the client has received a corticosteroid injection also aimed to reduce inflammation. The client is allowed to remove the orthosis for periods of gentle ROM exercises and hygiene.

Evidence

Level I

- Tarbhai, K., Hannah, S., & von Schroeder, H. P. (2012). Trigger finger treatment: A comparison of 2 splint designs. *Journal of Hand Surgery, 37*(2), 243-249.

  ○ The authors compared an MCP blocking orthosis with a DIP blocking orthosis for relief of symptoms and pain in clients with trigger finger. Subject comfort with the MCP joint blocking splint allowed for longer periods of usage. This study did not include patients with triggering of the thumb. However, the authors suggest that using a thumb MCP joint blocking splint may help patients with trigger thumb as well. There were positive outcomes in 77% of subjects.

Level II

- Colburn, J., Heath, N., Manary, S., & Pacifico, D. (2008). Effectiveness of splinting for the treatment of trigger finger. *Journal of Hand Therapy, 21*(4), 336-343.

  ○ This study demonstrated the effectiveness of providing patients with trigger finger an MCP blocking orthosis for reduction of symptoms. There was a significant reduction in symptoms and number of triggering events after using an MCP blocking orthosis on other fingers for a period of 6 weeks.

Level III

- Valdes, K. (2012). A retrospective review to determine the long-term efficacy of orthotic devices for trigger finger. *Journal of Hand Therapy, 25*(1), 89-96.

  ○ This retrospective study looked at patients treated with orthotic intervention for the treatment of trigger fingers. The study followed the patients 1 year after receiving orthotic intervention and found that 87% required no further intervention for the condition. Orthotic intervention had contributed to resolution of symptoms. The study provides clear evidence on the benefit of orthotic intervention for the condition of triggering.

Biomechanical Principles to Consider With Hand-Based Orthoses

In addition to the basic biomechanical principles discussed in Chapter 1, the practitioner should be aware of the following concepts pertinent to hand-based orthosis designs:

- The arches of the hand must be well supported. This is accomplished by molding the low-temperature thermoplastic material (LTTM) carefully in the palm to accommodate for the natural volar concavity of the proximal and distal transverse arches (Figure 8-17).

- If directed by the referring physician, use the three-point fixation concept within the orthosis because it can help to minimize the deforming forces that occur with metacarpal shaft fractures. Apply gentle volar pressure on the apex of the fracture, along with dorsal pressure proximal and distal to the fracture site (see Figure 8-4). This will optimize the stability of the fracture within the orthosis. Active digit flexion and extension should be encouraged within the orthosis to promote gliding of the extensor and flexor tendons across the metacarpal(s).

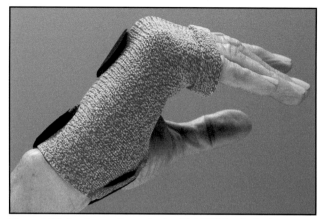

Figure 8-18. An ulnar gutter orthosis with MCP joints in flexion.

- The MCP joint(s) in the orthosis should be placed in 60 to 70 degrees of flexion whenever possible to maintain the length of the collateral ligaments and prevent joint stiffness. Similarly, the PIP and DIP joints should be positioned in full extension.

- For proximal phalanx fractures, use of an orthosis to block the MCP in flexion while allowing for active PIP joint flexion and extension exercises during the healing process will promote active movement/gliding of the extensor and flexor tendons across the fracture site. This will help minimize tendon adhesions and the development of an extensor lag at the PIP joint and tendon adhesions.

Hand-Based Orthotic Designs

The specific design selected for these orthoses will depend on the diagnosis, the client's current functional needs, the specific indications requested by the referring physician, and the practitioner's clinical judgement. The practitioner must consider the anatomy of the hand and how the orthosis will influence these structures when determining the most appropriate orthosis design.

ULNAR GUTTER ORTHOSIS

The ulnar gutter orthosis design covers the ulnar aspect of the hand and includes the MCP joints in flexion; it may or may not include the PIP or DIP joints. This orthosis typically includes both the fourth and fifth metacarpals and immobilizes and offers protection to the metacarpals and MCP, PIP, and DIP joints (Figure 8-18). This orthosis is often used to stabilize metacarpal fractures of the ulnar digits.

RADIAL GUTTER ORTHOSIS

The radial gutter orthosis design covers the radial aspect of the hand and, similar to the ulnar design, includes

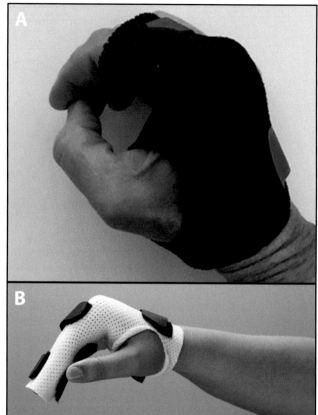

Figure 8-19. A radial gutter orthosis with (A) MCP joints in flexion but PIP and DIP joints are free and (B) MCP joints in flexion and PIP and DIP joints in extension.

the MCP joints in flexion and may or may not include the PIP and DIP joints (Figure 8-19). This orthosis typically includes both the second and third metacarpals and immobilizes and protects the MCP, PIP, and DIP joints. This orthosis is often used to stabilize a second or third metacarpal fracture.

VOLAR HAND-BASED ORTHOSIS

This hand-based resting orthosis design is placed on the volar aspect of the hand and digits. The client's clinical condition and referring physician's preference will dictate which digits are included and the joint position (Figure 8-20).

DORSAL HAND-BASED ORTHOSIS

This orthosis design is on the dorsal aspect of the hand and digits. Similar to the volar design, the client's clinical condition and referring physician's preference will dictate which digits are included and the joint position (Figure 8-21). This design is commonly used to block full MCP and/or PIP joint extension but allow for active flexion of these joints.

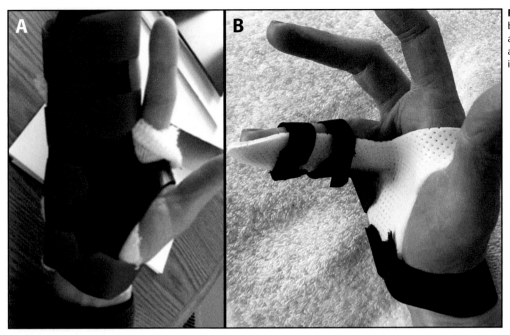

Figures 8-20. Volar hand-based orthosis with (A) fourth and fifth digits in extension and (B) fourth and fifth digits in a safe position.

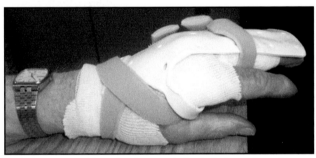

Figure 8-21. Dorsal-based orthosis with the digits in a safe position.

Orthotic Fabrication Steps

Orthotic fabrication begins after the practitioner has determined which design is most suited to the client's condition and specific needs, physician's referral, and clinical judgement.

Refer to the instructional video for detailed step-by-step instructions.

1. Pattern making
   ◦ Volar or dorsal orthosis (Figure 8-22)
   ◦ Radial gutter orthosis (Figure 8-23)
   ◦ Ulnar gutter orthosis (Figure 8-24)
   ◦ Anti-claw orthosis (Figure 8-25)
   ◦ Trigger finger orthosis (Figure 8-26)

2. Material selection

   A variety of factors are important to consider when selecting an appropriate LTTM for hand-based orthoses. In general:

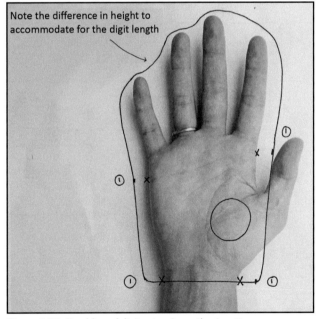

Figure 8-22. Hand-based digit extension orthosis pattern.

◦ 1/12- or 1/16-inch thickness is suitable for most hand-based designs.

◦ The material must have the ability to conform exceptionally well to the contours of the palm, MCP joints, and phalanges.

◦ Choose a material with memory for conditions that will require frequent adjustments (due to wound care needs, the presence of postsurgery or postinjury edema, the presence of pins).

Refer to Chapter 3 for an overview of LTTM characteristics.

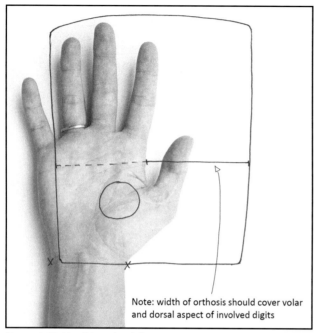

Figure 8-23. Hand-based radial gutter pattern.

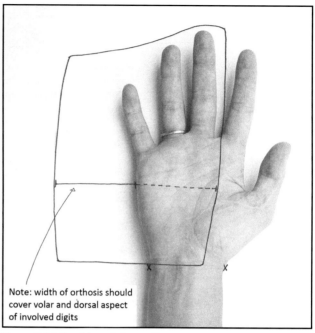

Figure 8-24. Hand-based ulnar gutter pattern.

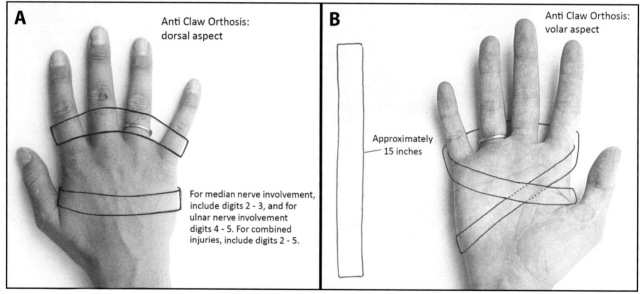

Figure 8-25. Anti-claw orthosis pattern. (A) Dorsal view and (B) volar view.

3. Client positioning

4. Molding techniques

5. Finishing techniques: edges and strapping

6. Orthosis check-out

   ◦ Can the client move his or her wrist fully in all directions in the orthosis?

   If no, adjust the proximal edge of the orthosis so it clears the wrist crease. Be sure to clear the edge just distal to the ulnar head and the radial styloid to avoid impingement in these areas.

   ◦ For orthoses that allow for movement of the MCP and PIP joints, can the client move these joints fully?

   If no, ensure that the distal edge of the orthosis clears the joint crease:

   - *Distal palmar crease for MCP movement*

   - *PIP joint crease for PIP joint movement*

   ◦ For dorsal hand-based orthoses, are the bony prominences protected (MCP, PIP, and DIP joints)?

   If no, check to ensure that the LTTM is molded well over these prominences. Padding can be added for

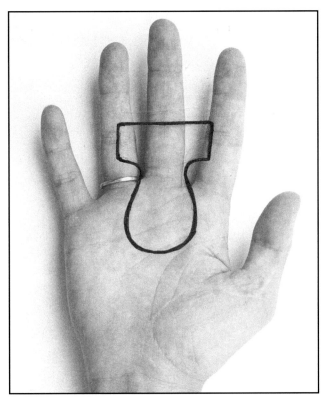

Figure 8-26. Trigger finger orthosis pattern.

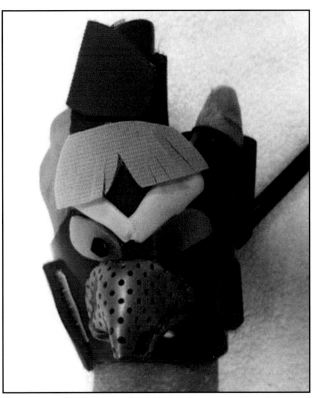

Figure 8-27. Special bird orthosis design for young client. (Reprinted with permission from Maria Candida Miranda Luzo.)

comfort if needed, but padding may increase pressure underneath the LTTM if sufficient space is not molded out to accommodate the padding.

- For radial gutter designs, can the client move his or her thumb easily within the orthosis?

  If no, flare the thumb hole edges to allow the thumb to move easily. Pay particular attention to the thumb carpometacarpal (CMC) joint and ensure that this area is cleared/flared well.

- For radial and ulnar gutter designs, is the orthosis secure on the hand?

  If no, place a strap on the proximal aspect of the orthosis with care taken to place it around the thumb CMC joint. This helps to secure the orthosis and prevent distal migration.

- Are the corners of the orthosis rounded and smooth?

  If no, round and smooth all corners of the orthosis.

- Are the straps secure and strap edges rounded?

  If no, ensure that the Velcro hook (Velcro BVBA) on the orthosis is secure and large enough to provide adequate surface area for the Velcro loop to adhere securely.

- Are all indentations and pattern marks removed?

  If no, use a heat gun to smooth the LTTM. Rubbing alcohol can be used to remove wax pencil marks. Ink

cannot be removed, so refrain from using this when drawing your pattern on the LTTM.

- Remove the orthosis after 5 to 10 minutes and observe the skin. Are there any reddened areas?

  If yes, adjust the orthosis by flaring and smoothing edges and/or flaring material away from bony prominences.

- Review the purpose and care of the hand-based orthosis with the client. Does he or she understand why he or she is wearing it? When he or she should wear it? How to take care of it?

  If no, discuss the wearing schedule and care of the orthosis with the client before he or she leaves the clinic and provide clear written instructions to take home with him or her (refer to the Appendix at the end of the chapter).

SPECIAL CONSIDERATIONS

When working with a pediatric population, consider using brightly colored LTTM to optimize compliance and involve the children in the process (Figures 8-27 and 8-28). Consider including the wrist to ensure the orthosis is secure on the hand. Older clients might benefit from the use of lighter, thinner materials to optimize comfort and minimize the potential for development of pressure areas over bony prominences and thinning skin. Contrasting

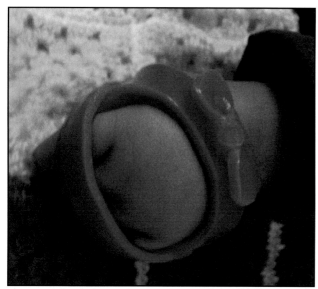

Figure 8-28. Special design for a pediatric client needing an anti-claw orthosis. (Reprinted with permission from Maria Candida Miranda Luzo.)

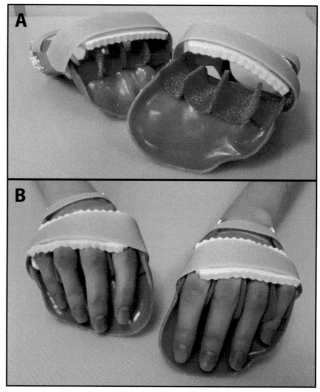

Figure 8-29. Bright-colored, hand-based orthoses with contrasting straps and finger separators. (Reprinted with permission from Anna Ovsyannikova.)

colors with LTTM and straps may help clients with visual impairments handle the orthosis more easily (Figure 8-29). Use of cotton stockinette under the orthosis and judicious use of padding over bony prominences will help optimize comfort.

HELPFUL ORTHOSIS FOR EXERCISES

One very useful hand-based orthosis, known as a *blocking orthosis*, holds the MCP joints in extension while allowing the client with stiff PIP and DIP joints the ability to actively exercise these joints. This orthosis can easily be made from a simple rectangle of material fashioned circumferentially around the hand, leaving the PIP and DIP joints (Figure 8-30).

Box 8-2 outlines helpful hints for hand-based orthotic fabrication.

Summary

- Knowledge of the key anatomical structures affected by a hand-based orthosis will help the practitioner understand how the orthosis will influence these structures, as well as assist him or her in determining the most appropriate orthotic design and wearing schedule.

- The goals of a hand-based orthosis and the specifics of each individual wearing schedule will vary depending on the client's needs and the diagnosis.

- The arches of the hand must be supported well and the LTTM conformed correctly to ensure that this is achieved.

- Special populations, such as pediatric and geriatric clients, may require specific orthotic designs or adaptations to achieve the best outcomes.

- Each orthosis must be molded to the individual anatomy for the best fit. Post-fabrication critique and check out help identify areas for modification and optimize client comfort.

In Your Client's Shoes

As a practitioner, it is very important to appreciate the effect that a hand-based orthosis will have on your client's performance of ADL. Some designs, specifically hand-based orthoses that include digits II and III, may significantly limit the client's ability to use his or her affected hand for prehensile tasks such as writing with a pen or opening a water bottle. You should experience how it feels to wear an orthosis for an extended period of time. This experience will enable you to be client centered when using orthoses as an intervention strategy in your practice. You must consider how to instruct your client on the importance of the wearing schedule and the benefits of compliance for maximum benefits.

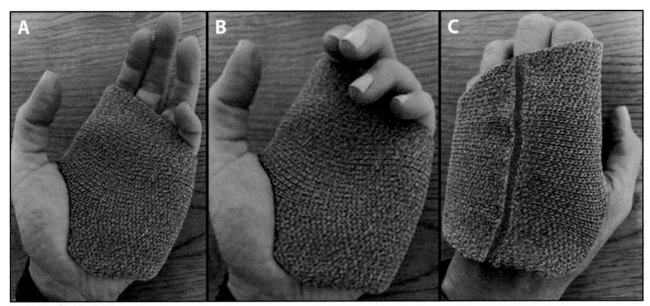

Figures 8- 30. A blocking orthosis for exercises. (A) Volar view extension. (B) Volar view active flexion of the digits. (C) Dorsal view.

Box 8-2. Helpful Hints

- Each client is an individual, and the selected orthosis must match the individual's needs, size, and functional demands.

- LTTM with memory is important when frequent readjustments of the orthosis are required (e.g., clients with edema or tendon injury). This makes remolding the orthosis easier and is cost efficient.

- It is very important to ensure that the orthosis is secure on the hand. A strap placed on the proximal aspect of the orthosis just distal to the wrist can help optimize security of the orthosis. Molding the LTTM around the thumb (make a hole for the thumb and flare it around the thenar eminence) can also help secure the orthosis on the hand.

- Inclusion of the wrist in the orthosis may increase the mechanical advantage and lessen the force needed to position the MCP joints comfortably in the orthosis.

- The use of soft strapping material with straps that are located between the digits and digit web spaces can optimize comfort.

- For dorsal or volar orthotic designs that include the PIP and DIP joints, position the straps directly over the joints to ensure that they are positioned in extension (unless a different position is necessary).

Suggested Reading

Adams, J., Hammond, A., Burridge, J., & Cooper, C. (2005). Static orthoses in the prevention of hand dysfunction in rheumatoid arthritis: A review of the literature. *Musculoskeletal Care, 3*(2), 85-101.

Brauns, A., Van Nuffel, M., De Smet, L., & Degreef, I. (2017). A clinical trial of tension and compression orthoses for Dupuytren contractures. *Journal of Hand Therapy, 30*(3), 253-261.

Catalano, L. W., Gupta, S., Ragland, R., Glickel, S. Z., Johnson, C., & Barron, A. (2006). Closed treatment of nonrheumatoid extensor tendon dislocations at the metacarpal joint. *Journal of Hand Surgery, 31*, 242-245.

Chan, R. K. (2002). Splinting for peripheral nerve injury in upper limb. *Hand Surgery, 7*(2), 251-259.

Chinchalkar, S. J., & Pipicelli, J. G. (2009). Addressing extensor digitorum communis adherence after metacarpal fracture with the use of a circumferential fracture brace. *Journal of Hand Therapy, 22*(4), 377-381. doi:10.1016/j.jht.2009.06.005

Colburn J., Heath N., Manary, S., & Pacifico, D. (2008). Effectiveness of splinting for the treatment of trigger finger. *Journal of Hand Therapy, 21*(4), 336-343.

Coppard, B. M., & Lohman, H. (2014). *Introduction to orthotics: A clinical reasoning and problem-solving approach* (4th ed.). St. Louis, MO: Elsevier Mosby.

Davison, P. G., Boudreau, N., Burrows, R., Wilson, K. L., & Bezuhly, M. (2016). Forearm-based ulnar gutter versus hand based thermoplastic splint for pediatric metacarpal neck fractures: A blinded, randomized trial. *Plastic Reconstructive Surgery, 137*(3), 908-916. doi:10.1097/01.prs.0000479974.45051.78

Dell, P. C., & Sforzo, C. R. (2005). Ulnar intrinsic anatomy and dysfunction. *Journal of Hand Therapy, 18*(2), 198-207.

DiBenedetti, D. B., Nguyen, D., Zografos, L., Ziemiecki, R., & Zhou, X. (2011). Prevalence, incidence, and treatments of Dupuytren's disease in the United States: Results from a population-based study. *Hand, 6*(2), 149-158. doi:10.1007/s11552-010-9306-4

Fufa, D. T., Chuang, S. S., & Yang, J. Y. (2014). Prevention and surgical management of postburn contractures of the hand. *Current Review of Musculoskeletal Medicine, 7*(1), 53-59. doi:10.1007/s12178-013-9192-9

Gulabi, D., Avci, C. C., Cecen, G. S., Bekler, H. I., Saglam, F., & Merih, E. (2014). A comparison of the functional and radiographical results of Paris plaster cast and ulnar gutter splint in the conservative treatment of fractures of the fifth metacarpal. *European Journal of Orthopedic Traumatology, 24*(7), 1167-1173. doi:10.1007/s00590-013-1290-2

Gülke, J., Leopold, B., Grözinger, D., Drews, B., Paschke, S., & Wachter, N. J. (2018). Postoperative treatment of metacarpal fractures—Classical physical therapy compared with a home exercise program. *Journal of Hand Therapy, 31*(1), 20-28.

Harding, I. J., Parry, D., & Barrington, R. L. (2001). The use of a moulded metacarpal brace versus neighbor strapping for fractures of the little finger metacarpal neck. *Journal of Hand Surgery (British and European Volume), 26*(3), 261-263.

Huisstede, B. M., Hoogvliet, P., Coert, J. H., Fridén, J., & European HANDGUIDE Group. (2014). Multidisciplinary consensus guideline for managing trigger finger: Results from the European HANDGUIDE Study. *Physical Therapy, 94*(10), 1421-1433.

Jacobs, M. A., & Austin, N. M. (2014). *Orthotic intervention for the hand and upper extremity* (2nd ed.). Baltimore, MD: Lippincott Williams & Wilkins.

Jerosch-Herold, C., Shepstone, L., Chojnowski, A. J., Larson, D., Barett, E., & Vaughan, S. P. (2011). Night-time splinting after fasciectomy or dermofasciectomy for Dupuytren's contracture: A pragmatic, multi-centre, randomized controlled trial. *BMC Musculoskeletal Disorders, 12*, 136.

Kemler, M. A., Houpt, P., van der Horst, C. M. (2012). A pilot study assessing the effectiveness of postoperative splinting after limited fasciectomy for Dupuytren's disease. *Journal of Hand Surgery, 37*(8), 733-737.

Larson, D., & Jerosch-Herold, C. (2008). Clinical effectiveness of postoperative splinting after surgical release of Dupuytren's contracture: A systematic review. *BMC Musculoskeletal Disorders, 9*, 104. doi:10.1186/1471-2474-9-104

McNemar, T. B., Howell, J. W., & Chang, E. (2003). Management of metacarpal fractures. *Journal of Hand Therapy, 16*(2), 143-151.

Poolman, R. W., Goslings, J. C., Lee, J. B., Statius Muller, M., Steller, E. P., & Struijs, P. A. (2005). Conservative treatment for closed fifth (small finger) metacarpal neck fractures. *Cochrane Database Syst Rev, 3*, CD003210.

Rennie, H. J. (1996). Evaluation of the effectiveness of a metacarpophalangeal ulnar deviation orthosis. *Journal of Hand Therapy, 9*, 371-377.

Sweet, S., & Blackmore, S. (2014). Surgical and therapy update on the management of Dupuytren's disease. *Journal of Hand Therapy, 27*(2), 77-84.

Tarbhai, K., Hannah, S., & von Schroeder, H. P. (2012). Trigger finger treatment: A comparison of 2 splint designs. *Journal of Hand Surgery, 37*(2), 243-249.

Valdes, K. (2012). A retrospective review to determine the long-term efficacy of orthotic devices for trigger finger. *Journal of Hand Therapy, 25*(1), 89-96.

Test Your Knowledge

SHORT ANSWER

1. Describe the three hand arches that are important to consider when fabricating a hand-based orthosis.

2. Explain the difference in the anatomy between the CMC joints of digits II and III and the CMC joints of digits IV and V.

3. Identify the recommended safe position of the MCP and IP joints in a hand-based orthosis and discuss the rationale behind it.

4. List the movements that a client should be able to perform without difficulty when wearing a hand-based orthosis.

5. Describe two different hand-based designs and discuss the rationale for each one.

6. List the appropriate orthotic design and LTTM suitable for the following:
   ○ A 60-year-old male who underwent surgery for Dupuytren's contracture
   ○ A 15-year-old young man with a stable fourth metacarpal shaft fracture
   ○ A 70-year-old woman with longstanding RA who has ulnar drift of her MCP joints

MULTIPLE CHOICE

7. Following an injury to the third and fourth metacarpal bones, in which position is the MCP joint most stable?
   a. Full extension
   b. Full flexion
   c. 20 degrees of flexion
   d. Full hyperextension

8. What is the benefit of positioning the hand in a safe position in a hand-based orthosis?
   a. It helps to minimize pain following injury.
   b. It helps to minimize edema following injury or surgery.
   c. It helps to decrease the risk of reinjury.
   d. It helps to minimize the risk of joint contractures.

9. What is the term used to describe a fracture to the fifth metacarpal neck?
   a. Bennett's fracture
   b. Colles' fracture
   c. Boxer's fracture
   d. Smith's fracture

10. What is a risk following fracture to a digit proximal phalanx?

   a. Nonunion of the bone due to poor blood supply

   b. Adherence of the flexor and/or extensor tendons over the bone

   c. Loss of wrist mobility

   d. Rotation of the bone at the fracture site

11. What is the purpose of an ulnar claw hand orthosis?

   a. The orthosis helps to facilitate healing of the injured nerve.

   b. The orthosis helps to rebalance the muscle forces across the MCP joints and prevent joint contractures.

   c. The orthosis helps to reposition the MCP joints and proximal phalanges in better alignment to facilitate hand function.

   d. The orthosis helps to protect healing wounds following surgery.

12. What is an advantage of a dorsally based hand orthosis design?

   a. It allows the client to flex his or her involved digits while in the orthosis.

   b. It positions the MCP and PIP joints in a safe position easier than a volarly based design.

   c. It allows the client to extend his or her involved digits while in the orthosis.

   d. It does not require as much LTTM as compared with a volarly based design.

13. What hand-deforming position is commonly seen following a dorsal hand burn?

   a. MCP ulnar deviation

   b. Zig-zag deformity

   c. Claw hand

   d. Wrist flexion contracture

CASE STUDIES

Case Study 1

Frank is an 18-year-old, right-hand–dominant man who sustained a boxer's fracture on his right dominant hand 4 days ago after punching a wall at school. His fracture is stable. He lives at home with his parents and younger sister. He is a senior in high school and is concerned that he will have trouble using his computer and playing video games.

He presents for therapy with a prescription that reads:
Right stable boxer's fracture

1. *Evaluate and treat*

2. *Provide right-hand–based protective orthosis for full-time wear; leave PIP joints free*

3. *Provide instructions on edema control and orthotic use*

Your assessment:

Frank presents to therapy for his evaluation and custom hand-based orthosis for his right hand. Your evaluation reveals the following:

- Moderate swelling and bruising on the dorsal aspect of the right hand

- Difficulty flexing and extending the fifth digit PIP joint (MCP joint movement not formally assessed); all other joints of the right upper extremity are within normal limits

- Reports of pain at 8/10 on 0 to 10 VAS at rest

- No impairment in sensation right hand

Using different clinical reasoning approaches, answer the following questions about this client and the prescribed orthosis.

Procedural Reasoning

1. What client factors are important to consider when determining the most suitable orthotic design for this client?

2. Which immobilization orthotic design would be most appropriate for this client? Why?

3. What LTTM properties are important to consider? List them here.

4. Describe the instructions you would give this client on:

   ◦ How to care for the orthosis

   ◦ Wearing schedule

   ◦ Precautions

   ◦ Exercises/activities

Pragmatic Reasoning

5. What resources are available to fabricate this orthosis (time, materials, expertise)?

6. Are you able to clearly document the need for this orthosis?

7. Does evidence-based practice support the use of this orthosis for this client's diagnosis?

Interactive Reasoning

8. What are the client's goals and valued occupations?

9. What impact will the client's injury and use of the orthosis have on his ADL?

Conditional Reasoning

10. What factors will influence this client's compliance to the wearing schedule of this orthosis?

Narrative Reasoning

11. How does this condition and, more specifically, this orthotic intervention affect this client's valued occupations?

12. What activities is this client most concerned about?

Ethical Reasoning

13. Does the client understand the need for the orthosis?

14. Does the client have the resources to be able to pay for the orthosis (as applicable)?

15. What other options are available to this client if he lacks the resources necessary to pay for the orthosis?

16. Write one short-term goal (1 to 2 weeks) and one long-term goal (6 to 8 weeks) for this client.

Case Study 2

Janine is a very pleasant 66-year-old woman who underwent a palmar fasciectomy on her nondominant left hand 2 days ago to treat her Dupuytren's disease. Her referral reads:

Left palmar fasciectomy:

1. *Provide custom hand-based orthosis*

2. *Provide dressing change and home instruction for edema control, gentle digit ROM, and wound care*

Your assessment:

Janine presents in therapy with a postoperative dressing in place with her fourth and fifth digits in extension and her wrist free. She is doing well overall and is thrilled to see her fingers "straight again." She is complaining of moderate pain in her palm and reports some tingling in her fourth and fifth fingertips. She lives alone in a single-story apartment and has no one to assist her with shopping, driving, cooking, or other household tasks. She is retired and spends her time volunteering at her church, playing bridge, and spending time with her grandchildren.

Using different clinical reasoning approaches, consider the following questions about this client and the prescribed orthosis. Some questions may be directed more toward the client and some questions may be directed more toward you as the practitioner for reflection.

Procedural Reasoning

1. What client factors are important to consider when determining the most suitable orthotic design for this client?

2. Which immobilization orthotic design would be most appropriate for this client? Why?

3. What LTTM properties are important to consider?

4. Describe the instructions you would give this client on:
   ◦ How to care for the orthosis
   ◦ Wearing schedule
   ◦ Precautions
   ◦ Exercises/activities

Pragmatic Reasoning

5. What resources are available to fabricate this orthosis (time, materials, expertise)?

6. Are you able to clearly document the need for this orthosis?

7. Does evidence-based practice support the use of this orthosis for this client's diagnosis?

Interactive Reasoning

8. What are the client's goals and valued occupations?

9. What impact will the client's injury, and use of the orthosis, have on her ADL?

Conditional Reasoning

10. What factors will influence this client's compliance to the wearing schedule of this orthosis?

Narrative Reasoning

11. How does this injury and, more specifically, this orthotic intervention affect this client's valued occupations?

12. What activities is this client most concerned about?

Ethical Reasoning

13. Does the client understand the need for the orthosis?

14. Does the client have the resources to be able to pay for the orthosis (as applicable)?

15. What other options are available to this client if she lacks the resources necessary to pay for the orthosis?

16. Write one short-term goal (1 to 2 weeks) and one long-term goal (6 to 8 weeks) for this client.

Appendix

STUDENT ASSIGNMENTS

1. Define all of the key terms used in this chapter.

2. As an occupational therapy practitioner, you must provide your client with detailed instructions for wearing and caring for his or her orthosis. This document must be required for the client's official records and insurance payments. Select one of the hand-based orthotic designs from this chapter and prepare a client-centered handout for wearing this orthosis. Base your client description on one of the two case studies in this chapter. Include the following in the handout:
   ◦ A description/name of the orthosis
   ◦ An outline of the wearing schedule (remember this will vary depending on the client's condition)

- A description of how to clean and care for the orthosis
- Instructions on what the client should be aware of when wearing the orthosis (red areas on skin, pain, increased swelling, etc.)
- Contact information and follow-up instructions

3. Prepare a case study of a client requiring a hand-based orthosis. Use one of the evidence-based resources cited in the chapter to support your orthotic intervention. Summarize the research and explain the outcomes of the study.

4. As an occupational therapy practitioner, it will be interesting and informative for you to spend an extended period wearing an orthosis to appreciate the impact that an orthosis will have on your client's daily occupations. Wear a hand-based orthosis designed by your lab partner for a 24-hour period. Take note of how this feels to have one body part immobilized. Elaborate in paragraphs on the following:

   - Describe the orthosis, material used, positioning, and typical diagnosis for this particular orthosis. (Which arm was splinted, when did you wear it, what did you do with it on?)
   - Comfort and ease of use: Is it easy to take on and off? Does the orthosis fit under clothing? Are there any pressure areas? What needs to be modified and how?

- Personal and public image: Does the orthosis attract attention in public? Does the orthosis attract attention in your family? How did this make you feel, even as a class assignment?

- Functionality: How were you able to function with the orthosis? Was the position helpful or harmful? What would the typical wearing schedule be for a client with the typical need for this orthosis? What instructions should be given to the typical client with the need for this orthosis?

- How does this change your appreciation of what your clients are experiencing with their orthoses?

5. Complete the check-out form on the next page.

Multiple Choice Answer Key

7. b
8. d
9. c
10. b
11. b
12. a
13. c

Hand-Based Orthosis Check-Out Form

*(This can be used for faculty to evaluate students' completed orthoses,
as well as for students to reference when evaluating their own completed orthosis.)*

Fabricate one of the orthotic designs for a hand-based orthosis on your classmate and complete the following check-out form:

Name of Orthosis:

Purpose of Orthosis:

Design/Function

_____ The hand and digits are positioned correctly for condition.

_____ The thenar area is cleared adequately to allow for full thumb motion.

_____ The orthosis effectively immobilizes the MCP, PIP, and DIP joints (as applicable).

_____ The orthosis allows for full wrist motion.

_____ The hand arches are supported: distal and proximal transverse arches, longitudinal arch.

_____ The orthosis does not cause impingement or pressure areas.

_____ The orthosis clears all bony prominences.

Straps/Orthosis Appearance

_____ The straps are in the correct position.

_____ The straps are secure and corners rounded.

_____ The orthosis edges are smooth and corners rounded.

_____ The proximal edge is flared.

_____ The orthosis is free of fingerprints, pattern marks, or indentations.

CHAPTER 9

Digit-Based Orthoses

Key Terms

Boutonniere deformity	Flexion contracture	Serial cast or serial orthosis
Buddy strapping or taping	Fracture reduction	Short arc motion (SAM) protocol
Camptodactyly	Intra-articular joint injuries	Swan neck deformity
Dislocations	Mallet finger	Total end range time (TERT)
Extension lag	Pseudo-boutonniere	Tuft fracture

Learning Outcomes

Upon completion of this chapter, you will be able to:

1. Describe the common clinical conditions that require a digit-based orthosis.

2. Describe the basic goals for prescribing a digit-based orthosis.

3. Identify pertinent anatomical structures and biomechanical principles involved in a digit-based orthosis and apply these concepts to orthotic design and fabrication.

4. Identify common clinical conditions of the digits that require immobilization with an orthosis.

5. Identify the most commonly selected orthotic designs for digit-based orthoses and describe the rationale for choosing one design over another.

6. After reviewing the instructional videos:

   a. Outline the steps involved in the fabrication of a digit-based orthosis.

   b. Complete the molding and fabrication steps of a digit-based orthosis.

   c. Evaluate the fit and function of a completed digit-based orthosis and identify and address all areas needing adjustment.

7. Identify elements of a client education program following provision of a digit-based orthosis.

8. Describe special considerations of digit-based orthotic design and fabrication for pediatric and special needs clients.

Schofield, K., & Schwartz, D. *Orthotic Design and Fabrication
for the Upper Extremity: A Practical Guide* (pp 167-189).
© 2019 Taylor & Francis Group.

Introduction

The hands and digits are involved in most of our daily functional tasks, and any injury or disability can significantly affect our ability to manipulate objects and perform fine motor tasks. The complex and intricate anatomy of the digits deserves special attention and understanding because improper immobilization methods may prevent a client from regaining full finger motion and strength or lead to permanent finger deformities. The digits often swell after an injury, whether it involves the bones, joints, soft tissue structures, or any combination of these. Reduction of this edema is critical to the management of finger injuries. Orthoses for the digits must take into account the optimal position of healing of each critically involved structure. The practitioner must regularly evaluate each digit-based immobilization orthosis for proper fit and positioning as edema is reduced and passive joint range of motion (ROM) is recovered. This chapter will highlight orthoses for common clinical and pathological conditions involving the digits, including orthoses that protect healing structures as well as functional orthoses that prevent and correct deformities. Orthoses for the thumb are covered in Chapter 5.

A digit-based orthosis will often interfere with complete functional use of the hand, making it challenging for clients to heed the wearing protocols. However, because the consequences of not wearing an orthosis may be serious, the practitioner must educate clients about the importance of doing so. Knowledge of the anatomical structures affected by each specific digit-based orthosis will help practitioners understand how the orthosis will influence these structures, educate their clients on the importance of the orthosis for healing and protection, and assist them in determining appropriate orthosis designs and wearing schedules.

Goals for Use of a Digit-Based Immobilization Orthosis

The goals of a digit-based orthosis will vary depending on each individual client's needs and the specifics of the clinical condition. Practitioners treating clients with injuries to the finger, such as fractures, sprains, ligament injuries, or other pathologies, must recognize the benefits that immobilization orthoses can offer their clients. These benefits include relief from pain, stability, prevention or correction of deformity, positioning during healing, and improved functional ability. It is critical to perform an ongoing assessment of the client's current status, particularly in relation to his or her functional ability. Custom-made finger orthoses may require adaptations to meet the client's changing needs. Inflamed or injured swollen joints require rest and immobilization; however, prolonged immobilization may lead to loss of ROM due to joint stiffness. The use of orthoses may help prevent the development of soft tissue and joint contractures and may improve function, allowing the client to maintain independence (Box 9-1).

When fabricating a digit-based immobilization orthosis, the practitioner must consider the specific clinical condition or diagnosis and the expected clinical outcome following orthotic use, then use sound clinical reasoning to select the most appropriate design. As discussed, the particular design chosen depends on multiple factors. The orthosis can be placed volarly or dorsally depending on the involved structures and the client's needs (Figures 9-1A and 9-1B). The orthosis might be placed dorsally over the middle phalanx and volarly over the distal phalanx. A tip protector can be fabricated to protect the fingertip after injury or amputation (Figure 9-1C). The orthosis might be a circumferential design encompassing both volar and dorsal

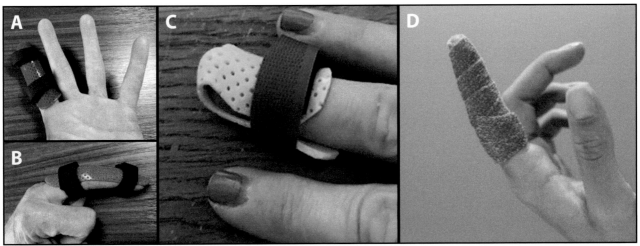

Figure 9-1. (A) A volar-based digit orthosis is placed on the volar surface of the finger. (B) A dorsal-based digit orthosis is placed on the dorsal surface of the finger. (C) A tip protector orthosis is placed on the tip of the finger. (D) A circumferential digit orthosis.

sides of the digit or be an oval shape over the middle and proximal phalanges (Figure 9-1D). There are many unique approaches to orthoses for the digits.

Clinical Conditions and Wearing Schedules

This section describes common clinical conditions where a digit-based orthosis might be prescribed and the current evidence supporting this orthosis as an appropriate intervention strategy. Readers are encouraged to review the references provided for additional details regarding each clinical condition and search current research databases for updated evidence as it becomes available.

ARTHRITIC CONDITIONS

Similar to issues in the other joints of the upper extremity, both rheumatoid arthritis (RA) and osteoarthritis (OA) can affect the digits with decreased motion, pain, joint instability, and weakness (Figure 9-2). Radiographic evidence of both RA and OA demonstrates significant changes in bony alignment and structure.

Rheumatoid Arthritis

As discussed in Chapter 3, RA is an autoimmune disease that commonly affects the wrist and small joints of the hand and digits and usually occurs bilaterally. The most commonly seen finger deformities from RA are swan neck and boutonniere.

Clients with RA will likely have additional joint involvement, such as the wrist, thumb, and MCP joints, which may require the fabrication of orthoses that address these joints. However, often the first complaints may involve only the digits, and use of digit-based orthoses can assist in

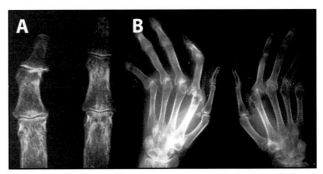

Figure 9-2. (A) X-ray of a finger showing signs of OA. (B) X-ray of a finger joint showing signs of RA.

protecting the involved joints and potentially minimizing further deformity.

Swan Neck Deformity

Swan neck deformity is characterized by hyperextension of the PIP joint and flexion of the DIP joint. Clients with RA commonly have swan neck deformity, along with other deformities of the hand and fingers (Figure 9-3). This deformity can be either fixed, meaning it is not possible to passively correct the deformity, or flexible, meaning it is possible to passively correct the deformity. This can severely affect the client's ability to actively flex the PIP joint and make it difficult to grasp larger objects. Finger orthoses are typically provided for clients with swan neck deformities when the finger is passively correctable, even if all of the digits are affected, and studies have demonstrated that these orthoses do improve function.

Practitioners may fabricate custom-made orthoses from thermoplastic materials or order them through several commercial companies. The orthosis is typically made from two connected oval-shaped rings that are joined at an angle to each other that corresponds to the joint axis of the PIP joint. This design prevents full PIP joint extension but

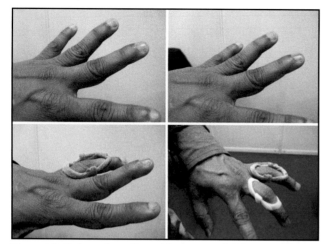

Figure 9-3. Orthoses for a client with a swan neck deformity of digits.

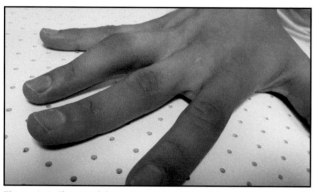

Figure 9-4. Client with boutonniere deformity. (Reprinted with permission from Anna Ovsyannikova.)

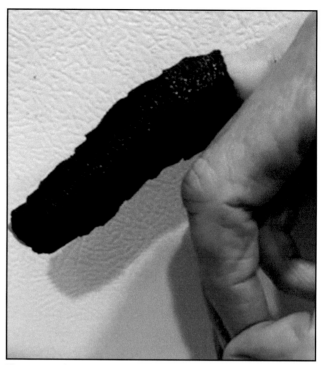

Figure 9-5. Client wearing an orthosis for boutonniere deformity.

allows the client to actively flex his or her PIP joint within the orthosis.

When fabricating the orthosis, the ovals should encompass as much of the length of the proximal and middle phalanges as possible for leverage and to optimize mechanical advantage of the orthosis.

Some clients may present with hyperlaxity of the PIP joints and appear to have a swan neck deformity. However, if the condition is not permanent nor disabling, there is no need to intervene, and orthotic intervention is not necessary.

Boutonniere Deformity

A **boutonniere deformity** consists of flexion of the PIP joint and hyperextension of the DIP joint. It is caused by an interruption of the central slip of the extensor tendon where the lateral slips separate and the head of the proximal phalanx pops through the gap like a finger through a button hole; thus the name from *boutonnière,* which is French for *button hole.* The deformity prevents full extension of the digit and interferes with the ability to grasp and release objects, place the hand in a pocket or flat on the table, or even don gloves (Figures 9-4 and 9-5). An orthosis is used to keep the PIP joint straight. Boutonniere deformity in

clients with RA is caused by inflammation of the joints, bone erosion, joint destruction, and damage to surrounding ligaments and tissues. As will be discussed later in the chapter, boutonniere deformity may also occur as a result of an injury to extensor mechanism in zone III. Although the mechanism of injury for a boutonniere deformity caused by RA is different from that caused from injuries to the extensor mechanism in zone III, the orthotic management is similar, but the wearing schedule may differ.

Osteoarthritis

OA is a wear-and-tear degenerative condition where the cartilage lining the articular joint surfaces is affected by repeated stress on the joints as a client ages or from repetitive stress. As discussed in Chapter 5, the thumb carpometacarpal joint is the most common joint affected by OA in the hand. The second most common site of OA in the hand is the DIP joint. It is subject to considerable stress during prehensile tasks, which can lead to degenerative changes with aging. It is a common condition, affecting up to 20% of men and women over the age of 40 years. OA may affect only one joint in the body, but it is more common to have the condition on both sides.

A specially designed digit-based orthosis can help with both RA and OA symptoms by supporting the painful finger joint in a resting and comfortable position to reduce pain and provide joint stability during activities of daily living (ADL) tasks. The specific goals of an orthosis for this condition are pain reduction, joint protection during ADL, and optimizing functional use of the affected hand by stabilizing the finger joints.

Wearing Schedule

Similar to the recommended wearing schedule for a thumb immobilization orthosis, the recommended wearing schedule of the digit-based immobilization orthosis for clients with arthritis is to wear as needed during periods of inflammation, swelling, and pain. Clients should be encouraged to remove the orthosis periodically to perform gentle ROM exercises and hygiene. When the inflammatory episode has resolved or diminished, clients can reduce orthosis use. For some clients, wearing the orthosis only during activities or only at night may be the appropriate schedule. Use clinical reasoning and discussion with clients to develop individual treatment plans.

Evidence

Level II

- Kennedy, D., Fiona, W., Carlisle, K., Honeyfield, L., Satchithananda, K., & Vincent, T. (2014). Splinting of the distal interphalangeal joint reduces pain and improves extension at the joint: Results from the splint-OA study. *Journal of Hand Therapy, 27*(3), e1.

  ○ This is an abstract describing a prospective, radiologist-blinded, controlled trial of custom splinting of the DIP joint conducted with 26 subjects with symptomatic hand OA. All subjects had at least two affected DIP joints. A custom gutter splint was worn on consecutive nights for 3 months, with clinical assessment and measurement of joint deviation by digital plain radiograph at baseline and after 3 months. The average pain (primary outcome measure) and worst pain scores in the intervention joint were significantly lower at 3 months compared with baseline. Short-term DIP joint splinting is a safe, simple, inexpensive treatment modality that reduces DIP joint pain and improves joint extension.

- Li-Tsang, C. W., Hung, L. K., & Mak, A. F. (2002). The effect of corrective splinting on flexion contracture of rheumatoid fingers. *Journal of Hand Therapy, 15*(2), 185-191.

  ○ The authors looked at 22 clients with arthritis and compared the effects of dynamic versus static orthoses to improve function and deformity. Both groups of clients demonstrated improved function and grip strength and decreased contractures. The orthoses were designed for PIP **flexion contracture** management and were worn for a minimum of 6 hours per day.

Level V

- Adams, J., Hammond, A., Burridge, J., & Cooper, C. (2005). Static orthoses in the prevention of hand dysfunction in rheumatoid arthritis: A review of the literature. *Musculoskeletal Care, 3*(2), 85-101.

  ○ The authors conducted a literature review to examine the evidence for immobilization orthoses as an intervention for clients with RA. They cite the results of several studies that indicate that orthoses contribute to decreased pain and inflammation, increased joint stability, and improved function. The authors also attempt to explain how the immobilization orthoses function in relation to the disease process of RA. They mention the limitations of the studies, including the lack of randomized clinical trials and the variability of the disease and its effects on individuals.

- Beasley, J. (2012). Osteoarthritis and rheumatoid arthritis: Conservative therapeutic management. *Journal of Hand Therapy, 25*(2), 163-172.

  ○ This Level V paper states that the goal of an orthosis worn during periods of acute inflammation in the joint helps to reduce joint friction and prevent excessive joint loading limiting joint motion. Excessive movement in unstable arthritic joints can cause increased discomfort and lead to further instability. The author refers to additional studies that have reported that wearing an orthosis decreases pain and increases function during daily activities in patients with arthritis.

- Van der Giesen, F. J., Nelissen, R. G., van Lankveld, W. J., Kremers-Selten, C., Peeters, A. J., Stern, E. B., … Vliet Vlieland, T. P. (2010). Swan neck deformities in rheumatoid arthritis: A qualitative study on the patients' perspectives on hand function problems and finger splints. *Musculoskeletal Care, 8*(4), 179-188.

  ○ This literature review looks at three specific splint designs for deformities commonly seen in clients with RA: ulnar drift, swan neck, and boutonniere. The authors examine the evidence for the use of orthoses in the treatment of each of these deformities and recommend early intervention with orthoses when the deformities are still flexible and easily corrected. They propose an evidence-informed approach to the treatment of clients with RA in which clinicians use their clinical experience and examine the available evidence to make treatment choices.

MIDDLE AND DISTAL PHALANGEAL FRACTURES

Fractures can occur in any of the finger bones (proximal, middle, or distal phalanges). Maintenance of **fracture reduction** (setting of the fractured segments together) is a primary goal of orthotic treatment and may dictate postinjury management, such as limitation of early mobilization of the digit. Use of a custom fabricated digit-based immobilization orthosis is often prescribed to stabilize and protect the bones during the healing process, either with conservative management or following surgery. A hand-based orthosis might be used for proximal phalangeal fractures, especially when multiple digits are involved. (See Chapter 7

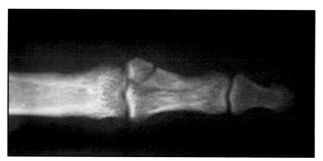

Figure 9-6. X-ray of a middle phalanx fracture.

for more details on orthotic management of proximal phalangeal fractures.) Often, a middle or distal phalangeal fracture can be managed with a digit-based immobilization orthosis. Typically, treatment of nondisplaced fractures of the middle phalanges requires immobilization for 6 to 8 weeks in joint extension. The physician may initially prescribe a digit-based immobilization orthosis to immobilize and protect the fracture or following cast removal for protection. An orthosis provides protection while the client works on regaining joint mobility (Figure 9-6).

Wearing Schedule

The appropriate wearing schedule of a digit-based immobilization orthosis for clients with fractures of the phalanges is full-time for protection and support until the fracture has healed. The preferred positioning for optimal healing is with the PIP and DIP joints in extension. This protects the length of the collateral ligaments, which may shorten if the joints are positioned in flexion. As discussed, fracture healing may take as long as 6 to 8 weeks. An immobilization orthosis might also be used following cast removal and is worn for protection while the client regains finger mobility. The client may be permitted to remove the orthosis for periods of gentle ROM exercises and hygiene if the fracture is stable.

Evidence

Level V

- Cannon, N. M. (2003). Rehabilitation approaches for distal and middle phalanx fractures of the hand. *Journal of Hand Therapy, 16*(2), 105-116.
  - This Level V paper highlights the importance of communication with the referring physician to appreciate the exact location of the fracture site and understanding each type of fracture, fixation, and the course of fracture healing to best handle the clinical picture of affected tissues, edema, and adhesions in the healing finger.
- Hardy, M. A. (2004). Principles of metacarpal and phalangeal fracture management: A review of rehabilitation concepts. *Journal of Orthopaedic and Sports Physical Therapy, 34*(12), 781-799.

  - The author explains the bone-healing process and outlines the various fixation methods for fracture stability. The author also stresses the need for intervention techniques that address the soft tissue injuries related to the bony injuries. Early controlled motion protocols that manage edema, wounds, scarring, and motion are critical. Two important data facts must be obtained from the referring physician: the date of the fracture and the method of fixation. The fracture date starts the bone-healing timetable, and the method of fixation helps to clarify when and how to begin motion. The goals of therapy are to begin early mobilization yet maintain fracture stability.

TUFT FRACTURE

A **tuft fracture** refers to a crush-type injury to the tip of the distal phalanx, resulting in multiple fracture fragments and a very painful fingertip. The tip of the finger should be immobilized in a fingertip protector orthosis for 2 to 3 weeks to allow for healing, but circumferential types of orthoses should be avoided because they may be restrictive and tight (see Figure 9-1C).

FINGER JOINT INJURIES: PROXIMAL INTERPHALANGEAL JOINT COLLATERAL LIGAMENT SPRAIN

Finger sprains are injuries that cause a stretching and tearing of the ligaments of the fingers. The most common causes of finger sprains are sports injuries and falls on the hand. Finger sprains are classified as grades I, II, and III, with grade III being the most significant injury, including a disruption of the ligament fibers and joint instability (Box 9-2).

Wearing Schedule

Grade I collateral ligament injuries of the PIP joint are treated initially by immobilization and edema control. When edema and pain are reduced, **buddy strapping or taping** is commonly used to protect the injured joint, but allow flexion and extension (Figure 9-7). Buddy strapping are fabricated from either Velcro strips (Velcro BVBA) and/or low-temperature thermoplastic material (LTTM). They are applied over the proximal phalanx and over the middle phalanx of the injured digit and the adjacent digit, allowing for motion at both the PIP and DIP joints. A layer of gauze can be placed between the digits to prevent the breakdown of the skin. Apply the buddy strapping loosely to avoid cutting off the blood flow and sensory input to the digit. It is important to have the client perform isolated DIP flexion exercises while wearing the buddy strapping to promote gliding of the lateral bands and the flexor digitorum profundus tendon.

Box 9-2. Classifications of Sprains

- Grade I: Mild sprain with stretching of ligaments with few torn fibers and no loss of joint stability. There may be mild pain with or without swelling.

- Grade II: A greater number of injured ligament fibers with possible joint laxity and usually with marked pain and swelling. There may also be bruising (black and blue) around or in the joint.

- Grade III: Most of the ligament fibers are torn with marked pain, swelling, and bruising, or there is complete disruption (completely torn), resulting in joint instability.

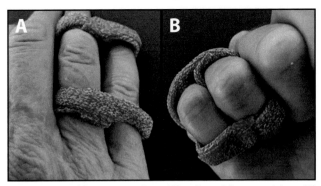

Figure 9-7. Buddy strapping for a PIP collateral ligament injury. (A) Dorsal view and (B) in flexion.

Acute grade II injuries can be treated conservatively with immobilization in slight flexion of the PIP joint for comfort. Physicians commonly prescribe a digit-based extension block orthosis to allow for active flexion but protected remobilization, depending on stability of the joint. The arc of motion can be gradually increased to full extension over 3 to 4 weeks. Buddy strapping might be applied while wearing the extension block orthosis. The orthosis is discontinued after 4 weeks, but buddy tape use is allowed with active flexion and extension and return to full function over 6 to 8 weeks.

Surgery is the typical treatment for grade III injuries to restore joint stability and alignment. Restricted motion with a dorsal extension block orthosis and buddy strapping would be an appropriate postoperative treatment protocol.

Evidence

Level V

- Chinchalkar, S. J., & Gan, B. S. (2003). Management of proximal interphalangeal joint fractures and dislocations. *Journal of Hand Therapy, 16*(2), 117-128.

  ○ This Level V paper proposes an assessment method for the management of complex finger PIP joint injuries based on the directional forces causing the injury and the associated soft tissue structures involved. The rehabilitation program is guided by understanding the injury-causing forces and the associated structures. Common complications and their management are also discussed.

- Leggett, J., & Meko, C. (2006). Acute finger injuries: Part II. Fractures, dislocations, and thumb injuries. *American Family Physician, 73*(5), 827-834.

  ○ The authors discuss various finger and joint injuries and appropriate evaluation methods, primary treatment, and interventions. This article provides an informative review of different injuries to the fingers and has excellent diagrams outlining the anatomy of each injured part.

PROXIMAL INTERPHALANGEAL JOINT FLEXION CONTRACTURES

Differences in the volar surface and dorsal surface of the PIP joint's unique anatomy may contribute to the development of PIP joint flexion contractures following injury. The volar plate of the PIP is made up of strong fibrocartilaginous material and contributes to the stability of the volar joint capsule while also preventing dorsal **dislocations**. Any injury of this structure or close to this structure limits PIP extension because of scar tissue. The scar tissue shortens the fibers of the volar plate and helps to pull the joint into increased flexion.

Wearing Schedule

The most common orthotic treatment for a PIP joint flexion contracture is the **serial cast or serial orthosis**. This refers to a PIP extension orthosis (from LTTM or plaster of Paris) fabricated with the joint held in maximum extension and worn continuously for several days or up to 1 week without removal by the client. When the client returns to the clinic, the orthosis is removed, and joint passive stretching along with modalities (physical agent modalities such as moist heat, paraffin wax, or ultrasound) are performed. The orthosis is remolded in an effort to maintain any new gains and increased PIP extension. The key points for success are maximizing the extension within the orthosis without causing tissue breakdown and also maximizing the uninterrupted duration of wear. The amount of time the joint is held in this position is known as the **total end range time (TERT)**. The LTTM should have memory if it is to be reused every time.

Evidence

Level II

- Glasgow, C., Fleming, J., Tooth, L. R., & Hockey, R. L. (2012). The long-term relationship between duration of treatment and contracture resolution using dynamic orthotic devices for the stiff proximal interphalangeal joint: A prospective cohort study. *Journal of Hand Therapy, 25*(1), 38-47.

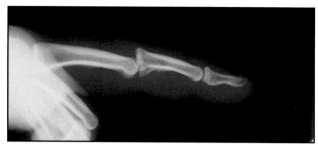

Figure 9-8. X-ray of a dorsal PIP joint dislocation.

Glasgow, C., Fleming, J., Tooth, L. R., & Peters, S. (2012). Randomized controlled trial of daily total end range time (TERT) for Capener splinting of the stiff proximal interphalangeal joint. *American Journal of Occupational Therapy, 66*(2), 243-248.

- ○ The authors looked at the TERT of orthotic wear for 22 clients with extension deficits of the PIP joint who received a dynamic PIP extension orthosis. They then compared the finger ROM in clients who wore the orthosis for 6 to 12 hours per day versus the finger ROM in clients who wore the orthoses for 12 to 16 hours per day. The authors found that most of the clients were unable to adhere to the longer splint wearing regimen of 12 to 16 hours per day. However, wearing a dynamic PIP extension orthosis does help clients regain finger motion, but clients' personal factors and ADL demands need to be taken into account when prescribing a time-based wearing protocol for the orthosis.

- • Prosser, R. (1996). Splinting in the management of proximal interphalangeal joint flexion contracture. *Journal of Hand Therapy, 9*(4), 378-386.

  - ○ The author conducted a study on 20 patients with PIP flexion contractures who received a dynamic orthosis that applied a 250 g force to the distal end of the middle phalanx. Each participant in the study was instructed to wear the orthosis for 8 to 12 hours per 24 hours for 8 weeks, followed by a 2- to 3-week weaning period. Statistical analysis showed that the time of orthotic intervention was the only statistically significant factor affecting outcome. Dynamic splinting was an effective form of treatment for PIP flexion contracture.

- • Flowers, K. R., & LaStayo, P. (1994). Effect of total end range time on improving passive range of motion. *Journal of Hand Therapy, 7*(3), 150-157.

  - ○ The authors of this randomized, clinical trial tested the theory of TERT to see if the amount of passive ROM gained from using an orthosis was related to the amount of time spent in the end-range position. For this purpose, the authors looked at two groups of patients with PIP flexion contractures. One group

of patients wore digital extension casts for 6 days and subsequent casts for 3 days, whereas the other group of patients wore the initial digital extension casts for 3 days and the subsequent casts for 6 days. The results showed that there is a relationship between gains in passive ROM and the amount of time a stiff joint is held in its maximal end-range position.

Level III

- • Uğurlu, Ü., & Özdoğan, H. (2016). Effects of serial casting in the treatment of flexion contractures of proximal interphalangeal joints in patients with rheumatoid arthritis and juvenile idiopathic arthritis: A retrospective study. *Journal of Hand Therapy, 29*(1), 41-50.

  - ○ The authors of this retrospective study sought to evaluate the outcomes of serial casting in the treatment of PIP joint flexion contractures in patients with RA and juvenile idiopathic arthritis. They analyzed the records of 18 patients treated with serial casting. The changes in the finger joints were studied and compared statistically using t-tests. A total of 49 fingers were serially casted with plaster of Paris over a 14-year period. This intervention resulted in significant (26.8 degrees; $P < .001$) reduction in the PIP joint extension loss. Small but statistically significant losses in flexion were associated with these gains ($P < .001$). The authors conclude that, although this was a small retrospective study, serial casting is an effective method to correct flexion contractures in PIP joints in selected patients with arthritis.

VOLAR AND DORSAL PROXIMAL INTERPHALANGEAL JOINT DISLOCATIONS

The most commonly dislocated (separated) joint in the hand is the PIP joint (Figure 9-8). The direction of dislocation is named for the distal bone segment: A dorsal dislocation refers to dorsal displacement of the middle phalanx, whereas a volar dislocation refers to volar displacement of the middle phalanx. A dorsal dislocation is more common than a volar dislocation and can injure the volar plate or cause an avulsion fracture of the middle phalanx.

Wearing Schedule

The treatment following a dorsal dislocation after reduction or realignment of the bone and joint surface is to hold the PIP in an immobilization orthosis in about 30 degrees of flexion for 2 to 4 weeks to allow healing. This position prevents the PIP joint from dislocating with active extension. A dorsal extension block orthosis or a circumferential orthosis is typically fabricated for this condition, and active flexion of the PIP joint is permitted (see Figure 9-1B).

Table 9-1

EXTENSOR TENDON AND FINGER JOINT INJURIES AND ORTHOTIC MANAGEMENT

EXTENSOR TENDON ZONE	ORTHOSIS	WEARING SCHEDULE
I and II (mallet injury)	DIP extension	Full-time for 6 to 8 weeks or per physician orders
III (PIP joint injury)	PIP extension or short arc motion (SAM) protocol	4 to 6 weeks SAM protocol: Gradual increased active flexion with extension orthosis used in between exercises for 6 weeks
Swan neck deformity	Dorsal extension block to PIP joint, allow full flexion	Functional orthosis: Wear full-time as needed during activities
Boutonniere deformity	PIP in full extension	Acute (within 3 weeks of injury): 6 to 8 weeks Chronic (more than 3 weeks past injury): Work toward full PIP extension, then treat as acute injury

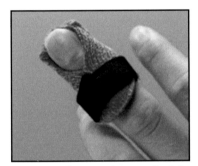

Figure 9-9. Client wearing an orthosis for a mallet injury of the middle finger.

The treatment following a volar dislocation is to hold the PIP joint in full extension in an orthosis for 6 weeks. A volar-based or circumferential orthosis is typically fabricated for this condition.

COMPLEX INJURIES OF THE PROXIMAL INTERPHALANGEAL JOINT

Intra-articular joint injuries are considered complex injuries that involve a fracture of the proximal phalanx on the PIP joint surface. The PIP joint may become unstable if more than 30% of the articular surface is involved. These types of fractures often require surgery and/or dynamic traction orthotic management. This is an advanced orthotic fabrication skill and is not covered in this textbook.

INJURIES TO THE DORSAL DIGITS

Injuries to the dorsal digits, including lacerations, bites, blows, and crush injuries, involve the extensor mechanism and are classified by the extensor tendon zones (Table 9-1).

Box 9-3. Classification of Mallet Injuries

- Type 1: Closed with or without avulsion fracture
- Type 2: Open laceration at or proximal to the DIP joint with loss of tendon continuity
- Type 3: Deep abrasion with loss of skin, subcutaneous cover, and tendon substance
- Type 4:
  ○ Transepiphyseal plate fracture in children
  ○ Hyperflexion injury with fracture of the articular surface of 20% to 50%
  ○ Hyperextension injury with fracture of the articular surface usually greater than 50% and with early or late palmar subluxation of the distal phalanx

Zones I and II

A Zone I injury or **mallet finger** occurs as a result of disruption to the extensor tendon at its attachment on the distal phalanx, causing a flexion deformity of the DIP joint (Figure 9-9). This injury can lead to development of swan neck deformity if left untreated. Disruption of the terminal extensor tendon across the DIP joint transfers all of the extension force to the PIP joint during active extension. This then causes the lateral bands to displace dorsally over the PIP joint, causing a swan neck deformity.

Mallet finger is classified into four types based on its severity (Box 9-3). Zone II injuries occur over the middle phalanx. In this area, the lateral bands are moving in a volar-to-dorsal direction and are merging with fibers of the

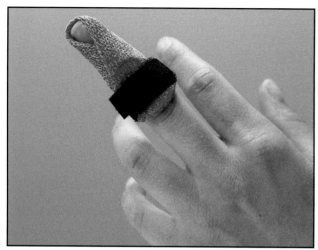

Figure 9-10. Additional orthosis for treatment of a mallet injury.

central slip. These are usually partial lacerations and may be treated like a zone I injury.

Wearing Schedule

Closed mallet fingers or type 1 injuries can be treated with an immobilization orthosis positioning the DIP joint in full extension or slight hyperextension for 6 to 8 weeks, which may include an additional 2 weeks of nighttime use (Figure 9-10). The client must be educated on the importance of keeping the DIP joint extended for the entire treatment period. Active ROM at the PIP joint is allowed.

After 6 to 8 weeks, the fingers should be examined again. If the client can actively extend the DIP joint, orthotic use can be reduced to high-risk times such as sleeping, manual work, or athletic performance. Orthotic management of mallet injuries can be successful even 3 months after injury. Type 2 to 4 zone I and II injuries with associated fractures should be treated surgically.

Other considerations include:

- Take special care to avoid skin blanching, which may lead to skin necrosis if the DIP joint is splinted in slight hyperextension or neutral extension.

- No convincing evidence demonstrates that any splint design is more effective than another.

- The evidence generally supports the continuous wearing of most splints for approximately 6 weeks.

- The choice of splinting material is important to the management of skin problems. A choice of alternative splinting material or lining may be required for sensitive skin and to limit maceration (i.e., skin breakdown due to prolonged exposure to moisture).

- There are recommendations to use a small strip of waterproof or elastic tape positioned from the volar surface of the PIP joint and pull up and over the dorsal finger to the dorsal PIP joint. This tape supports the distal phalanx in the desired extended position, and any orthosis can be molded over. This ensures that the finger is maintained in extension during skin checks and if the client seeks to change from one orthosis to another orthosis.

Evidence

Level I

- Handoll, H. H., & Vaghela, M. V. (2004). Interventions for treating mallet finger injuries. *Cochrane Database of Systematic Reviews*, (3), CD004574.

  ○ This systematic review looked at the effectiveness of various orthotic designs used in orthotic management of mallet fingers, studying the results of four randomized clinical trials. The authors noted various flaws in the different studies, which compared various types of orthoses, both commercially available and custom-made, and surgical intervention. Flaws included small sample sizes and lack of blinding for assessors of data. Conclusions from the review indicate that no one orthotic intervention is superior to others, but each mallet orthosis must be strong enough for prolonged use, typically 6 to 8 weeks, followed by 4 weeks of nighttime use.

- Valdes, K., Naughton, N., & Algar, L. (2015). Conservative treatment of mallet finger: A systematic review. *Journal of Hand Therapy, 28*(3), 237-246.

  ○ The authors of this systematic review examined the evidence from four randomized clinical trials on conservative treatment of mallet finger injuries. Interventions included the use of casting, AlumaFoam (Hartmann USA), thermoplastic, and commercially available stack orthoses. Conclusions include a recommended immobilization duration of about 6 to 8 weeks, with additional weeks of immobilization in cases of persistent lags. Limitations were small sample sizes and the lack of functional outcome measures.

Level II

- O'Brien, L. J., & Bailey, M. J. (2011). Single blind, prospective, randomized controlled trial comparing dorsal aluminum and custom thermoplastic splints to stack splint for acute mallet finger. *Archives of Physical Medicine and Rehabilitation, 92*(2), 191-198.

  ○ The authors of this clinical trial compared the use of a commercial orthosis, the stack orthosis, with dorsal and custom thermoplastic splinting in clients with acute mallet finger injuries. This was a multicenter, randomized, controlled trial including 64 patients. The interventions included the prefabricated stack splint as the control, a dorsal padded aluminum splint, and a custom-made thermoplastic thimble splint. All splints were worn for 8 weeks continuously, with a 4-week graduated withdrawal and exercise program. The results indicate that there was no difference in the primary outcome of **extension lag** between groups at 12 or 20 weeks;

however, the stack and dorsal splints had significant rates of treatment failure compared with none in the thermoplastic group. The authors note that because these orthoses for mallet fingers must be worn continuously for 6 to 8 weeks, and compliance correlates with favorable outcomes, custom-made thermoplastic splints may have the most favorable outcomes.

Level V

- Howell, J., Hirth, M., van Strien, G., Bassini, L., & Devan, D. Mallets around the globe: Does one best method for immobilization and mobilization exist? *ASHT Times, 20*(4), 12-15.

  ◦ The five authors from different parts of the world investigated the current evidence to find support for a specific immobilization treatment of mallet fingers or zone I extensor tendon injuries. They found a general consensus that immobilization is the key intervention. However, there was no consensus on the method or type of immobilization orthosis, whether the PIP needed to be included along with the DIP joint, the optimum duration of wear, the best outcome measures to use, and a specific definition of success, among other issues.

  The authors summarized the best available evidence in the following treatment recommendations:

  - Immobilization of 6 to 12 weeks

  - Skin breakdown and joint pain and stiffness may be issues

  - Later surgical intervention may be an option

  - 20% of all patients have a minimal extension lag

  - A 0.5-mm gap equals a 10-degree lack of terminal extension at the DIP joint

Zones III and IV

Injuries to the dorsum of the digit in zones III and IV affect the part of the extensor mechanism known as the *central slip*. The injury can be closed or open, and the central slip may avulse with or without a bony fragment. A boutonniere deformity may occur as a result of this injury, even 10 to 14 days after the initial injury. Absent or weak active extension of the PIP joint is a positive finding, along with DIP joint hyperextension. Active extension is retained at first by the lateral bands, but the head of the proximal phalanx eventually pushes through the central slip, resulting in volar migration of the lateral bands. This results in loss of extension at the PIP joint and hyperextension at the DIP joint (see Figure 9-4).

Closed injuries to zones III and IV require splinting for 4 to 6 weeks of the PIP joint in extension with the DIP joint left free (Box 9-4).

Box 9-4. Clinical Test for a Boutonniere Deformity

- Place the finger in 90 degrees of flexion at the PIP joint.

- Ask client to extend the PIP joint against resistance.

- The ability to extend against resistance is an indication of central slip continuity.

The term **pseudo-boutonniere** refers to a finger that presents with a PIP flexion contracture but has no DIP joint involvement, meaning the DIP joint can be passively flexed. In a true boutonniere deformity, the lateral bands transmit force toward PIP flexion and DIP hyperextension, and the DIP joint cannot be passively flexed.

Wearing Schedule

Orthotic management for injuries to zones III and IV of the digital extensor mechanism consists of immobilization of the PIP joint in maximum extension for 6 to 8 weeks (see Figure 9-8). A critical component to the therapy program is to leave the DIP joint free in the orthosis and instruct the client in active DIP flexion exercises. This movement helps to stretch the taut oblique retinacular ligament, which will in turn reduce its moment arm, contributing to PIP joint flexion.

Sometimes, static immobilization of the PIP joint is followed by dynamic mobilization to prevent extension lag. Extension lag refers to the lack of full *active* joint extension at the PIP joint, even when passive ROM might be complete. Box 9-5 includes treatment protocols for management of boutonniere deformity.

Considerations

The selection of orthotic design may be determined by the expertise of the clinician in orthotic fabrication and/or the protocol requested by the surgeon. Early DIP joint mobilization exercises are recommended unless the lateral bands are involved. Early active ROM regimes may decrease the incidence of extension lag and adhesions. Regular follow-up in hand therapy is required to monitor and manage possible complications.

Evidence

Level IV

- Page, G., Kahanov, L., & Eberman, L. E. (2014). Active boutonnière deformity in a collegiate football player: A case review. *Athletic Training and Sports Health Care, 6*(5), 237-240.

  ◦ This case report details the treatment of an athlete with an active boutonniere deformity, disruption of

Box 9-5. Management of the Boutonniere Deformity

- Treatment protocol for an acute boutonniere deformity (within 3 weeks past injury). Conservative management of the acute boutonniere deformity consists of the following:
  - PIP joint immobilization at 0 degrees extension for 6 to 8 weeks
  - Initiate active ROM of the PIP joint at 6 to 8 weeks.
  - Use the orthosis in between exercises and at night.
  - Gradually increase flexion activities while monitoring extension lag of the PIP joint.
  - Discharge the orthosis when active ROM is full and client has regained full functional use of the hand.
- Treatment protocol for a chronic boutonniere deformity (more than 3 weeks past injury):
  - Achieve full passive PIP extension using dynamic, static progressive, or serial static splints or casts.
  - With the PIP supported in full extension, perform aggressive DIP flexion exercises to stretch the oblique retinacular ligament and regain DIP flexion.

the central slip causing PIP flexion and DIP hyperextension. The case refers to the injury as an active or acute boutonniere because full PIP extension was maintained both actively and passively. The immediate treatment was full PIP and DIP joint extension for 4 weeks, followed by buddy taping and an oval ring–type PIP joint extension block during activities. The authors stress the importance of full-time splint use immediately, followed by nighttime use if necessary and exercises for active DIP flexion.

Short Arc Motion Protocol for Repaired or Closed Zone III and Zone IV Injuries

The **short arc motion (SAM) protocol** is a rehabilitation treatment protocol for clients following a surgically repaired central slip injury in zones III and IV. Using this protocol, the client receives two orthoses: (1) an immobilization orthosis with the PIP in 0 degrees of extension, and (2) a template exercise orthosis molded to allow 30 degrees of PIP flexion and 20 degrees of DIP flexion (Figure 9-11). The client performs active flexion with the template orthosis and active PIP extension to 0 degrees. The template is remolded each week to allow additional PIP and DIP flexion. Box 9-6 provides a summary of the SAM protocol.

Evidence

Level II

- Evans, R. B. (2010). Early active short arc motion for the closed central slip injury. *Journal of Hand Therapy,* 23(4), e15-e16.
  - The author describes a study of 36 digits with PIP volar dislocations and central slip ruptures treated with a SAM protocol instead of 4 to 6 weeks of PIP joint immobilization. Treatment included PIP extension splinting with active DIP flexion exercises

and regular changes of the PIP positioning in the splint with active motion up to 40 degrees of PIP joint flexion. Results of the study indicate that central slip repairs can tolerate early motion protocols with careful monitoring of positioning and exercises.

Level V

- Evans, R. B., & Thompson, D. E. (1992). An analysis of factors that support early active short arc motion of the repaired central slip. *Journal of Hand Therapy,* 5(4), 187-201.
  - The authors devised a protocol of treatment for repaired central slip ruptures at zone III to combat complications of tendon adherence, extensor tendon lag, and lack of excursion, stiffness, and joint flexion. The exact positioning of the wrist and MCP, PIP, and DIP joints are defined as they relate to tendon excursion, force application, and controlled stress.

FINGERTIP AMPUTATIONS AND TIP INJURIES

Orthoses are commonly provided to protect the sensitive fingertip after amputation or injury. Take care to ensure that strappings are not too restrictive to affect blood flow and sensory input. The orthosis might be a volar, dorsal circumferential, or cap design. The orthosis may require modifications as edema decreases (see Figure 9-1C).

Wearing Schedule

An orthosis to protect the fingertip might be worn full-time except for periods of exercise and desensitization activities. The orthosis should not be too bulky as to interfere with ADL.

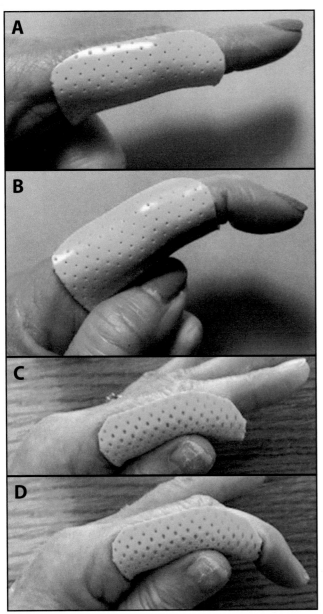

Figure 9-11. SAM protocol for central slip repairs. (A) DIP extension, (B) DIP flexion, (C) PIP extension, and (D) PIP flexion in template orthosis.

Evidence

Level V

- Lemmon, J. A., Janis, J. E., & Rohrich, R. J. (2008). Soft-tissue injuries of the fingertip: Methods of evaluation and treatment. An algorithmic approach. *Plastic and Reconstructive Surgery, 122*(3), 105e-117e.

  ○ This article presents a straightforward assessment of fingertip injuries and reconstructive procedures. The anatomy of the fingertip is presented, and terminology and treatment options are discussed based on the type of injury and the finger involved.

Box 9-6. Summary of SAM Protocol

THREE ORTHOSES

1. PIP and DIP immobilized at 0 degrees extension between exercises
2. Exercise template orthosis with 30 degrees of PIP flexion and 20 degrees of DIP flexion
3. Exercise orthosis with PIP in 0 degrees of extension and DIP free

EXERCISES

- Finger flexion to the template orthosis with active extension to 0 degrees, 10 to 20 reps every 1 to 2 hours
- Modify exercise orthosis and increase flexion by 10 degrees every week

6 WEEKS

- Orthosis at night only and intermittently during the daytime

Biomechanical Concepts of Digit-Based Immobilization Orthoses

Digit-based immobilization orthoses represent a lever system where an individual joint (the PIP or DIP joint) comprises the fulcrum, or axis, and the lever arms cover the proximal and distal bones. The practitioner should follow some basic biomechanical principles when designing finger orthoses to optimize effectiveness and comfort:

- Allow full flexion at the uninvolved MCP joint.

- Make the orthosis as long as possible to optimize mechanical advantage and leverage. For example, oval orthoses for swan neck deformities should span the full length of the proximal and middle phalanges to support the PIP joint fully and prevent hyperextension.

- Fully support the tip of the finger but do not let the orthosis extend past the tip unless it is protecting a pin.

- Mold the orthosis so that it fits the contours of the digit and strap it in place snugly, but do not compress the digital nerves or blood supply.

- Always match strapping to the size of the finger. Completely cover the adhesive hook Velcro with the strapping material. This will prevent the Velcro from snagging on clothing or blankets and will make the straps more secure on the orthosis. The straps should be strategically placed to provide optimal support and

Box 9-7. Digit-Based Orthotic Designs

- Volar: Used for protection and rest
- Dorsal: Used to limit full active extension
- Circumferential:
  - Used for protection and rest and edema control
  - Used to promote full PIP joint extension
- Oval:
  - Function
  - Used to limit full extension and/or flexion
- Fingertip protector: Protects fingertip with high sensitivity or after amputation

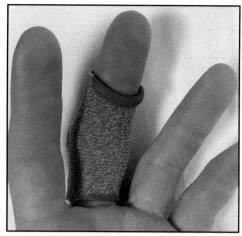

Figure 9-12. A circumferential design covers the volar and dorsal surfaces of the digit. (Reprinted with permission from Anna Osvyannikova.)

comfort and be as wide as possible to distribute forces over a large area. Typically, 1-inch strapping may be cut in half lengthwise. Straps are placed over the bones and not the joints. Two straps are often sufficient to secure finger-based designs. Be sure to round strap corners.

Digit-Based Orthotic Designs

There are many different designs for digit-based orthoses. The specific design will depend on the individual client's clinical condition, current functional needs, specific indications requested by the referring physician, and practitioner preference. The practitioner must consider the anatomy of the digit and involved structures and how an orthosis will influence these structures when determining the most appropriate orthosis design. Other factors to consider include the specific joints involved (PIP and/or DIP joints), the client's size, materials available, and whether a volar, dorsal, or circumferential design is the best option.

This section reviews each design, its main uses, and its advantages and disadvantages. Common designs for digit-based orthoses include the volar, dorsal, and circumferential designs, but some orthoses incorporate both volar and dorsal material, whereas other designs are oval shaped. Box 9-7 reviews the different types of digit-based immobilization orthotic designs.

VOLAR DESIGN

A volar-based digital immobilization orthosis immobilizes the PIP and may also include the DIP joints. This design is commonly used following middle and distal phalangeal fractures (see Figure 9-1A).

CIRCUMFERENTIAL DESIGN

This design immobilizes both volar and dorsal aspects of the digit and can be used for many different injuries (Figure 9-12).

This design can also be used to rest and protect the entire finger following any type of injury or inflammatory period. This design may be more comfortable and feel more protective to a client with a very painful and swollen digit.

DORSAL EXTENSION BLOCK DESIGN

The digit-based dorsal extension block orthosis rests on the dorsal aspect of the proximal, middle, and distal phalanges or any part of these bones. This might also be called an *extension block orthosis*. This design is used to limit full extension while the joint recovers from an injury. Full active flexion is allowed (see Figure 9-1B).

OVAL DESIGN

A figure-of-8 or oval design is an orthosis that positions the PIP joint in slight flexion to prevent hyperextension while allowing full flexion. This is used primarily in fingers with laxity or hyperextensibility of the PIP joint. Keeping the finger in slight flexion adds stability to the joint, aiding functional activities (Figures 9-13).

FINGERTIP PROTECTOR

Fingertip protectors are caps of LTTM used to protect the fingertip after injury or when the fingertip is hypersensitive to touch. These orthoses can be made with or without straps and should be checked for fit regularly because they can become loose if edema decreases in the finger (see Figure 9-1C).

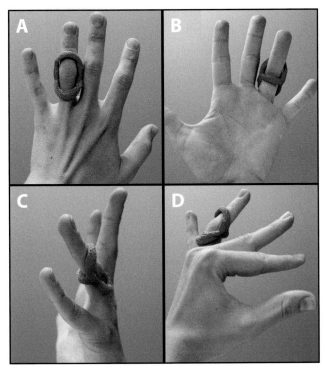

Figure 9-13. Views of the anti-swan neck orthosis for hyperextension of the PIP joint. (A) Dorsal, (B) volar, (C) ulnar, and (D) radial.

VOLAR AND DORSAL COMBINED

A design often used by clinicians to treat mallet injuries is called a *volar-dorsal design*. This starts as a small rectangle of LTTM with one hole punched out. The finger is placed through the hole in the material with the dorsal surface over the middle phalanx and the volar portion under the distal phalanx to support it in slight hyperextension. Care must be taken to avoid stretching the hole as the finger goes through.

Orthotic Fabrication Steps

Orthotic fabrication begins after the practitioner has determined which design is most suited to the client's condition, specific needs, and physician referral specifications. The process begins with designing the pattern, followed by selecting the LTTM, positioning the client, molding the LTTM to the client, fitting and adjusting the orthosis, applying straps, and ending with evaluating the orthosis for fit and comfort. The final step in this process is educating the client on the purpose, wearing schedule, and care of the orthosis.

Refer to the instructional video for detailed step-by-step instructions.

1. Pattern making
   - Simple finger immobilization orthosis
   - Mallet orthosis
   - Anti-swan neck orthosis (figure-of-8, oval design)

Box 9-8. Material Characteristics for Digit-Based Orthoses

- Thickness: Choose 1/12 or 1/16 inch.
- Choose materials with drapability to match contours of fingers.
- Choose materials with memory when frequent adjustments will be needed.
- Choose materials with perforations to help ventilate the skin.
- Be sure to smooth all edges to avoid rubbing in between fingers.

2. Material selection
   - A variety of factors are important to consider when selecting an appropriate LTTM. These include material thickness, degree of conformability and stretch, presence of memory, and material color (Box 9-8).

3. Client positioning
   - The client should be seated with the elbow resting comfortably on table, preferably near the splint pan.
   - The practitioner should have easy access to the client's extremity; often, the corner of the table allows for the best access.
   - The client's digits should be relaxed to allow the material to conform.

4. Molding techniques

5. Finishing techniques: edges and strapping

6. Orthosis check-out
   - Can the client fully flex and extend joints not included in the orthosis? (With the figure-of-8 or anti-swan neck orthosis, check to see if the client can flex the PIP joint but not fully extend the PIP joint.)

     If no, the orthosis is too long or the proximal edge is not flared adequately.
   - Can the client move his or her hand and wrist in all directions without the orthosis interfering with this motion?

     If no, the orthosis is too long or the proximal edge is not flared adequately.
   - Does the client complain of discomfort when moving his or her hand and adjacent fingers in the orthosis?

     If yes, locate the area(s) of discomfort. Some possible solutions:
     - *Flare the distal edge and proximal edges of the orthosis.*
     - *Smooth and round all rough edges.*

Box 9-9. Special Considerations for Special Populations

- Be aware of the weight of the material and choose accordingly.
- Match thinner materials to smaller body parts.
- Explain the orthotic wearing schedule to the client and the caregiver.
- Make sure the client understands how to don and doff the orthosis, and when to wear it.
- Match strap width to body part. Cut straps in half lengthwise or even into thirds for small body parts.

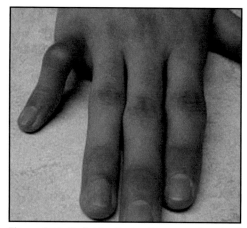

Figure 9-14. Pediatric client with camptodactyly of the little finger. (Reprinted with permission from Jill Peck-Murray.)

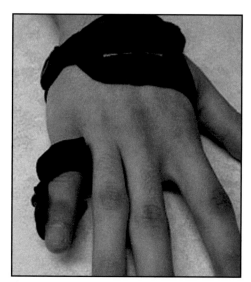

Figure 9-15. Pediatric client with a digit-based orthosis. (Reprinted with permission from Jill Peck-Murray.)

○ Are the corners of the orthosis rounded and smooth?

If no, round and smooth all corners of the orthosis.

○ Are the straps secure and edges rounded?

If no, adjust the straps: No Velcro should be exposed. The straps should be matched to the size of the digit.

○ Are all indentations and pattern marks removed?

If no, use a heat gun to smooth the LTTM. Rubbing alcohol can be used to remove wax pencil marks. Ink cannot be removed, so refrain from using this when drawing your pattern on the LTTM.

○ Remove the orthosis after 5 to 10 minutes and observe the skin. Are there any reddened areas? Does the fingertip feel numb?

If yes, adjust the orthosis by flaring and smoothing edges and/or flaring material away from bony prominences.

○ Review the purpose and care of the digit-based immobilization orthosis with the client. Does he or she understand why he or she is wearing it? When he or she should wear it? How to take care of it?

If no, discuss the wearing schedule and care of the orthosis with the client before he or she leaves the clinic and provide clear written instructions to take home with him or her (refer to the Appendix at the end of the chapter).

SPECIAL CONSIDERATIONS

Box 9-9 outlines special considerations when fabricating digit-based immobilization orthoses for special populations.

Pediatric Clients

Camptodactyly refers to a condition of nontraumatic PIP joint flexion contractures apparent at birth (type I) or later in adolescence (type II) or associated with other syndromes (type III). The condition may be caused by a variety of factors, including positioning in the intrinsic minus position due to nerve palsies and/or increased tone, volar soft tissue shortening, volar capsular tightness, or extrinsic flexor tendon tightness. The condition is most common in the little finger but may also affect the ring and middle fingers. It occurs in females more than in males. Conservative treatment may consist of stretching and the use of orthoses to position the PIP joint in maximal end-range extension. Postoperative management also involves the use of PIP extension orthoses or, if the MCP joint is included in the orthotic design, a hand-based orthosis (Figures 9-14 and 9-15).

Box 9-10. Helpful Hints

- Use thinner materials (1/12 and 1/16 inch) depending on size of client's digit.
- Consider the optimal position of healing of each joint along with the purpose of the orthosis.
  - Mallet injury: DIP extension or hyperextension
  - PIP dorsal dislocation: PIP flexion block
  - PIP volar dislocation: PIP in 0 degrees of extension
  - Anti-swan neck: PIP flexion block
- Match straps to size of digits.
- Make sure uninvolved joints are free to move.
- Use Coban (3M) or strappings to keep in place.
- Use Dycem (Dycem Ltd) inside orthosis to prevent slippage.
- Use tape directly on finger to place fingertip in slight hyperextension before applying mallet orthosis.

Evidence

Level IV

- Netscher, D. T., Staines, K. G., & Hamilton, K. L. (2015). Severe camptodactyly: A systematic surgeon and therapist collaboration. *Journal of Hand Therapy, 28*(2), 167-175.
  - The authors propose a logical treatment plan based on corresponding components of preoperative and intraoperative evaluations of camptodactyly. They conducted a retrospective cohort study design and reviewed 18 consecutively operated digits in 12 patients with camptodactyly affecting the PIP joint. There were five girls and eight boys, averaging 8 years of age (range, 9 months to 15 years) at surgery. They report that their findings indicate that surgery corrected flexion contractures, with a mean postoperative flexion contracture of 3 degrees (range, 0 to 25 degrees) at a mean follow-up of 11 months (range, 3 to 32 months). A total of 15 of the 18 digits achieved full active PIP extension. The authors suggest using a detailed clinical assessment to guide surgical treatment followed by focused therapy to improve flexion contractures in digits with moderate to severe camptodactyly. The authors emphasize that hand therapy is essential to maintain postsurgical treatment of camptodactyly.

Box 9-10 presents helpful hints for the fabrication of digit-based orthoses.

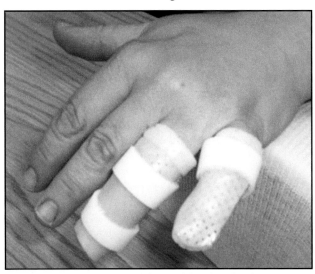

Figure 9-16. Geriatric client with bilateral digit-based orthoses.

Summary

- Knowledge of the key anatomical structures of the digit and how these are affected by a digit-based immobilization orthosis will help the practitioner in determining the most appropriate orthotic design and wearing schedule.
- The goals of a digit-based immobilization orthosis and the specifics of each individual wearing schedule will vary depending on the client's needs and the clinical condition.
- A digit-based immobilization orthosis represents a first-class lever system.
- Digit-based immobilization orthoses can be fabricated using a volar, dorsal, oval, or circumferential design. The design chosen depends on the client's clinical condition, current functional needs, specific indications requested by the referring physician, and practitioner preference.
- Special populations such as pediatric and geriatric clients may require specific orthotic designs or adaptations to achieve the best outcomes with orthoses (Figure 9-16).
- Each orthosis must be molded to the individual anatomy for the best fit. Post-fabrication critique and checkout help identify areas for modification and optimize client comfort.

In Your Client's Shoes

As a practitioner, it is very important to appreciate the effect that an orthosis will have on your client's daily occupations. The digit-based orthosis will most likely interfere with many, if not all, of your client's ADL. You should experience how it feels to wear an orthosis for an extended period of time by wearing one yourself. Now try to complete your normal ADL and instrumental ADL! This experience will enable you to be client centered when using orthoses as an intervention strategy in your practice. You must consider how to instruct your client on the importance of the wearing schedule and the benefits of compliance for maximum benefits.

Suggested Reading

Adams, J., Hammond, A., Burridge, J., & Cooper, C. (2005). Static orthoses in the prevention of hand dysfunction in rheumatoid arthritis: A review of the literature. *Musculoskeletal Care, 3*(2), 85-101.

Beasley, J. (2012). Osteoarthritis and rheumatoid arthritis: Conservative therapeutic management. *Journal of Hand Therapy, 25,* 163-172.

Blazar, P. E., & Steinberg, D. R. (2000). Fractures of the proximal interphalangeal joint. *Journal of the American Academy of Orthopaedic Surgeons, 8*(6), 383-390.

Cannon, N. M. (2003). Rehabilitation approaches for distal and middle phalanx fractures of the hand. *Journal of Hand Therapy, 16*(2), 105-116.

Chan R. K. (2002). Splinting for peripheral nerve injury in upper limb. *Hand Surgery, 7*(2), 251-259.

Chinchalkar, S. J., & Gan, B. S. (2003). Management of proximal interphalangeal joint fractures and dislocations. *Journal of Hand Therapy, 16*(2), 117-128.

Cook, S., Daniels, N., & Woodbridge, S. (2017). How do hand therapists conservatively manage acute, closed mallet finger? A survey of members of the British Association of Hand Therapists. *Hand Therapy, 22*(1), 13-25.

Coppard, B. M., & Lohman, H. (2014). *Introduction to orthotics: A clinical reasoning and problem-solving approach* (4th ed.). St. Louis, MO: Elsevier Mosby.

Evans, R. B. (1994). Early active short arc motion for the repaired central slip. *Journal of Hand Surgery, 19,* 991-997.

Evans, R. B. (1995). Immediate active short arc motion following extensor tendon repair. *Hand Clinics, 2*(3), 483-512.

Evans, R. B. (2010). Early active short arc motion for the closed central slip injury. *Journal of Hand Therapy, 23*(4), e15-e16.

Evans, R. B., & Thompson, D. E. (1992). An analysis of factors that support early active short arc motion of the repaired central slip. *Journal of Hand Therapy, 5*(4), 187-201.

Flowers, K. R., & LaStayo, P. (1994). Effect of total end range time on improving passive range of motion. *Journal of Hand Therapy, 7*(3), 150-157.

Glasgow, C., Fleming, J., Tooth, L. R., & Hockey, R. L. (2012). The long-term relationship between duration of treatment and contracture resolution using dynamic orthotic devices for the stiff proximal interphalangeal joint: A prospective cohort study. *Journal of Hand Therapy, 25*(1), 38-47.

Glasgow, C., Fleming, J., Tooth, L. R., & Peters, S. (2012). Randomized controlled trial of daily total end range time (TERT) for Capener splinting of the stiff proximal interphalangeal joint. *American Journal of Occupational Therapy, 66*(2), 243-248.

Griffin, M., Hindocha, S., Jordan, D., Saleh, M., & Khan, W. (2012). Management of extensor tendon injuries. *Open Orthopaedics Journal, 6*(1), 36-42.

Handoll, H. H., & Vaghela, M. V. (2004). Interventions for treating mallet finger injuries. *Cochrane Database of Systematic Reviews,* (3), CD004574.

Hardy, M. A. (2004). Principles of metacarpal and phalangeal fracture management: A review of rehabilitation concepts. *Journal of Orthopaedic and Sports Physical Therapy, 34*(12), 781-799.

Hirth, M., van Strien, G., Bassini, L., & Devan, D. (2014). Mallet fingers around the globe: Does one best method for immobilisation and mobilisation exist? *ASHT Times, 20*(4), 12-15.

Jacobs, M. A., & Austin, N. M. (2014). *Orthotic intervention for the hand and upper extremity* (2nd ed.). Baltimore, MD: Lippincott Williams & Wilkins.

Kennedy, D., Fiona, W., Carlisle, K., Honeyfield, L., Satchithananda, K., & Vincent, T. (2014). Splinting of the distal interphalangeal joint reduces pain and improves extension at the joint: Results from the splint-OA study. *Journal of Hand Therapy, 27*(3), e1.

Kjeken, I., Smedslund, G., Moe, R. H., Slatkowsky-Christensen, B., Uhlig, T., & Hagen, K. B. (2011). Systematic review of design and effects of splints and exercise programs in hand osteoarthritis. *Arthritis Care & Research, 63*(6), 834-848.

Leggett, J. C., & Meko, C. J. (2006). Acute finger injuries: Part I. Tendons and ligaments. *American Family Physician, 73*(5), 810-816.

Leggett, J. C., & Meko, C. J. (2006). Acute finger injuries: Part II. Fractures, dislocations, and thumb injuries. *American Family Physician, 73*(5), 827-834.

Lemmon, J. A., Janis, J. E., & Rohrich, R. J. (2008). Soft-tissue injuries of the fingertip: methods of evaluation and treatment. An algorithmic approach. *Plastic and Reconstructive Surgery, 122*(3), 105e-117e.

Li-Tsang, C. W., Hung, L. K., & Mak, A. F. (2002). The effect of corrective splinting on flexion contracture of rheumatoid fingers. *Journal of Hand Therapy, 15*(2), 185-191.

Netscher, D. T., Staines, K. G., & Hamilton, K. L. (2015). Severe camptodactyly: A systematic surgeon and therapist collaboration. *Journal of Hand Therapy, 28*(2), 167-175.

O'Brien, L. J., & Bailey, M. J. (2011). Single blind, prospective, randomized controlled trial comparing dorsal aluminum and custom thermoplastic splints to stack splint for acute mallet finger. *Archives of Physical Medicine and Rehabilitation, 92*(2), 191-198.

Page, G., Kahanov, L., & Eberman, L. E. (2014). Active boutonnière deformity in a collegiate football player: A case review. *Athletic Training and Sports Health Care, 6*(5), 237-240.

Porter, B. J., & Brittain, A. (2012). Splinting and hand exercise for three common hand deformities in rheumatoid arthritis: A clinical perspective. *Current Opinion in Rheumatology, 24*(2), 215-221.

Prosser, R. (1996). Splinting in the management of proximal interphalangeal joint flexion contracture. *Journal of Hand Therapy, 9*(4), 378-386.

Ugurlu, Ü., & Özdogan, H. (2016). Effects of serial casting in the treatment of flexion contractures of proximal interphalangeal joints in patients with rheumatoid arthritis and juvenile idiopathic arthritis: A retrospective study. *Journal of Hand Therapy, 29*(1), 41-50.

Valdes, K., Naughton, N., & Algar, L. (2015). Conservative treatment of mallet finger: A systematic review. *Journal of Hand Therapy, 28*(3), 237-246.

Valdes, K., & Marik, T. (2010). A systematic review of conservative interventions for osteoarthritis of the hand. *Journal of Hand Therapy, 23,* 334-351.

Van der Giesen, F. J., Nelissen, R. G., van Lankveld, W. J., Kremers-Selten, C., Peeters, A. J., Stern, E. B., ... Vliet Vlieland, T. P. (2010). Swan neck deformities in rheumatoid arthritis: A qualitative study on the patients' perspectives on hand function problems and finger splints. *Musculoskeletal Care, 8*(4), 179-188.

Varney, A. C. (2013). Hand fractures. In C. Cooper (Ed.), *Fundamentals of hand therapy: Clinical reasoning and treatment guidelines for common diagnoses of the upper extremity* (2nd ed., pp. 361-382). St. Louis, MO: Mosby.

Vipond, N., Taylor, W., & Rider, M. (2007). Postoperative splinting for isolated digital nerve injuries in the hand. *Journal of Hand Therapy, 20*(3), 222-231.

Test Your Knowledge

SHORT ANSWER

1. Identify the anatomical landmarks associated with a digit-based orthosis.

2. Describe the extensor zones of the digits and the appropriate orthosis for an injury at each zone.

3. Describe the pulley system of each digit.

4. List the movements of the digits and the muscles that perform these movements.

5. Draw the extensor mechanism in a simplified format or line drawing.

6. Draw the flexor tendons in a simplified format or line drawing.

7. Describe the orthotic wearing schedule for a mallet injury and for a boutonniere injury.

8. List the different orthotic designs for a mallet orthosis.

9. Identify the anatomical landmarks associated with a digit-based orthosis.

10. Describe the biomechanical principles that apply to a digit orthosis.

11. Describe the SAM protocol for a zone III injury.

12. List the appropriate orthotic design and LTTM suitable for the following:

    ◦ A 45-year-old woman with drooping of the ring finger DIP joint

    ◦ A 16-year-old boy with a collateral injury of his middle finger PIP joint

    ◦ A 35-year-old man with an inability to straighten the PIP joint

    ◦ A 27-year-old woman with a laceration on the lateral side of the little finger

MULTIPLE CHOICE

13. What type of lever system does a digit-based orthosis represent?

    a. Third-class

    b. First-class

    c. Second-class

    d. Fourth-class

14. What will occur if the lever system represented by a digit-based orthosis is not balanced?

    a. The digit will lock into a flexed position.

    b. The digits will not be able to move fully.

    c. The elbow will not be able to flex fully.

    d. The digit will not be supported properly.

15. Which of the following anatomic structures would not be included in a digit-based immobilization orthosis?

    a. The olecranon

    b. The middle phalanx

    c. The volar plate

    d. The collateral ligaments

16. What is the recommended method of preventing pressure on a bony prominence when fabricating a digit-based orthosis?

    a. Pad the area after molding the orthosis.

    b. Flare the thermoplastic material away from the area after molding the orthosis.

    c. Pad the area prior to molding the orthosis.

    d. Make the forearm component of the orthosis as long as possible.

17. What movement should the client not be able to do while wearing a digit-based orthosis for a boutonniere deformity?

    a. Flex the PIP joint

    b. Flex the thumb IP joint

    c. Flex the wrist

    d. Extend the wrist

18. What will the client experience if the straps are not properly positioned on his or her mallet orthosis?

    a. The client will be able to move the thumb fully.

    b. The client will be able to flex the PIP joint.

    c. The client will be able to flex the DIP joint.

    d. The client will have difficulty getting the orthosis on and off.

19. Why is it important to clear the distal palmar crease completely when fabricating a digit-based orthosis?

    a. This allows for full MCP flexion in the orthosis.

    b. This allows for full PIP and DIP joint mobility in the orthosis.

    c. This allows for full wrist mobility in the orthosis.

    d. This allows for full extension of the digits in the orthosis.

20. What is the primary advantage of the dorsal digit-based orthosis design?

    a. It allows for more sensory input in the finger.

    b. It prevents digital extension.

    c. It allows for more digital mobility.

    d. It is easier to fabricate than volar designs.

21. Why might a practitioner choose a circumferential digit-based design over a volar or dorsal design?

    a. When a client needs edema control as well as support.

    b. When a client has difficulty putting the orthosis on.

    c. When a client needs light support for function.

    d. When a client needs to wear the orthosis only at night.

CASE STUDIES

Case Study 1

James is a 43-year-old, right-hand–dominant auto mechanic who lost the tip of his left middle finger distal to the DIP joint while working on a car engine. He was seen in the emergency room, where the wound was closed with sutures. The tip was not able to be replanted because it was extremely dirty. James was referred to a specialist for further treatment and suture removal. There, he received a prescription for a visit to therapy for desensitization and a custom-fitted orthosis. James states that he is in a great deal of discomfort and keeps bumping his finger on objects. He is reluctant to look at the injured hand.

James presents for therapy with a prescription that reads:

Middle finger tip amputation, right hand:

1. *Evaluate and treat.*

2. *Provide tip orthosis.*

3. *Sensory reeducation and desensitization.*

Your assessment:

James presents to therapy for his evaluation and for a custom-fitted tip protector orthosis for the sensitive left middle finger. The left middle finger displays mild erythema and swelling throughout. Active ROM is limited: MCP extension/flexion is 0/60, and PIP extension/flexion is 20/60. No motion is noted at the DIP joint, which is swollen and painful. Pain was evaluated using the visual analog scale and rated as 8/10 and throbbing. James lives with his wife and two children and hopes to be able to return to work, but only when he is ready.

Using different clinical reasoning approaches, answer the following questions about this client and the prescribed orthosis.

Procedural Reasoning

1. What client factors are important to consider when determining the most suitable orthotic design for this client?

2. Which digit-based immobilization orthotic design would be most appropriate for this client? Why?

3. What LTTM properties are important to consider?

4. Describe the instructions you would give this client on:
   - How to care for the orthosis
   - Wearing schedule
   - Precautions
   - Exercises/activities

Pragmatic Reasoning

5. What resources are available to fabricate this orthosis (time, materials, expertise)?

6. Are you able to clearly document the need for this orthosis?

7. Does evidence-based practice support the use of this orthosis for this client's diagnosis?

Interactive Reasoning

8. What are the client's goals and valued occupations?

9. What impact will the client's injury and use of the orthosis have on his ADL?

Conditional Reasoning

10. What factors will influence this client's compliance to the wearing schedule of this orthosis?

Narrative Reasoning

11. How does this condition and, more specifically, this orthotic intervention affect this client's valued occupations?

12. What activities is this client most concerned about?

Ethical Reasoning

13. Does the client understand the need for the orthosis?

14. Does the client have the resources to be able to pay for the orthosis (as applicable)?

15. What other options are available to this client if he lacks the resources necessary to pay for the orthosis?

16. Write one short-term goal (1 to 2 weeks) and one long-term goal (6 to 8 weeks) for this client.

Case Study 2

Steven is a 43-year-old, right-hand–dominant professor of English studies at a local university who injured his right digit II at the DIP joint while playing with his children in the park. Steven states he caught a wildly thrown ball and it hit his finger. He was seen at the local urgent care center because he could not straighten the tip of his finger. Steven was diagnosed with a right digit II or index mallet injury. He now presents for therapy with a prescription that reads:

Right mallet, digit II:

1. *Evaluate and treat.*

2. *Provide appropriate orthosis.*

3. *Active ROM exercises.*

Your assessment:

Steven's right digit II is flexed at the DIP joint, and Steven is unable to active extend it. He has not been compliant with the urgent care physician's support and wrap and removed it to take a shower. The digit is not swollen or red. PIP and MCP flexion and extension of the involved digit are within normal limits. Steven denies any numbness, tingling, or other sensory symptoms in his right digit.

Steven is a single father with two middle school–aged children. He is concerned about being able to perform his routine of household ADL, including caring for the children, preparing meals, supervising after-school activities, shopping, and completing other chores around the house. He is not as concerned about his work activities because he mostly gives lectures and reads student papers and assignments.

Using different clinical reasoning approaches, consider the following questions about this client and the prescribed orthosis. Some questions may be directed more toward the client, and some questions may be directed more toward you as the practitioner for reflection.

Procedural Reasoning

1. What client factors are important to consider when determining the most suitable orthotic design for this client?

2. Which digit-based immobilization orthotic design would be most appropriate for this client? Why?

3. What LTTM properties are important to consider?

4. Describe the instructions you would give this client on:
   ◦ How to care for the orthosis
   ◦ Wearing schedule
   ◦ Precautions
   ◦ Exercises/activities

Pragmatic Reasoning

5. What resources are available to fabricate this orthosis (time, materials, expertise)?

6. Are you able to clearly document the need for this orthosis?

7. Does evidence-based practice support the use of this orthosis for this client's diagnosis?

Interactive Reasoning

8. What are the client's goals and valued occupations?

9. What impact will the client's injury and use of the orthosis have on his ADL?

Conditional Reasoning

10. What factors will influence this client's compliance to the wearing schedule of this orthosis?

Narrative Reasoning

11. How does this injury and, more specifically, this orthotic intervention affect this client's valued occupations?

12. What activities is this client most concerned about?

Ethical Reasoning

13. Does the client understand the need for the orthosis?

14. Does the client have the resources to be able to pay for the orthosis (as applicable)?

15. What other options are available to this client if he lacks the resources necessary to pay for the orthosis?

16. Write one short-term goal (1 to 2 weeks) and one long-term goal (6 to 8 weeks) for this client.

Appendix

STUDENT ASSIGNMENTS

1. Define all of the key terms used in this chapter.

2. Draw the dorsal mechanism on a glove.

3. Draw the volar pulley system on a glove.

4. As an occupational therapy practitioner, you must provide your client with detailed instructions for wearing and caring for his or her orthosis. This document must be required for the client's official records and insurance payments. Select one of the digit-based orthotic designs from this chapter and prepare a client-centered handout for wearing this orthosis. Base your client description on one of the two case studies in this chapter. Include the following in the handout:
   ◦ A description/name of the orthosis
   ◦ An outline of the wearing schedule (remember this will vary depending on the client's condition)
   ◦ A description of how to clean and care for the orthosis
   ◦ Instructions on what the client should be aware of when wearing the orthosis (red areas on skin, pain, increased swelling, etc.)
   ◦ Contact information and follow-up instructions

5. Prepare a case study of a client requiring a digit-based immobilization orthosis. Use one of the evidence-based resources cited in the chapter to support your orthotic intervention. Summarize the research and explain the outcomes of the study.

6. As an occupational therapy practitioner, it will be interesting and informative for you to spend an extended period wearing an orthosis to appreciate the effect that an orthosis will have on your client's daily occupations. Wear a digit-based orthosis designed by your lab partner for a 24-hour period. Take note of how it feels to have one body part immobilized. Elaborate in paragraphs on the following:

   ○ Describe the orthosis, material used, positioning, and typical diagnosis for this particular orthosis. (Which digit was splinted, when did you wear it, what did you do with it on?)

   ○ Comfort and ease of use: Is it easy to take on and off? Does the orthosis fit under clothing? Are there any pressure areas? What needs to be modified and how?

   ○ Personal and public image: Does the orthosis attract attention in public? Does the orthosis attract attention in your family? How did this make you feel, even as a class assignment?

   ○ Functionality: How were you able to function with the orthosis? Was the position helpful or harmful? What would the typical wearing schedule be for a client with the typical need for this orthosis? What instructions should be given to the typical client with the need for this orthosis?

   ○ How does this change your appreciation of what your clients are experiencing with their orthoses?

7. Complete the check-out form on the next page.

Multiple Choice Answer Key

13. b

14. d

15. a

16. c

17. a

18. c

19. a

20. b

21. a

Digit-Based Orthosis Check-Out Form

*(This can be used for faculty to evaluate students' completed orthoses,
as well as for students to reference when evaluating their own completed orthosis.)*

Fabricate one of the orthotic designs for a digit-based orthosis on your classmate and complete the following check-out form:

Name of Orthosis:

Purpose of Orthosis:

Design/Function

_____ The digit is in the correct position.

_____ Uninvolved joints can move freely: MCP, PIP or DIP.

_____ The orthosis supports the appropriate length of the digit.

_____ The orthosis is half the width of the digit.

Straps/Orthosis Appearance

_____ The straps are in the correct position.

_____ The Velcro hook is secure and covered completely.

_____ The orthosis edges are smooth with rounded corners.

_____ The proximal edge is flared slightly.

_____ The orthosis does not cause impingement or pressure areas.

_____ The orthosis is free of fingerprints, pen marks, or indentations.

Part Three

ADVANCED ORTHOTIC CONCEPTS

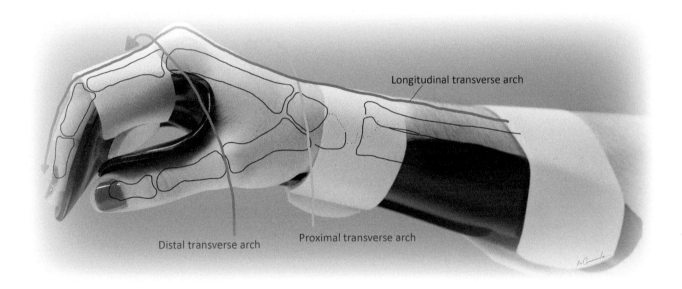

Longitudinal transverse arch

Distal transverse arch

Proximal transverse arch

CHAPTER 10

Orthoses for Tendon Management

Key Terms

Adhesion	Gliding	Pulley ring
Dorsal blocking orthosis	Immediate controlled active motion (ICAM)	Relative motion orthosis or yoke orthosis
Duran (modified)		
Early active motion	Intrinsic healing	Vincula
Excursion	Juncturae tendinum	Wide awake local anesthesia no tourniquet (WALANT)
Extrinsic healing	Kleinert	

Learning Outcomes

Upon completion of this chapter, you will be able to:

1. Describe the healing process for flexor and extensor tendons following surgical repair.

2. Describe the orthoses used for flexor and extensor tendon rehabilitation.

3. Identify pertinent anatomical structures and biomechanical principles involved in the fabrication of a dorsal blocking orthosis and apply concepts to orthotic design and fabrication.

4. Design patterns for orthoses for flexor tendon and extensor tendon rehabilitation protocols.

5. After reviewing the instructional videos:

   a. Outline the steps involved in the fabrication of a dorsal blocking orthosis.

   b. Outline the steps involved in the fabrication of a relative motion orthosis.

   c. Complete the molding and fabrication steps of the above orthoses.

   d. Evaluate the fit and function of a completed orthosis for flexor or extensor tendon management and identify and address all areas needing adjustment.

6. Identify elements of a client education program following provision of a dorsal blocking and relative motion orthosis.

Schofield, K., & Schwartz, D. *Orthotic Design and Fabrication for the Upper Extremity: A Practical Guide* (pp 193-210).

Figure 10-1. (A) Flexor tendons zones. (B) Extensor tendons zones.

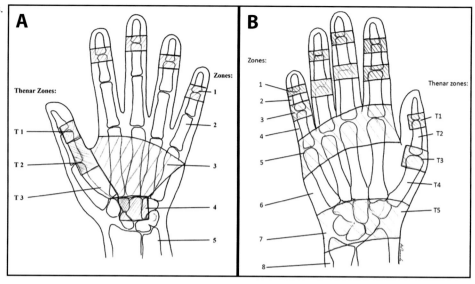

Introduction

Specialized rehabilitation protocols, including custom orthoses, are necessary following injury and surgical repair of the extrinsic flexor and extensor tendons due to the intricate anatomical structures through which these tendons move and glide. Tendon injuries on the volar and dorsal hand and forearm are commonly associated with concurrent soft tissue injury and postoperative edema and require proper surgical technique and supervised therapeutic interventions, including specific orthotic designs. This chapter will provide a brief discussion on flexor and extensor tendon anatomy and tendon healing, biomechanical principles, and the common rehabilitation approaches used following tendon injury and repair. Readers are encouraged to seek additional resources on tendon injuries and postoperative management.

Tendon Anatomy and Healing

A thorough understanding of tendon anatomy, wound-healing principles, and the importance of controlled movement and stress application to a healing tendon is critical. In order for the practitioner to optimize functional outcomes following repair of tendon injuries, several factors must be considered, including the design, fabrication, application, and modification of orthoses used during rehabilitation. These principles should also be considered throughout the recovery period because the client's condition may change and require additional interventions.

FLEXOR TENDON ANATOMY

The flexor tendons in the hand enter the hand under the transverse carpal ligament, within the carpal tunnel. The four tendons of the flexor digitorum profundus (FDP) lie deep to the four tendons of the flexor digitorum superficialis (FDS) and the flexor pollicis longus (FPL) tendon. The FDP tendons continue deep to the FDS tendons in the palm and digits. The FDS tendon splits into two slips at the level of the proximal phalanx, and both slips converge to insert onto the base of the middle phalanx. The FDP runs between the two slips of the FDS and courses distally and inserts onto the base of the distal phalanx. The FDS flexes the metacarpophalangeal (MCP) and proximal interphalangeal (PIP) joints; the FDP flexes the distal interphalangeal (DIP) joint and assists in PIP and MCP joint flexion. The FPL is part of the deep layer of muscles in the forearm and is the sole muscle that flexes the thumb interphalangeal (IP) joint.

As the FDS and FDP run under the transverse carpal ligament and into the palm from their origin in the forearm, they are surrounded by a synovial bursa. This bursa is filled with synovial fluid that provides lubrication and nutrition to the tendons and allows the tendons to glide without friction. In the digits, the FDS and FDP run together in a synovial sheath that is surrounded by a series of pulleys (see Figure 2-31). These pulleys position the FDS and FDP close to the axis of joint motion during active movement and optimize flexion of the PIP and DIP joints. If the pulleys are damaged, they might also need surgical repair, and therapists will fabricate a "**pulley ring**" of thermoplastic material to protect this repair. The A2 and A4 pulleys have been identified as being the most important to prevent bowstringing of the tendons, and these may be repaired when injured, requiring additional protection.

EXTENSOR TENDON ANATOMY

Chapter 2 provides a detailed description of extensor tendon anatomy from the fingertips proximally to the MCP joints (zones I through IV). This section will describe the anatomy of the extensor tendons in zones V through VII (Figure 10-1; Box 10-1).

Box 10-1. Tendon Zones of Injury

FLEXOR TENDON ZONES

- Zone 1: Insertion of FDS on middle phalanx to insertion of FDP on distal phalanx
- Zone II: Area where FDS and FDP travel together in the tendon sheath from the A1 pulley to the insertion of the FDS; commonly referred to as *no man's land* (see Chapter 8)
- Zone III: Area between distal border of carpal tunnel to the A1 pulley
- Zone IV: Area where the flexor tendons are covered by the transverse carpal ligament (carpal tunnel)
- Zone V: Proximal border of the transverse carpal ligament to the musculotendinous junction in the forearm

EXTENSOR TENDON ZONES

- Zone I: Insertion of the ED tendon on the distal phalanx
- Zone II: Distal to the insertion of the central slip on the middle phalanx to the area where the lateral bands converge to form the common terminal extensor tendon
- Zone III: Central slip over the PIP joint
- Zone IV: Area over proximal phalanx
- Zone V: Area over MCP joints, including sagittal bands, common extensor tendon, and part of the juncturae tendinae
- Zone VI: Area over the metacarpal shafts, juncturae tendinum, and common extensor tendon
- Zone VII: Area of extensor retinaculum and all six dorsal compartments under it; includes all wrist, thumb, and digit extensor tendons

The extrinsic extensor tendons to the digits and thumb run on the dorsal aspect of the wrist under the extensor retinaculum (see Chapter 1) and course distally to the digits. These include the extensor digitorum (ED), extensor indicis proprius, extensor digiti minimi, extensor pollicis longus, extensor pollicis brevis, and abductor pollicis longus. The wrist extensors also run under the extensor retinaculum and include the extensor carpi radialis longus, extensor carpi radialis brevis, and extensor carpi ulnaris.

The **juncturae tendinum** (tendinous slips that connect the ED tendons) are located just proximal to the MCP joints and help to stabilize the ED tendons over the MCP joints during active finger flexion and assist in extension of adjacent digits. These structures are important to consider when designing orthoses following extensor tendon repair.

ZONES OF INJURY

The volar and dorsal aspects of the hand and wrist are divided into distinct flexor and extensor tendon zones of injury. There are five flexor zones and seven extensor zones. These zones help identify locations of the specific anatomical structures and help guide the practitioner in determining the most suitable rehabilitation regime for the client, including the type and design of the orthosis needed. For flexor and extensor zones, the odd-numbered zones are located over joints (DIP, PIP, MCP, and wrist), and the even-numbered zones over the shafts of the bones (distal, middle, and proximal phalanges; metacarpals; radius and ulna).

TENDON HEALING

After surgical repair, tendons heal by two primary means: **intrinsic** and **extrinsic healing**. Intrinsic healing occurs as a result of nutrition from the synovial fluid surrounding the tendon within the sheath and formation of new tendon cells at the repair site. Extrinsic healing occurs as a result of blood supply from the **vincula** (small vessels arising from the digital arteries) and deposition of collagen cells on the outside of the tendon at the repair site. The application of early controlled movement of a tendon following repair is thought to facilitate intrinsic healing and limit the amount and organization of collagen deposition at or near the repair site, thus minimizing **adhesion** development.

Tendon healing can be classified in three stages: early, intermediate, and late. The strength of the tendon repair (the amount of force the tendon can withstand without rupture), referred to as *tensile strength*, is at its weakest from 0 to 3 weeks following repair (early stage) and becomes progressively stronger from weeks 3 to 6 as more collagen is laid down at the repair site (intermediate stage). It is not until the late stage (week 12 and beyond) that the tendon can withstand normal tensile forces. It is during this phase that the tendon continues to remodel in response to the forces placed on it. Collectively, the first 3 weeks should be aimed at protecting the tendon from undo stress and excessive movement, followed by more controlled stress (initiation of active movement to increase excursion and force) on

Box 10-2. Goals of Orthotic Intervention Following Tendon Injuries and Repair

- Protect newly repaired tendons from stress and excessive movement to promote healing.
- Promote early protected active and/or passive movement of newly repaired tendons to prevent development of adhesions and joint contractures.
- Promote early protected active and/or passive movement of repaired tendons to facilitate optimal healing and tensile strength.

the tendon from weeks 3 to 6. Six weeks post-tendon repair and beyond is characterized by progressive tendon gliding exercises and graded application of resistance to facilitate remodeling and improve tensile strength.

Goals for Use of Orthoses Following Tendon Injury and Repair

The goal of an orthosis following injury and repair of either a flexor or extensor tendon will vary depending on the individual client and his or her condition, the physician orders, and the expected functional outcomes. Box 10-2 presents a summary of the goals of orthotic intervention following tendon repair.

Tendon Rehabilitation Approaches

Thorough knowledge of the different rehabilitation protocols that are typically used following surgical tendon repair is essential to a practitioner when fabricating an orthosis as part of a tendon rehabilitation program. In particular, the practitioner must know the location or zone of injury (see discussion earlier in this chapter), the strength of the repair, the number of suture strands used at the repair site, and involvement of other structures such as a nerve or artery. Close communication with the referring surgeon is essential to guide the rehabilitation program and optimize the client's outcomes. Further, the practitioner must account for specific client factors that may influence the rehabilitation regime chosen (e.g., age, presence of edema, wound-healing complications, ability to adhere to a strict rehabilitation protocol, or injury to other structures) and adjust the orthosis and regime components accordingly.

FLEXOR TENDON PROTOCOLS

This section describes the three most common rehabilitation protocols used following flexor tendon injury and repair. Orthotic intervention is critical following repair in all zones of injury. Although the protocols differ, the design of the orthosis used is essentially the same. The differences are as follows:

- The position of the joint(s) in the orthosis
- The length of time the orthosis is used
- The exercises the client performs within the orthosis

Typically, the client will be seen in the first week following surgery. The bulky postoperative bandaging is removed by the clinician, and wound care needs are addressed. Then, new dressings are applied and kept in place with a stockinette sleeve. The low-temperature thermoplastic material (LTTM) orthosis can be molded directly over this sleeve (Figure 10-2A through D).

Immobilization

Immobilization is a protocol that is typically used for children younger than 10 years and for those clients who cannot adhere to a detailed rehabilitation regime due to impaired cognition or other factors that may affect compliance. The affected hand and wrist are immobilized in a **dorsal blocking orthosis** or extension restriction orthosis with the wrist, MCP, PIP, and DIP joints included for 3 to 4 weeks. The wrist is positioned between 0 and 10 degrees of extension (check with referring physician), the MCP joints at 40 to 50 degrees of flexion, and the PIP/DIP joints in extension (Figure 10-3). A custom orthosis or a cast may be used, depending on the client's particular needs. Following the initial immobilization period, the orthosis may be modified to bring the wrist to neutral or slight extension, and passive and/or active tendon gliding exercises can begin (Table 10-1). Development of adhesions (scar tissue at the site of repair, causing loss of gliding and movement of the involved tendon[s] and joint stiffness) is common during the immobilization period, especially if there is concurrent injury to other structures such as a bone fracture.

Early Passive Motion

Early passive motion is an approach that was developed over 35 years ago in an attempt to address the frequent development of dense adhesions specifically within zone II (see Box 10-1). This approach involves early passive movement of the repaired tendon(s) to minimize development of scar adhesions and facilitate tendon healing. This protocol was initially based on the theory that 3 to 5 mm of tendon gliding and excursion can decrease the risk of adhesion development. The **Kleinert** and modified **Duran** protocols are based on this theory. A dorsal blocking, extension restriction orthosis is used with the wrist in 10 degrees of extension (wrist position may depend on the surgeon's

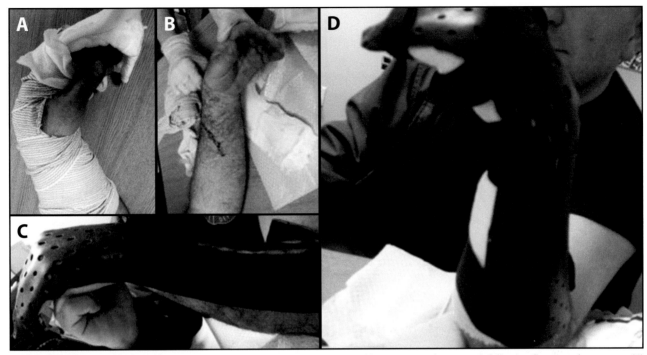

Figure 10-2. (A) Client seen post-flexor tendon surgery in bulky dressings. (B) Addressing wound care needs following flexor tendon surgery. (C) Applying the dorsal blocking orthosis for a flexor tendon injury. (D) Dorsal blocking orthosis positions client in wrist and MCP joint flexion.

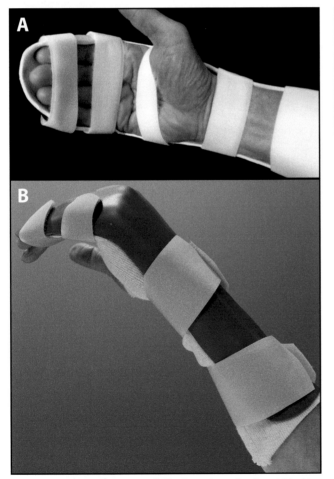

Figure 10-3. (A) Volar view and (B) ulnar view of a dorsal blocking orthosis in wrist and MCP joint flexion.

Table 10-1	
EARLY PASSIVE MOTION EXERCISES	
All of these exercises are done within the dorsal blocking orthosis 10 times every 1 to 2 hours during the day.	
PIP flexion and extension with the DIP joint relaxed	Figures 10-4A, B
DIP joint flexion and extension with the PIP joint relaxed	Figure 10-4C
Combined PIP and DIP joint flexion with the MCP in extension	Figure 10-4D
Combined MCP, PIP, and DIP joint flexion	Figure 10-4E
Active PIP and DIP joint extension to the limits of the dorsal block orthosis	Figure 10-4F

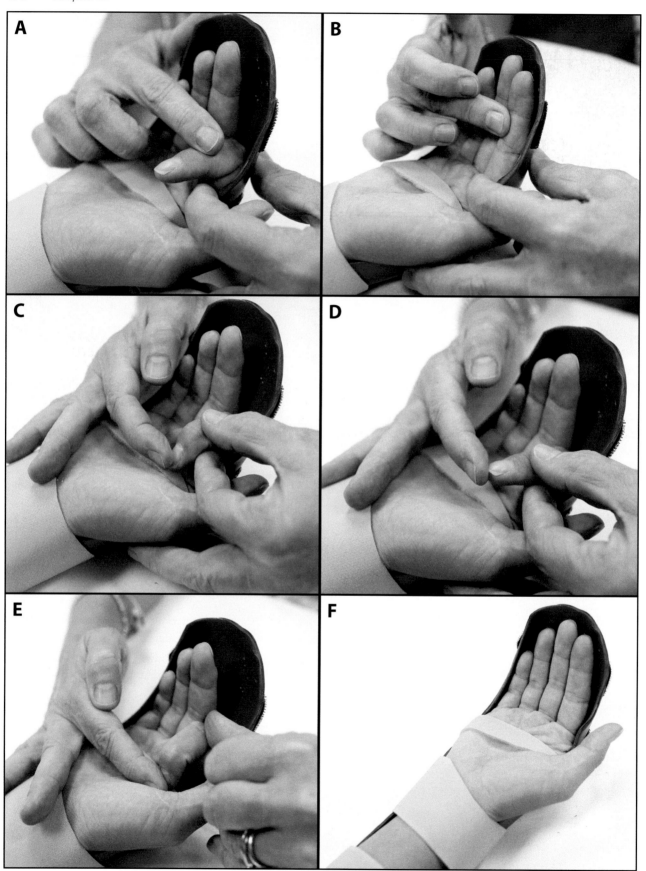

Figure 10-4. Exercises for flexor tendon rehabilitation postsurgery. (A) PIP joint flexion and extension with the DIP joint relaxed. (B) DIP joint flexion and extension with the PIP joint relaxed. (C) Combined PIP and DIP joint flexion with the MCP in extension. (D) Combined MCP, PIP, and DIP joint flexion. (E) Combined MCP, PIP, and DIP joint flexion. (F) Active PIP and DIP joint extension to the limits of the dorsal block orthosis.

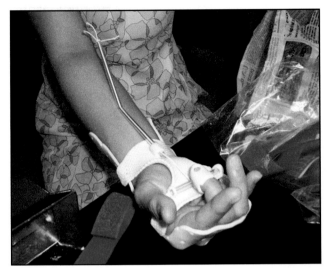

Figure 10-5. Elastic thread holding finger in flexion within the Kleinert orthosis.

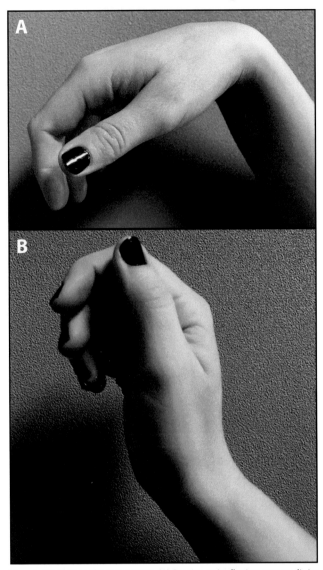

Figure 10-6. Tenodesis exercises. (A) Passive wrist flexion causes digits to passively extend. (B) Active wrist extension creates passive digit flexion and positioning of the thumb to allow for prehension.

preference), the MCP joints at 50 degrees of flexion, and the PIP/DIP joints in full extension. The client performs passive digit flexion exercises within the orthosis 10 to 20 times per hour during the day (see Table 10-1). The Modified Duran protocol uses a strap to position the IP joints in extension between exercises and at night. The Kleinert protocol also includes elastic traction on the involved digit(s) that holds the digit(s) in flexion, and the client performs active extension against the resistance of the elastic traction followed by passive flexion (Figure 10-5). Although both protocols are used in current clinical practice, the Modified Duran protocol is generally favored over the Kleinert protocol due to the heightened risk of PIP flexion contractures with the latter regime. The choice of rehabilitation approach ultimately depends on the referring surgeon's preference.

Early Active Motion

Early active motion is an approach to tendon rehabilitation that differs from both the early passive motion and immobilization regimes. The most notable difference is initiation of early active contraction of the muscle-tendon unit to achieve more natural gliding and excursion at the repair site. This regime requires a strong surgical repair (at least four strands, sometimes six), an experienced practitioner, a motivated and compliant client, and minimal edema. Clients who present with concurrent injury to other structures (such as a fracture, nerve, or artery) are generally not suitable candidates for this protocol. It is ultimately the referring surgeon's decision to initiate active motion following tendon repair. A variety of orthoses are used with this approach. The easiest and most common is a dorsal blocking orthosis with the wrist positioned in neutral to slight extension, the MCP joints at 50 to 60 degrees of flexion, and the PIP/DIP joints in full extension (see Figure 10-3). The client performs prescribed active and passive exercises within the orthosis and removes it for tenodesis exercises

(Figure 10-6). Another protocol features a hinged dorsal blocking orthosis, which allows limited movement at the wrist. This enables the client to perform the tenodesis exercises within the orthosis (Figure 10-7).

Evidence

Level III

- Frueh, F. S., Kunz, V. S., Gravestock, I. J., Held, L., Haefeli, M., Giovanoli, P., & Calcagni, M. (2014). Primary flexor tendon repair in zones 1 and 2: Early passive mobilization versus controlled active motion. *Journal of Hand Surgery, 39*(7), 1344-1350.

  ○ This retrospective study compared flexor tendon repairs in zones I and II using early passive mobilization and early active motion protocols. A total of 159 digits were available for analysis. A statistically

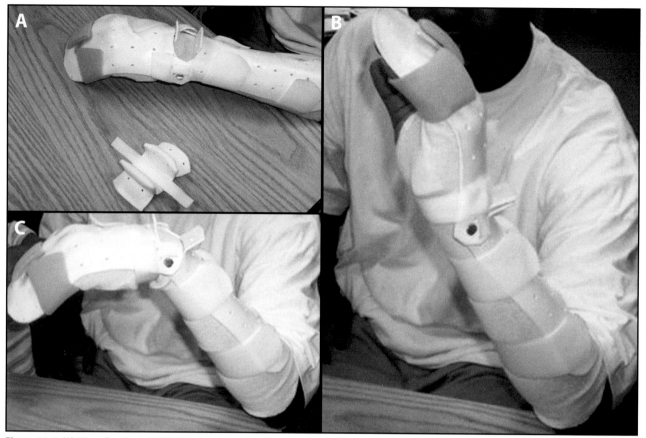

Figure 10-7. (A) Hinged orthosis. (B) Wrist extension within hinged orthosis. (C) Wrist flexion within hinged orthosis.

significant difference was found in the total active motion group at 4 weeks. At 12 weeks, however, there was no significant difference between the groups in total active motion. The authors recommend further study to examine whether faster return of motion is associated with return to work earlier as compared with the early passive motion protocol.

Level IV

- Starr, H. M., Snoddy, M., Hammand, K. E., & Seiler, J. G. (2013). Flexor tendon repair rehabilitation protocols: A systematic review. *Journal of Hand Surgery, 38*, 1712-1717.

  ○ This systematic review analyzed 34 studies of flexor tendon rehabilitation protocols ranging from Level I to IV. Orthoses were used in each study. Wrist flexion ranged from 0 to 30 degrees and MCP flexion from 40 to 90 degrees, and PIP/DIP was in full extension. Wearing time ranged from 3 to 6 weeks. Early passive motion protocols had reduced risk of tendon ruptures but higher risk of adhesions and decreased joint motion as compared with early active motion protocols. Combining elements of each protocol to optimize outcomes is common

practice. With better suture technique and more defined rehabilitation protocols, the authors note that early active motion may provide more optimal outcomes with better postoperative motion.

EXTENSOR TENDON PROTOCOLS

This section describes the three common rehabilitation regimes and orthoses that can be used following injury and surgical repair of extensor tendon injuries in zones V through VII: immobilization, early passive extension, and controlled active extension using the relative motion orthosis. Orthoses used for zones I through IV are discussed in Chapter 9.

Immobilization

The immobilization approach, similar to that used with flexor tendon injuries, may be used in instances where a more complicated mobilization approach is not appropriate, such as with young clients, clients with cognitive deficits, or where compliance is a concern. Evidence does suggest that these injuries can tolerate immobilization well, but recovery and return to full function may take longer as compared with a regime that involves early tendon

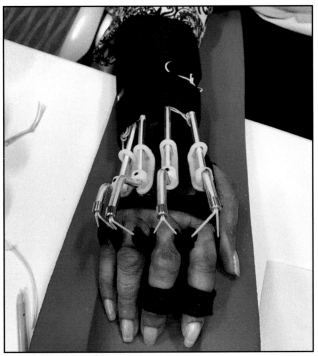

Figure 10-8. MCP dynamic extension orthosis following repair of the extensor tendons in zone V.

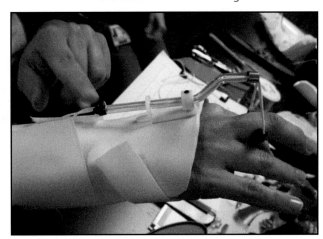

Figure 10-9. Dynamic MCP extension mobilization orthosis with flexion block.

mobilization. An orthosis (either an immobilization orthosis or a dynamic orthosis) may be used to immobilize the wrist and involved digit(s). The position of the joints in the orthosis can vary according to surgeon preference, location of the repair, and concurrent injury to other structures, such as bone, ligament, or nerve. The orthosis is typically worn for 4 weeks full-time, with intermittent wear during the day and at night for an additional 2 to 4 weeks.

Early Passive Extension

The early passive extension approach is used for multiple tendon injuries; injuries involving bone, ligament, or other structures; and tendon injuries at the extensor retinaculum because adhesions are common. The orthosis used is typically a dynamic or mobilization orthosis that positions the wrist in extension and holds the digits in extension at rest, allowing for controlled MCP flexion (usually 30 to 40 degrees for the first 3 weeks) and passive extension with the assistance of an outrigger and rubber bands or springs (Figures 10-8 and 10-9). Full MCP flexion is blocked with a volar orthosis or a stop on the outrigger line. The client performs active flexion to the limits of the orthosis and passive extension regularly throughout the day. The amount of allowable MCP flexion is increased as the strength of the tendon repair improves. The orthosis is used for 5 to 6 weeks, although the MCP flexion block may be removed after a period of 3 weeks. Refer to Chapter 11 for a more detailed description of this and other mobilization orthoses.

Controlled Active Extension Using the Relative Motion Orthosis

The **relative motion orthosis or "yoke" orthosis** was initially described as one component of the orthotic management of postoperative rehabilitation of repaired extensor tendon injuries in zones V and VI. Known as the **immediate controlled active motion (ICAM)** protocol, the yoke component is worn together with a wrist extension immobilization orthosis. It is designed to hold one or two digits in relative extension compared with the adjacent digits. It can also be used as an exercise aid to facilitate either flexion or extension at the PIP joint of the affected digit depending on the position. The yoke orthosis is also appropriate for the management of sagittal band injuries and for postoperative management of tendon ruptures in clients with rheumatoid arthritis. It is appreciatively less bulky than other orthoses, more comfortable for the client, and easily worn during activities of daily living (ADL).

The goals of a relative motion orthosis for tendon injuries are to limit full flexion or extension at the MCP joints, limit full tendon excursion and thus protect a repair from excessive stress, and facilitate increased motion at the more distal PIP and DIP joints (blocking the MCP joint will help to transfer the force of muscle contraction more distally to these joints during active movement). To facilitate PIP extension, the orthosis holds the affected digit in about 15 degrees of MCP joint flexion in comparison to the adjacent digits and may be helpful with cases of MCP joint hyperextension, limited extensor tendon excursion, and IP joint stiffness/loss of extension (Figure 10-10). To facilitate PIP flexion, the orthosis holds the affected digit in about 15 degrees of MCP joint extension relative to the adjacent digits and is helpful when the client has difficulty flexing the PIP joint.

The reader is encouraged to seek additional resources for a complete overview of these protocols.

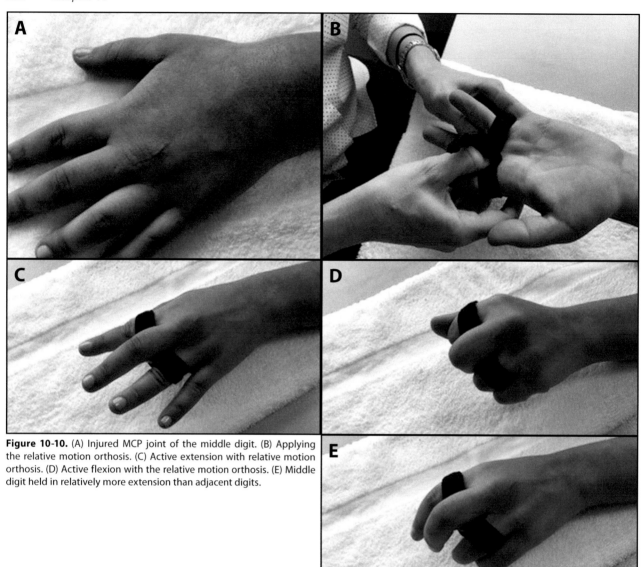

Figure 10-10. (A) Injured MCP joint of the middle digit. (B) Applying the relative motion orthosis. (C) Active extension with relative motion orthosis. (D) Active flexion with the relative motion orthosis. (E) Middle digit held in relatively more extension than adjacent digits.

Evidence

Level II

- Wong, A. L., Wilson, M., Girnary, S., Nojoomi, M., Acharya, S., & Paul, S. M. (2017). The optimal orthosis and motion protocol for extensor tendon injury in zones IV-VIII: A systematic review. *Journal of Hand Therapy, 30*(4), 447-456.

   ○ The authors conducted a systematic review to determine the optimal combination postoperative therapy protocol and choice of orthosis for rehabilitation of proximal extensor tendon injuries (zones IV to VIII). Their literature search included a systematic review of randomized clinical trials and cohort studies investigating extensor tendon rehabilitation from 1960 to 2016. The outcome measures considered included total active motion, grip strength, return to work, patient attrition, and patient-reported outcomes. The systematic review consisted of 11 studies in English of average quality. The authors reported that the studies' results and outcomes were difficult to compare due to differences in reporting. Here are their findings: Early total active motion and final grip strength were greater with dynamic extension orthoses and relative motion orthoses compared with immobilization orthoses. Four studies excluded patients who did not follow up, and the loss to follow-up was 12% to 33% in the other studies. Patient-reported outcomes were not comparable because they were only included in three studies and each used a different assessment tool. The authors concluded that only average-quality evidence supports the use of the early active motion protocol, but the best orthosis to deliver this protocol could not be determined.

Level III

- Svens, B., Ames, E., Burford, K., & Caplash, Y. (2015). Relative active motion programs following extensor tendon repair: A pilot study using a prospective cohort and evaluating outcomes following orthotic interventions. *Journal of Hand Therapy, 28*(1), 11-19.

  ○ The authors describe a two-center nonrandomized prospective trial of patients with extensor tendon injuries of zones IV, V, and VI who received a relative motion orthosis and wrist orthosis and followed the postoperative extensor tendon protocol described by Howell, Merritt, and Robinson (2005). One group of patients wore the orthosis for 4 weeks and one group wore the orthosis for 6 weeks. Results were similar for both groups and matched previously reported outcomes of other studies of the relative motion orthosis extensor protocol with no differences for the different length of orthotic wear.

- Hirth, M. J., Bennett, K., Mah, E., Farrow, H. C., Cavallo, A. V., Ritz, M., & Findlay, M. W. (2011). Early return to work and improved range of motion with modified relative motion splinting: A retrospective comparison with immobilization splinting for zones V and VI extensor tendon repairs. *Hand Therapy, 16*(4), 86-94.

  ○ This retrospective study compared treatment of extensor tendon injuries in zones V and VI using an immobilization protocol with treatment using the relative motion splint. Although range of motion measures were better for the relative motion group at 6 weeks, at 12 weeks, the results were comparable. The relative motion group completed rehabilitation in a shorter time period.

Level V

- Hirth, M. J., Howell, J. W., & O'Brien, L. (2016). Relative motion orthoses in the management of various hand conditions: A scoping review. *Journal of Hand Therapy, 29*, 405-432.

  ○ The authors reviewed 15 articles (Levels III and IV) on the use of the relative motion orthosis. The authors found that the relative motion orthosis was used for three different clinical applications: protective, exercise, and adaptive. The authors note that the majority of the current literature on the use of relative motion orthoses is for extensor tendon rehabilitation protocols and conservative management of sagittal band injuries. The use of the relative motion orthosis for other conditions is described in Level V articles.

UPDATES IN THE FIELD

Advances in surgical procedures lead to new developments in rehabilitation protocols. Tendon surgery now can be performed under local anesthesia without tourniquet (**wide awake local anesthesia no tourniquet [WALANT]** technique) by injecting epinephrine mixed with lidocaine to achieve vasoconstriction in the area of surgery. This allows the client to be awake throughout the proceedings. A key advantage of the WALANT technique is the creation of a bloodless field without the use of an arm tourniquet. The use of local anesthesia permits active motion intraoperatively, which is particularly helpful in tenolysis, flexor tendon repairs, and setting the tension on tendon transfers. With regard to flexor tendon repairs, this method allows the tendon to move actively during surgery to test tendon function intraoperatively and to ensure the tendon is properly repaired before leaving the operating table. The client can actually see his or her fingers achieve full flexion during the surgery, which may lead to improved compliance with the home exercise program and better outcomes.

This development has led to new rehabilitation instructions following surgery. Clients may be allowed to perform gentle active motion exercises, making one-half of a full fist immediately following the procedure. Make sure to adhere to the surgeon's guidelines for the postoperative protocol to follow with each individual client.

Biomechanical Concepts of Orthoses for Tendon Management

It is critical for a practitioner to consider the biomechanical and anatomical principles related to tendon movement when using orthoses to protect and facilitate optimal healing of repaired flexor or extensor tendons. Combined with a thorough knowledge of biomechanical concepts related to orthotic fabrication, this will assist the practitioner in designing an effective, comfortable orthosis.

The practitioner must accommodate the bony prominences of the wrist and hand when fabricating an orthosis following a tendon injury, particularly when the hand and wrist are placed in a flexed position (as with dorsal blocking orthoses). The following are important considerations:

- Bony prominences: The ulnar head; radial styloid; dorsal aspect MCP, PIP, and DIP joints; and thumb MCP and IP joints may be subject to compressive forces from the orthosis's straps and from the LTTM. Choosing a highly conforming material will optimize the client's comfort and the security of the orthosis (Figure 10-11). Placing either putty or a small piece of nonstick-coated LTTM over the bony prominences and molding the orthosis over this will create a "bubble" that will protect the bone from aggravating and shearing forces.

- Hand edema: As discussed earlier, the relative laxity of the skin on the dorsal aspect of the hand encourages development of edema in this area following injury. As

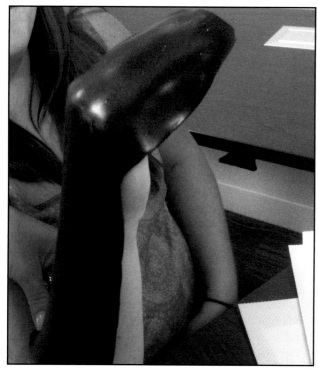

Figure 10-11. Dorsal blocking orthosis showing conformability of material.

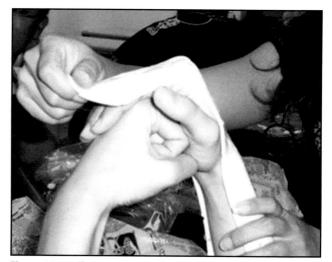

Figure 10-12. Client positioning during molding of a dorsal blocking orthosis.

a result, the hand typically falls into a position of comfort: MCP extension, PIP and DIP joint flexion, thumb adduction, and wrist flexion. Following flexor tendon injuries, it is important to position the MCP joints in at least 40 to 50 degrees of flexion and limit wrist flexion to 20 degrees. This helps to minimize the development of joint and soft tissue contractures and position the hand and wrist in a more functional position. Placing the PIP and DIP joints in full extension following both flexor and extensor tendon repairs will similarly discourage stiffness and joint contractures.

- Hand arches: Dorsal hand edema is common following tendon repair and can adversely affect all three hand arches. The proximal and distal transverse arches flatten with wrist flexion and MCP extension, and the longitudinal arch loses its curvature with MCP extension and PIP/DIP joint flexion posturing. Positioning the MCP joints in 40 to 50 degrees of flexion and limiting wrist flexion to 20 degrees will help to support the arches.

Orthotic Fabrication Steps

Orthotic fabrication begins after the practitioner has determined which design is most suited to the client's condition, specific needs, and physician referral specifications. The process begins with designing the pattern, followed by selecting the LTTM, positioning the client, molding the material to the client, fitting and adjusting the orthosis, applying straps, and ending with evaluating the orthosis for fit and comfort. The final step in this process is educating the client and other caregivers on the purpose, wearing schedule, and care of the orthosis.

Refer to the instructional videos for detailed step-by-step instructions.

DORSAL BLOCKING ORTHOSIS

The dorsal blocking orthosis can be made easily from a rectangular piece of material. Measure from the tip of the client's fingers (in MCP flexion and PIP/DIP extension) over the wrist and to about half the length of the forearm. The width just falls about one-half inch over the widest part of the MCP joints and the widest part of the forearm musculature.

The wrist tends to fall in flexion and the digits in extension due to gravity. Supporting the elbow on a table and having the client place his or her uninvolved fist in his or her palm during the molding process will help encourage better positioning of the wrist and digits (see Figure 10-11). Be sure to keep the MCP joints flexed and position the PIP and DIP joints in full extension.

Use a highly conforming material with drape and stretch to easily accommodate bony prominences (Figure 10-12). Place putty or coated LTTM over the ulnar head to create a "bubble" and mold the material over this. This will protect the bone from aggravating and shearing forces. A thickness of 1/8 inch is necessary for most adults.

Dorsal Blocking Orthosis Check-Out

- Can the client flex his or her elbow without the orthosis migrating distally?

  If no, the orthosis is too long or the proximal edge is not flared adequately.

- Are the wrist and MCP, PIP, and DIP joints positioned correctly?

  If no, the orthosis should be remolded.

- Are the corners of the orthosis rounded and smooth?

  If no, round and smooth all corners of the orthosis.

- Are the straps secure and correctly placed?

  If no, adjust the straps:

  ○ *The wrist strap should go in a circumferential fashion around the wrist; the ends should meet together. No Velcro should be exposed.*

  ○ *The proximal strap should be angled on the orthosis so it sits flat on the forearm.*

  ○ *The strap in the palm should be angled to accommodate for the distal transverse arch and be positioned just proximal to the distal palmar crease.*

  ○ *Straps over the PIP and DIP joints should hold these joints in full extension.*

- Are all indentations and pattern marks removed?

  If no, use a heat gun to smooth the LTTM. Rubbing alcohol can be used to remove wax pencil marks. Ink cannot be removed, so refrain from using this when drawing your pattern on the LTTM.

- Remove the orthosis after 5 to 10 minutes and observe the skin. Are there any reddened areas?

  If yes, adjust the orthosis by flaring and smoothing edges and/or flaring material away from bony prominences. Pay particular attention to the ulnar head and dorsal aspect of the MCP joints.

- Review the purpose and care of the orthosis with the client. Does he or she understand:

  ○ The purpose of the orthosis

  ○ The wearing schedule

  ○ Exercises to do within the orthosis

  ○ How to take care of the orthosis

  ○ How to don and doff correctly (if allowed)

  If no, discuss the wearing schedule and care of the orthosis with the client before he or she leaves the clinic and provide clear written instructions to take home with him or her (refer to the Appendix at the end of the chapter):

  ○ *Take a photo of the orthosis correctly positioned using a smart phone and send it to your client for reference along with written instructions on the wearing schedule.*

  ○ *Document all of your instructions to the client and maintain a copy of these in the client's chart.*

RELATIVE MOTION ORTHOSIS

Use a strip of thin material with stretch and elasticity about 1 inch wide and 8 inches long to create this orthosis. Some materials may need to be folded in half lengthwise or even tripled on themselves lengthwise to get enough rigidity and strength.

Wrap the material around the proximal phalanx adjacent to the involved digit and create a ring. Then, on the volar surface, wrap the material around the proximal phalanx of the adjacent digit on the other side of the involved digit. Press the material together over the volar surface of the involved digit and trim away any excess material. Position the client's hand in supination during the molding process and place pressure over the proximal phalanx of the repaired digit while molding the orthosis. This allows the practitioner to use gravity to assist in keeping the repaired digit in more extension than the adjacent digits (see Figure 10-10B).

Relative Motion Orthosis Check-Out

- Can the client fully flex all of his or her PIP and DIP joints in the orthosis?

  If no, flare the distal edge of the orthosis to allow for full unrestricted flexion and extension.

- Is the affected digit positioned in extension?

  If no, the orthosis should be remolded.

- Are the unaffected digits positioned in 10 to 15 degrees more flexion than the affected digit?

  If no, the orthosis should be remolded.

- Is the orthosis secure on the hand during movement?

  If no, apply a strap on the volar aspect of the proximal phalanges.

- Are all indentations and pattern marks removed?

  If no, use a heat gun to smooth the LTTM. Rubbing alcohol can be used to remove wax pencil marks. Ink cannot be removed, so refrain from using this when drawing your pattern on the LTTM.

- Remove the orthosis after 5 to 10 minutes and observe the skin. Are there any reddened areas?

  If yes, adjust the orthosis by flaring and smoothing edges.

- Review the purpose and care of the orthosis with the client. Does he or she understand:

  ○ The purpose of the orthosis

  ○ The wearing schedule

  ○ Exercises to do within the orthosis

  ○ How to take care of the orthosis

  ○ How to don and doff correctly (if allowed)

*If no, discuss the wearing schedule and care of the ortho-
sis with the client before he or she leaves the clinic and
provide clear written instructions to take home with him
or her (refer to the Appendix at the end of the chapter).*

- *Take a photo of the orthosis correctly positioned using
a smart phone and send it to your client for reference along with written instructions on the wearing
schedule.*

- *Document all of your instructions to the client and
maintain a copy of these in the client's chart.*

SPECIAL CONSIDERATIONS

Clients with edema will require frequent orthotic checkups to make sure the fit and positioning remain correct.
Choose materials with memory for ease with remolding
and consider alternate methods to secure the orthosis in
the early stages of rehabilitation, such as Coban wrap (3M),
cotton, or Ace bandages (3M). Consider cotton bandages in
the early stages to avoid excessive pressure on the tissues
from the dressings.

Presence of edema in the digits following tendon repair
can make it much more difficult for clients to perform their
prescribed exercises. Additionally, the extra fluid makes
tendon movement more difficult and, as a result, may place
more stress on the repair. It is advisable to wait at least 3 to
5 days after surgery to begin tendon mobilization exercises
to make time for the edema to subside.

Summary

- The goals of orthoses for tendon injuries and subsequent wearing schedules will vary depending on the
client's needs, diagnosis, and rehabilitation approach
used.

- Each client may require a specific orthotic design or
adaptation in order to achieve the best outcome with
his or her orthosis.

- Each orthosis must be molded to the individual anatomy for the best fit.

- Post-fabrication critique and check-out help identify
areas for modification and optimize client comfort.

In Your Client's Shoes

Using an orthosis after a tendon injury and surgical
repair will significantly affect your client's daily occupations for up to 8 weeks. Depending on the tendon(s)
involved, clients may require this orthosis be worn 24 hours
per day, whereas others may be permitted to remove it for
hygiene and during rest periods. Can you determine which
schedule matches each tendon rehabilitation approach
described in this chapter?

You should experience how it feels to wear this type of
orthosis for one of the schedules listed previously for a full
24-hour period. This experience will enable you to be client
centered when using orthoses as an intervention strategy
in your practice. You must consider how to instruct your
clients on the importance of wearing their orthoses exactly
as prescribed in order to prevent reinjuring their injured
tendon(s) and optimize their outcomes.

Reference

Howell, J. W., Merritt, W. H., & Robinson, S. J. (2005). Immediate controlled active motion following zone 4-7 extensor tendon repair.
Journal of Hand Therapy, 18, 182-190. doi:10.1197.j.jht.2005.02.011

Suggested Reading

Chesney, A., Chauhan, A., Kattan, A., Farrokhyar, F., & Thoma, A.
(2011). Systematic review of flexor tendon rehabilitation protocols in zone II of the hand. *Plastic Reconstructive Surgery, 127*,
1583-1592.

Chow, J. C., Sensinger, J., McNeal, D., Chow, B., Amirouche, F., &
Gonzalez, M. (2014). Importance of proximal A2 and A4 pulleys
to maintaining kinematics in the hand: A biomechanical study.
Hand, 9(1), 105-111.

Colditz, J. C., & Moore, R. S. (2007). *Under the skin: Relating tendon
anatomy of the hand to clinical questions* [Instructional Video
Series]. Available from https://handlab.com/medpro/hand-thera-
py-education-products/exam/under-the-skin-exam.html

Cooper, W., Khor, W., & Sivakumar, B. (2015). Flexor tendon repairs
in children: Outcomes from a specialist tertiary centre. *Journal of
Plastic, Reconstructive and Aesthetic Surgery, 68*, 717-723.

Coppard, B. M., & Lohman, H. (2014). *Introduction to orthotics: A
clinical reasoning and problem-solving approach* (4th ed.). St. Louis,
MO: Elsevier Mosby.

Frueh, F. S., Kunz, V. S., Gravestock, I. J., Held, L., Haefeli, M.,
Giovanoli, P., & Calcagni, M. (2014). Primary flexor tendon repair
in zones 1 and 2: Early passive mobilization versus controlled
active motion. *Journal of Hand Surgery, 39*(7), 1344-1350.

Hirth, M. J., Bennett, K., Mah, E., Farrow, H. C., Cavallo, A. V., Ritz,
M., & Findlay, M. W. (2011). Early return to work and improved
range of motion with modified relative motion splinting: A retrospective comparison with immobilization splinting for zones V
and VI extensor tendon repairs. *Hand Therapy, 16*(4), 86-94.

Hirth, M. J., Howell, J. W., & O'Brien, L. (2016). Relative motion orthoses in the management of various hand conditions: A scoping
review. *Journal of Hand Therapy, 29*, 405-432.

Howell, J. W., & Peck, F. (2013). Rehabilitation of flexor and extensor
tendon injuries in the hand: Current updates. *Injury, 44*, 397-402.

Jacobs, M., & Austin, N. (2014). *Orthotic intervention for the hand
and upper extremity: Splinting principles and process* (2nd ed.).
Baltimore, MD: Lippincott Williams & Wilkins.

Lalonde, D. (2014). Minimally invasive anesthesia in wide awake hand
surgery. *Hand Clinics, 30*(1), 1-6.

Lalonde, D., & Martin, A. (2013). Epinephrine in local anesthesia in finger and hand surgery: The case for wide-awake anesthesia. *Journal
of the American Academy of Orthopaedic Surgeons, 21*(8), 443-447.

Lied, L., Borchgrevink, G. E., & Finsen, V. (2017). Wide awake hand surgery. *Journal of Hand Surgery (Asian-Pacific Volume)*, 22(3), 292-296.

Mackin, E. J., Callahan, A. D., Skirven, T. M., Schneider, L. H., & Osterman, A. L. (Eds.). *Hunter, Mackin & Callahan's rehabilitation of the hand and upper extremity* (5th ed.). St. Louis, MO: Mosby.

Starr, H. M., Snoddy, M., Hammand, K. E., & Seiler, J. G. (2013). Flexor tendon repair rehabilitation protocols: A systematic review. *Journal of Hand Surgery*, 38, 1712-1717.

Svens, B., Ames, E., Burford, K., & Caplash, Y. (2015). Relative active motion programs following extensor tendon repair: A pilot study using a prospective cohort and evaluating outcomes following orthotic interventions. *Journal of Hand Therapy*, 28(1), 11-19.

Tang, J. B., Amadio, P.C., Boyer, M. I., Savage, R., Zhao, C., Sandow, M., … Wolfe, S. W. (2013). Current practice of primary flexor tendon repair: A global view. *Hand Clinics*, 29, 179-189.

Wong, A. L., Wilson, M., Girnary, S., Nojoomi, M., Acharya, S., & Paul, S. M. (2017). The optimal orthosis and motion protocol for extensor tendon injury in zones IV-VIII: A systematic review. *Journal of Hand Therapy*, 30(4), 447-456.

Test Your Knowledge

SHORT ANSWER

1. Identify all anatomical landmarks associated with a dorsal blocking orthosis.

2. Describe the purpose of using a dorsal blocking orthosis following a flexor tendon repair.

3. Describe the common hand and wrist position used with a dorsal blocking orthosis.

4. Describe how a relative motion orthosis protects a repaired extensor tendon.

MULTIPLE CHOICE

5. Which flexor tendon rehabilitation protocol uses elastic traction on the injured digit(s)?

   a. Kleinert

   b. Duran

   c. Immobilization

   d. Early active motion

6. What is the typical position of the hand and wrist in a dorsal blocking orthosis?

   a. Wrist flexion, MCP flexion, PIP/DIP flexion

   b. Wrist extension, MCP extension, PIP and DIP joint extension

   c. Wrist extension, MCP flexion, PIP and DIP joint flexion

   d. Wrist flexion, MCP flexion, PIP and DIP joint extension

7. When is immobilization following flexor tendon repair indicated?

   a. When there are multiple tendons involved.

   b. When there is concurrent injury to bone, ligament, and/or nerve.

   c. When the client is very young, old, or otherwise unable to follow detailed instructions.

   d. When there is significant swelling in the hand and wrist.

8. Which zone(s) of injury is a relative motion orthosis typically indicated for?

   a. Zone VII

   b. Zones III and IV

   c. Zones I and II

   d. Zones V and VI

9. Which flexor zone of injury is commonly referred to as no man's land?

   a. Zone II

   b. Zone I

   c. Zone V

   d. Zone III

10. How many flexor tendons are located within the carpal tunnel?

    a. 8

    b. 9

    c. 6

    d. 4

11. How are the annular pulleys arranged in the digits?

    a. The odd-numbered pulleys are over the joints; the even-numbered pulleys are along the shafts of the bones.

    b. The odd-numbered pulleys are along the shafts of the bones; the even-numbered pulleys are over the joints.

    c. All of the pulleys are located along the shafts of the proximal, middle, and distal phalanges. None are located at the MCP, PIP, or DIP joints.

    d. All of the pulleys are located at the digit joints: MCP, PIP, and DIP joints.

12. What is the purpose of moving a newly repaired tendon soon after surgery?

    a. It helps to reduce the swelling.

    b. It helps the tendon heal at a faster rate.

    c. It helps to minimize development of adhesions and facilitates tendon healing.

    d. It reduces the total wearing time of the orthosis after surgery.

CASE STUDIES

Case Study 1

Jane is a 35-year-old, right-hand–dominant woman who lacerated the FDS and FDP to her right second and third digits in zone II 3 days ago. Her surgeon has ordered a dorsal blocking orthosis and early passive motion protocol for her.

Her referral reads:

1. *Evaluate and treat.*

2. *Provide dorsal blocking orthosis.*

3. *Begin early passive motion.*

Your assessment:

Jane is seen for her first therapy appointment 3 days following surgery. Her postsurgical dressings were removed, and her wounds were cleaned and redressed. She reports mild pain in her hand and wrist, but overall she is doing well. She is concerned about how she will be able to care for her two young sons, aged 3 and 5 years, and about her ability to drive. She appears very motivated to participate in therapy and states she will do "whatever I have to do to get better."

Using different clinical reasoning approaches, answer the following questions about this client and the prescribed orthosis.

Procedural Reasoning

1. What client factors are important to consider when determining the most suitable orthotic design for this client?

2. Which positioning in the dorsal blocking immobilization orthosis would be most appropriate for this client? Why?

3. What LTTM properties are important to consider?

4. Describe the instructions you would give this client on:
   ◦ How to care for the orthosis
   ◦ Wearing schedule
   ◦ Precautions
   ◦ Exercises/activities

Pragmatic Reasoning

5. What resources are available to fabricate this orthosis (time, materials, expertise)?

6. Are you able to clearly document the need for this orthosis?

7. Does evidence-based practice support the use of this orthosis for this client's diagnosis?

Interactive Reasoning

8. What are the client's goals and valued occupations?

9. What effect will the client's injury and use of the orthosis have on her ADL?

Conditional Reasoning

10. What factors will influence this client's compliance to the wearing schedule of this orthosis?

Narrative Reasoning

11. How does this injury and, more specifically, this orthotic intervention affect this client's valued occupations?

12. What activities is this client most concerned about?

Ethical Reasoning

13. Does the client understand the need for the orthosis?

14. Does the client have the resources to be able to pay for the orthosis (as applicable)?

15. What other options are available to this client if she lacks the resources necessary to pay for the orthosis?

16. Write one short-term goal (1 to 2 weeks) and one long-term goal (6 to 8 weeks) for this client.

Case Study 2

Jack is an active 4-year-old boy who sustained a laceration to the dorsal aspect of his left nondominant hand while playing with scissors. The injury was in zone VI and involved all four ED tendons.

His referral reads:

1. *Evaluate and treat.*

2. *Provide orthosis.*

3. *Wound care and dressing changes.*

Your assessment:

Jack is seen in outpatient therapy with his mother and father. He is a happy little boy but is scared and does not want you to touch him. After some coaxing, you are able to remove his postsurgical dressings and put a clean dressing on his wound. His sutures are clean, and he has very little swelling.

Using different clinical reasoning approaches, consider the following questions about this client and the prescribed orthosis. Some questions may be directed more toward the client, and some questions may be directed more toward you as the practitioner for reflection.

Procedural Reasoning

1. What client factors are important to consider when determining the most suitable positioning in an orthosis for this client?

2. What LTTM properties are important to consider?

3. Describe the instructions you would give this client's parents on:
   ◦ How to care for the orthosis
   ◦ Wearing schedule
   ◦ Precautions
   ◦ Exercises/activities

Pragmatic Reasoning

4. What resources are available to fabricate this orthosis (time, materials, expertise)?

5. Are you able to clearly document the need for this orthosis?

6. Does evidence-based practice support the use of this orthosis for this client's diagnosis?

Interactive Reasoning

7. What are the client's goals and valued occupations?

8. What effect will the client's injury and use of the orthosis have on his ADL?

Conditional Reasoning

9. What factors will influence this client's compliance to the wearing schedule of this orthosis?

Narrative Reasoning

10. How does this injury and, more specifically, this orthotic intervention affect this client's valued occupations?

11. What activities is this client most concerned about?

Ethical Reasoning

12. Does the client understand the need for the orthosis?

13. Does the client have the resources to be able to pay for the orthosis (as applicable)?

14. What other options are available to this client if he lacks the resources necessary to pay for the orthosis?

15. Write one short-term goal (1 to 2 weeks) and one long-term goal (6 to 8 weeks) for this client.

Appendix

STUDENT ASSIGNMENTS

1. Define all of the key terms used in this chapter.

2. Select one of the orthosis designs from this chapter and prepare a client-centered handout for wearing this orthosis. Base your client description on one of the two case studies in this chapter. Include the following in the handout:

   ◦ A description/name of the orthosis

   ◦ An outline of the wearing schedule (remember that this will vary depending on the client's condition)

   ◦ A description of how to clean and care for the orthosis

   ◦ Instructions on what clients should be aware of when wearing the orthosis (red areas on skin, pain, swelling, etc.)

   ◦ Contact information and follow up instructions

3. Prepare a case study of a client requiring an orthosis following either a flexor or extensor tendon repair. Use one of the cited resources in the chapter to support your orthotic intervention. Summarize the research and explain the outcomes of the study.

4. As an occupational therapy practitioner, it will be interesting and informative for you to spend an extended period wearing an orthosis to appreciate the effect that an orthosis will have on your client's daily occupations. Wear a dorsal blocking orthosis designed by your lab partner for a 12-hour period, preferably through the night. Take note of how it feels to have one body part completely immobilized. Elaborate in paragraphs on the following:

   ◦ Describe the orthosis, material used, positioning, and typical diagnosis for this orthosis.

   ◦ Comfort and ease of use: Is it easy to take on and off? Are there any pressure areas that caused discomfort? What areas need to be modified? How would you do this?

   ◦ Personal and public image: Did the orthosis attract attention to your family members, roommates, children, and/or parents?

   ◦ Functionality: How was your function affected by this orthosis? Was the position helpful or harmful? What would the typical wearing schedule be for this type of orthosis?

   ◦ How does this change your appreciation of what your clients are experiencing with their orthosis?

5. Complete the check-out form on the next page.

Multiple Choice Answer Key

5. a

6. d

7. c

8. d

9. a

10. b

11. a

12. c

Dorsal Blocking Orthosis Check-Out Form

*(This can be used for faculty to evaluate students' completed orthoses,
as well as for students to reference when evaluating their own completed orthosis.)*

Fabricate one of the orthotic designs for a dorsal blocking orthosis on your classmate and complete the following check-out form:

Name of Orthosis:

Purpose of Orthosis:

Design/Function

_____ The wrist is positioned correctly according to protocol.

_____ The MCP joints are positioned in flexion (degree of flexion matches purpose of orthosis).

_____ The PIP joints are positioned correctly.

_____ The DIP joints are positioned correctly.

_____ The thumb is positioned correctly (for thumb tendon injuries).

_____ The hand portion supports all of the fingers.

_____ The orthosis is half the width of the forearm.

_____ The orthosis is at least two-thirds the length of the forearm.

_____ The orthosis does not migrate distally with elbow flexion.

_____ The orthosis does not cause impingement or pressure areas.

_____ The orthosis clears all bony prominences.

Straps/Orthosis Appearance

_____ The straps are in the correct position: forearm, wrist, fingers (and thumb as applicable).

_____ The straps are secure and corners rounded.

_____ The orthosis edges are smooth and corners rounded.

_____ The proximal edge is flared.

_____ The orthosis is free of fingerprints, pattern marks, or indentations.

CHAPTER 11

Orthoses for Mobilization

Key Terms

Creep
Dynamic orthoses
Elastic deformation
Fibroplasia
Force
Hard end feel
Inflammatory

Lever arm
Low-load prolonged stretch (LLPS)
Modified Weeks test
Outrigger
Plastic deformation
Scar maturation

Serial static
Soft end feel
Stages of healing
Torque
Torque angle curve
Total end range time (TERT)

Learning Outcomes

Upon completion of this chapter, you will be able to:

1. Recognize the indications, precautions, and contraindications for orthoses for mobilization.

2. Describe the clinical conditions and goals for prescribing a dynamic mobilization orthosis.

3. Describe the clinical conditions and goals for prescribing a static progressive mobilization orthosis.

4. Describe the clinical conditions and goals for prescribing a serial static mobilization orthosis.

5. Describe a typical wearing schedule for a dynamic, static progressive, or serial static orthosis for mobilization.

6. Discuss objective methods to select an appropriate orthosis for mobilization for a specific diagnosis or condition.

Introduction

Orthoses for mobilization are orthoses that place controlled **force** on a body part. These orthoses are an advanced intervention that many practitioners use to help their clients regain functional independence. They also include additional components, called **outriggers**, that are

Schofield, K., & Schwartz, D. *Orthotic Design and Fabrication for the Upper Extremity: A Practical Guide* (pp 211-225).
© 2019 Taylor & Francis Group.

Table 11-1

COMPARISON OF MOBILIZATION ORTHOSES

TYPE	DYNAMIC (see Figure 11-1)	STATIC PROGRESSIVE (see Figure 11-2)	SERIAL STATIC (see Figure 11-3)
Immobilization base	Yes	Yes	Yes
Outrigger	Yes	Yes	No
Components	Dynamic components for force application: rubber bands, elastic, coils, springs	Static components for force application: Velcro, static line, screws, gears, turnbuckles	None
Purpose	Mobilize joints, functional assist for weak/absent muscles	Used to increase passive joint range, or soft tissue length	Increase passive joint range or soft tissue length

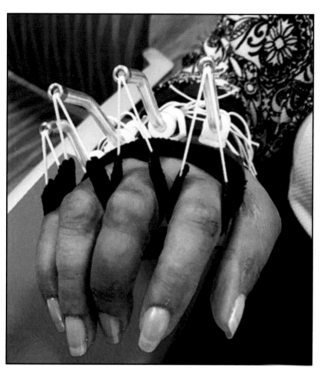

Figure 11-1. Dynamic extensor tendon orthosis.

secured to the thermoplastic base and hold the mechanism through which force or stress is applied to the body part. Outriggers are designed to offer support or force in a way that can be adjusted and may allow for movement of the specific body part while wearing the orthosis, depending on the specific goals and purpose. Orthoses for mobilization are commonly used to help clients regain passive range of motion (PROM) and/or to stretch tight or contracted soft tissue structures.

Types of Orthoses for Mobilization

Orthoses for mobilization are divided into three basic categories (Table 11-1):

1. **Dynamic orthoses**
2. Static progressive orthoses
3. **Serial static orthoses**

DYNAMIC ORTHOSES

Dynamic orthoses typically incorporate elastic components and/or coils or springs to put tension on a joint in order to increase ROM or act as a substitute for weak or absent muscles. Dynamic mobilization orthoses can have a variety of uses and functions (Figure 11-1). For example, they are often used to aid in functional activities, as with peripheral nerve injuries where muscles are weakened or paralyzed. The springs and/or coils of a mobilization orthosis can help substitute for the weak or paralyzed muscles as in cases of radial nerve palsy or ulnar nerve/median nerve palsy. The outriggers can also be used to mobilize stiff joints or pull fingers into better alignment.

STATIC PROGRESSIVE ORTHOSES

Static progressive orthoses are a type of mobilization orthosis that incorporate nonelastic components to apply force to a joint to hold it in its end-range position in order to improve joint PROM. Examples of these static components are string, turnbuckles (devices that allow for regulation of tension), gears, monofilaments, fishing lines, and Velcro (Velcro BVBA) hook and loop tape (Figure 11-2). Static

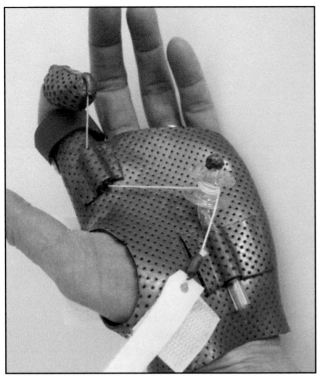

Figure 11-2. Static progressive orthosis for a stiff digit.

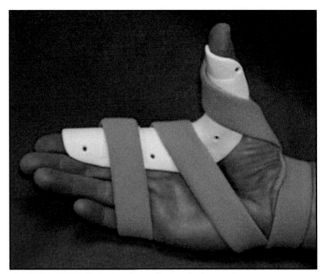

Figure 11-3. Serial static orthosis for a tight first web space.

progressive orthoses allow progressive changes in joint position as the PROM of the involved joint changes and improves over time.

SERIAL STATIC ORTHOSES

The use of serial static orthoses is a method of holding a stiff joint in its end-range position in order to increase PROM. Every few days, or even once per week, the practitioner removes the orthosis for additional treatment of heat, stretching, and exercise of the stiff or contracted joint before applying a new orthosis to the client in a new end-range position. Serial static orthoses are very useful in the treatment of stiff joints, such as a proximal interphalangeal (PIP) joint flexion contracture; the wrist following fractures or trauma due to extrinsic tightness; or a tight first web space, which can also occur after trauma or fractures (Figure 11-3).

When comparing the construction of dynamic and static progressive orthoses, it is apparent that both types of mobilization orthoses start with an immobilization base and have an outrigger attachment. Dynamic orthoses use dynamic components for force application, such as rubber bands, elastic, coils, and springs. Dynamic orthoses help to mobilize joints and allow movement within the orthosis. Conversely, static progressive orthoses are typically constructed with nonelastic components for force application, such as Velcro, static line, screws, gears, and turnbuckles. Static progressive orthoses are used to increase PROM. In

Box 11-1. Goals of Orthoses for Mobilization

- Remodel longstanding, dense, mature scar tissue
- Elongate soft tissue contractures
- Increase PROM
- Substitute for weak or absent muscle function
- Provide resistance for exercise
- Maintain intra-articular fracture reduction (a special type of dynamic orthosis places tension across the PIP joint when there is an intra-articular fracture; the orthosis helps to keep the fragments of bone in place)

the static progressive orthosis, as the tissue length changes, the client is able to readjust tension to a new maximum tolerable length and hold this tension on the stiff joint in its end-range position.

Goals for Use of Orthoses for Mobilization

Goals for using orthoses for mobilization are presented in Box 11-1.

Depending on the client's condition, the practitioner might fabricate either a dynamic, static progressive, or serial static orthosis to regain tissue length and joint ROM. For clients with nerve palsies or weakened muscles, a dynamic orthosis is the proper choice because these can be functional as well as corrective and allow the client to move his or her joints while wearing the orthosis.

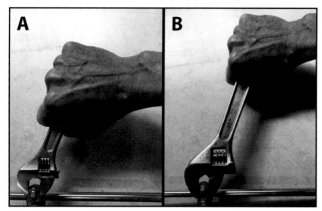

Figure 11-4. Torque example. (A) Wrench with short lever arm requires more force. (B) Wrench with longer lever arm requires less force.

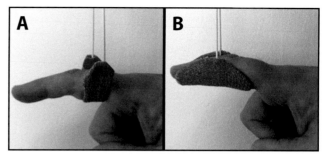

Figure 11-5. Finger cuff with (A) short lever arm and (B) long lever arm.

Biomechanical Concepts of Orthoses for Mobilization

The connective tissue in the body is capable of being stretched due to its viscoelastic qualities. While under tension, it can respond by reaching an either elastic or plastic deformation state. **Elastic deformation** means that the tissue reverts back to its original length when the force on it is removed. **Plastic deformation** means the tissue will maintain its new length even without the force. Orthoses can be used to apply this force to the tightened or shortened tissue to promote tissue growth and lead to tissue remodeling.

There are two types of loading conditions with the application of mobilizing orthoses: **creep** and stress relaxation. In creep-based loading, the force applied is constant and the displacement of the limb varies. The specific tension is applied through rubber bands or elastic thread, exerting a variable force on the body part. Dynamic orthoses may need to be worn for 6 to 12 hours daily in order to be effective.

In stress relaxation loading, the displacement is constant and the applied force varies. This is the principle of static progressive orthoses where clients are instructed to constantly adjust and readjust the tension on their stiff joints. The tissue reaches the plastic deformation state more quickly and the effects will last longer. The force from the static progressive orthosis holds the shortened tissue at its maximum tolerable length. As this tissue length changes, the design of the orthosis also allows for changes and adjustments over time.

Low-load prolonged stretch (LLPS), applied over a long duration to a stiff joint, has been shown to be more effective than a high load of stress applied to a stiff joint for a short duration. The increase in PROM gained from exposure to LLPS is directly proportional to the amount of time the joint is held in its end-range position. This concept is known as **total end range time (TERT)**.

One additional concept of orthoses for mobilization is the application of **torque**. Torque is the extent to which a force tends to cause rotation of an object around an axis, such as a bone around a joint. Torque can be defined simply as an equation: torque = amount of force × length of the **lever arm** (Figure 11-4). Torque is maximized by a long lever arm; the longer the lever arm, the less force required to generate sufficient torque to move or influence the joint. The amount of torque depends on the distance between the joint axis and the point of attachment of the mobilization assist as well as the amount of force applied to the body part. A longer lever arm means less torque or force is required to mobilize the body part. Less force on a stiff body part means a more comfortable or tolerable orthosis for the client, and hopefully increased compliance with the wearing protocol (Figure 11-5).

Indications and Contraindications for Orthoses for Mobilization

This section will cover the indications and contraindications for the use of orthoses for mobilization in clinical practice.

INDICATIONS

The indications for any of the three types of orthoses for mobilization include the following complex, and even not-so-complex, injuries: crush injuries, multiple fractures, scar tissue, stiffness, or any trauma that might occur resulting in joint stiffness. As the practitioner assesses the client's overall condition and prognosis, it might be apparent that orthoses for mobilization will be an important and beneficial intervention for regaining ROM and function in the future. First, one must consider in what **stage of healing** the injured extremity presents before it is appropriate to apply any type of force to correct stiffness or decreased joint ROM. Orthoses for mobilization can be part of the overall treatment plan. The correct choice of orthoses depends significantly on the stage of healing the client's tissue presents in at the time. Wounds of the body typically heal in a set pattern, known as the *three main stages of healing* (Box 11-2).

In stage 1, the **inflammatory** phase, initially all wounds and injuries cause an inflammatory reaction where edema and white blood cells invade the wound. This initial stage of healing can last less than 1 week but may take longer to resolve depending on the client's general health and the presence of complicating factors such as infections, number of tissues involved, and mechanism of injury. The first phase of healing requires protection and proper positioning for best healing of the injured part. The correct and most appropriate orthotic approach is typically immobilization to allow for rest and resolution of the edema.

During stage 2, the **fibroplasia** phase, the predominate cell type is the fibroblast, the cell that contributes to the collagen production for wound healing. The wound is full of new vascular growth and granulation tissue. This is laying the groundwork for the synthesis of new collagen tissue. The collagen tissue begins to synthesize and becomes stronger and more abundant. This phase of healing usually lasts about 4 to 6 weeks, with a reduction in edema and pain and the beginning of restoration of movement and function in the involved extremity. Orthoses that apply a low load of force or stress on involved joints to improve PROM may be applied during this phase.

Stage 3, the last phase of healing, termed the **scar maturation** phase or remodeling phase, is where the scar collagen fibers increase and mature and reorganize. It is in this phase that mobilization orthoses are most effective. However, take care to avoid the overly aggressive use of mobilizing forces and orthosis that go too far in terms of force application and positioning, which can lead right back to a renewal of the inflammatory process. The connective tissue of the body responds to low loads of prolonged stress. Practitioners can help to influence and promote the reorganization of this tissue to accommodate this stress and allow for patterns of joint motion critical to function.

CONTRAINDICATIONS

A practitioner considering using an orthosis for mobilization for any client must use sound clinical reasoning and a very careful assessment of the client's particular situation. There are some significant contraindications to applying orthoses for mobilization to a client. Of critical importance is the recognition and acknowledgement of the continued period of acute edema or inflammation, in which the tissue is still indicating it is not ready or able to tolerate any kind of stress or force. This must be resolved before any type of mobilization orthosis can be applied. Specific treatment protocols, such as for Dupuytren's disease, have not shown any real benefit to the use of any type of mobilization orthoses prior to surgical intervention. The practitioner must also recognize other client factors that may influence

Box 11-2. Stages of Healing

INFLAMMATORY PHASE

- Increased blood flow to area of injury; signs of inflammation, including erythema, heat, edema, and pain
- Use of orthoses to protect, support, position, and reduce pain and edema

PROLIFERATION OR FIBROPLASIA PHASE

- Formation of new granulation tissue with collagen and network of blood vessels; wound closure
- Active exercises and possibly light functional activities to help decrease edema and regain mobility

MATURATION OR REMODELING PHASE

- Final phase of wound healing when wound has closed; involves remodeling of collagen fibers to allow motion and gliding of tissues
- May need increased stretching and orthotic intervention to regain full ROM when limited by scar and shortening of soft tissue

the effectiveness of a mobilization orthosis, such as client appropriateness. These include factors such as the sensory status of the hand and the client's ability to follow directions and understand the principles involved.

Decision Making

Selecting the most appropriate mobilization orthosis for your client is an important decision that should be based on sound clinical reasoning and supporting evidence. The following information may help the practitioner make a decision in selecting an orthosis to help a client regain functional ROM in a stiff joint.

SOFT END FEEL VERSUS HARD END FEEL

When a client has a stiff joint or limited joint ROM, the practitioner can subjectively determine whether the specific joint has a **soft end feel** or a **hard end feel**. End feel is defined as the type of resistance that is felt when passively moving a joint through the end ROM. End feel is evaluated by applying pressure to the joint at the end of the available PROM. A soft end feel means the soft tissues give way with a small amount of pressure, whereas a hard end feel means firm pressure is required to mobilize the joint further than the limitation.

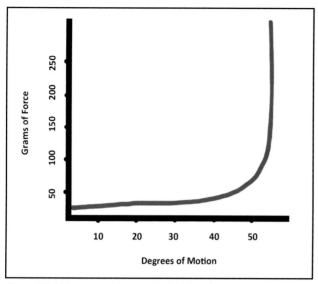

Figure 11-6. Torque angle curve slowly rising slope.

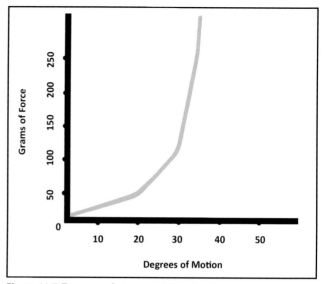

Figure 11-7. Torque angle curve rapidly rising slope.

Table 11-2

MODIFIED WEEKS TEST

CHANGE IN PROM	RECOMMENDED ORTHOSIS
About 20 degrees	No orthosis needed
About 15 degrees	Static orthosis
About 10 degrees	Dynamic orthosis
About 0 to 5 degrees	Static progressive orthosis

Adapted from Flowers, K. (2002). A proposed decision hierarchy for splinting the stiff joint, with an emphasis on force application parameters. *Journal of Hand Therapy, 17*(3), 158-162.

The soft end feel can be described as a joint with immature scar tissue in the joint structures, and the limitations in motion can be addressed with any type of mobilization orthosis. The hard end feel can be described as a joint with mature scar tissue that might respond best to serial static or static progressive orthoses, described earlier in this chapter.

TORQUE ANGLE CURVE

The amount of force directed to the stiff joint by the practitioner can be measured quantitatively through the use of a torque gauge and the results of the joint movement plotted on a graph, called the **torque angle curve** (Figures 11-6 and 11-7).

The torque angle curve graph will display one of two variations of slopes, either indicating a rapidly rising slope where a large amount of force is needed to mobilize the joint, or a slowly rising slope where a small amount of

force elicits movement of the stiff joint. The gentle slope describes tissue that is more compliant, and a steeper slope describes tissue that is stiffer and noncompliant. This is a more objective measure of joint stiffness than the assessment of hard versus soft end feel of a joint.

THE MODIFIED WEEKS TEST

The **modified Weeks test** is an assessment done prior to orthotic fabrication to help clarify what type of mobilization orthosis may be most appropriate for the client. A cold reading is taken of the stiff joint's PROM. Then the client's stiff joint is placed in a heated modality, such as a fluidotherapy unit or a heated whirlpool, so that the joint can be mobilized for 20 minutes. Afterward, the stiff joint is placed at its end-range position, with a tolerable overstretch and heat applied for another 10 minutes. The preconditioned reading is the PROM measurement taken immediately after these 30 minutes of heat and mobilization. The preconditioned reading is then compared with the cold reading.

The difference between the two PROMs can influence the orthotic selection according to the guidelines outlined in Table 11-2.

Clinical Conditions and Wearing Schedules

A growing body of literature and clinical trials support the use of mobilization orthoses for limitations of ROM and decreased function of the upper extremity (UE). In order to use an evidence-based approach when working with a client, before proceeding with a similar orthotic intervention, the practitioner should also compare his or her client with

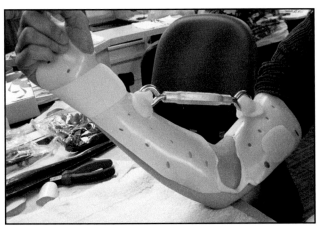

Figure 11-8. Static progressive elbow extension orthosis.

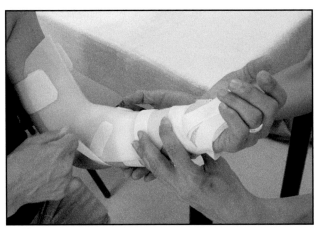

Figure 11-9. Static progressive supination orthosis.

the clients and diagnoses described in the clinical trials to see if those conditions and symptoms match those of the client. The practitioner must also discuss the intervention and findings on clinical outcomes with the client.

STATIC PROGRESSIVE ORTHOSES

The evidence for the use of static progressive orthoses is presented here, organized by UE joints: elbow, forearm, wrist, and fingers.

Orthoses for Mobilization of the Elbow

Multiple studies examine the role of static progressive orthoses and/or dynamic orthoses for the treatment of elbow stiffness (Figure 11-8). One of the more recently published articles is a systematic review by Veltman, Doornberg, Eygendaal, and van den Bekerom (2015) and includes eight elbow studies (one randomized clinical trial and seven retrospective studies). Six of these elbow studies incorporated the use of a static progressive orthosis for the treatment of elbow stiffness. Two studies incorporated the use of a dynamic orthoses. Both types of orthoses described in the studies were commercially available models. Although the recommended wearing schedule for the dynamic orthoses was 8 hours per day for 2 months, most clients used their dynamic orthoses much less than prescribed. On the other hand, clients receiving a static progressive orthosis were instructed to wear it either 30 minutes 4 times per day (four studies) or 15 to 20 hours per day (two studies). Despite the difference in wearing schedules in the static progressive treatment protocols, an equal amount of progress was demonstrated with shorter time frames in the four studies. When considering the fabrication of a dynamic or static progressive orthosis for a client, it is critical to consider the wearing schedule and anticipate which instructions your client is more likely to follow.

Orthoses for Mobilization of the Forearm

Research by Parent-Weiss and King (2006) and McGrath et al. (2009) looked at static progressive orthoses for clients lacking forearm rotation (Figure 11-9). One study used a commercially available orthosis, and the other study used a custom-made orthosis. Both groups of clients (a total of 66 from both studies) did well, gaining supination and pronation with similar wearing schedules of several hours per day for 3 to 4 months' duration.

Orthoses for Mobilization of the Wrist

Studies by Lucado, Li, Russell, Papadonikolakis, and Ruch (2008); Lucado and Li (2009); and McGrath et al. (2009) looked at static progressive orthoses for the wrist (Figure 11-10). A total of 80 clients were included in these three studies, and all three used commercially available orthoses with a similar wearing schedule of 30 to 60 minutes, three times per day. All clients gained increased wrist ROM in both flexion and extension. The McGrath et al. study included 47 clients who wore their orthoses for 30 to 60 minutes one to three times per day for an average of 10 weeks. The total arc of wrist motion increased by a mean of 35 degrees (range, 5 to 100 degrees). Average gain in wrist flexion was 18 degrees (range, 1 to 50 degrees), and average gain in wrist extension was 17 degrees (range, 3 to 50 degrees).

Lucado et al. (2008) described increased motion for clients following distal radius fractures, but also reported on improved Disabilities of the Arm, Shoulder and Hand scores and improved grip strength as well. This study looked retrospectively at 19 clients using a static progressive orthosis for wrist ROM for an average duration of use of 75 days. Wrist extension increased on average around 19 degrees, and wrist flexion increased an average of 12 degrees. McGrath et al. (2009) also reported that clients had improved satisfaction scores as a result of orthotic usage.

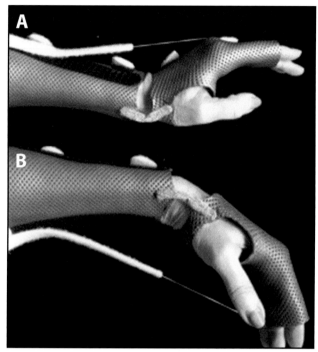

Figure 11-10. Static progressive wrist flexion/extension orthosis in (A) extension and (B) flexion.

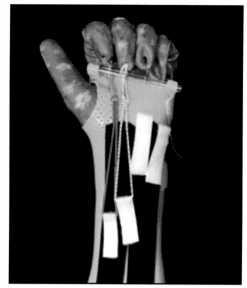

Figure 11-11. Orthosis for composite flexion of the digits with both dynamic and static progressive components.

Orthoses for Mobilization of the Fingers

Only a few studies have examined the use of static progressive orthoses for joints in the hand (Figure 11-11). A small-scale study by Benaglia, Sartorio, and Franchignoni (1999) describes treatment of PIP joint contractures in four volleyball players. Although this was a small sample size, the authors were able to use a custom-made static progressive orthosis to achieve significant improvement in ROM. A more recently published study by Wang, Erlandsson, Rui, and Li-Tsang (2014) looked at metacarpophalangeal (MCP) joint contractures in 31 clients. This study included TERT as an outcome measure and suggested that all clients keep a journal of orthotic wear. This is a great suggestion! These studies on the use of mobilization orthoses to improve stiffness of the finger joints are particularly relevant and important to us as hand therapists because the orthoses included were custom-made, original designs using low-temperature thermoplastic material (LTTM).

There are multiple studies providing evidence to support the commercially available static progressive orthoses system known as the *Joint Active System* (Joint Active Systems, Inc). Clients are instructed to place the static progressive orthosis on their involved body part and adjust the tension so that they can feel a pain-free stretch. They are directed to readjust this stretch every 5 minutes and continue to wear the orthosis for a total of 30 minutes. Clients are instructed to repeat this process for the opposite direction of motion if their ROM is limited in both directions. For example, both wrist flexion and wrist extension are limited. Clients are to wear the orthosis for 1 hour per day for the first week. Clients are

then to gradually increase usage up to three times per day by the third week. In addition, clients are instructed to always increase the tension on the affected body part every 5 minutes while wearing the orthotic device. The general approach using the Joint Active System is consistent with orthotic usage for a 30-minute stretch in each direction (flexion and extension or supination and pronation) three times per day.

DYNAMIC ORTHOSES

Dynamic orthoses for mobilization may be part of the rehabilitation or postoperative protocol for a number of clinical conditions of the UE. The following sections detail some of the more commonly seen postoperative orthoses for mobilization.

Extensor Pollicis Longus Laceration After Surgical Repair

As a repaired extensor pollicis longus tendon heals after surgery, a dynamic extensor tendon orthosis can assist the client to extend the thumb and aid function. Immobilization of the repaired tendon might result in increased scarring and limited glide and tendon excursion. With the help of a dynamic thumb extensor tendon orthosis, the client can pinch and release objects, prevent joint stiffness, and return to functional activities (Figure 11-12).

Postoperative Metacarpophalangeal Joint Arthroplasty

After surgical reconstruction and realignment of the MCP joints, dynamic orthoses help to maintain the implants in MCP joint extension while allowing limited and gentle active flexion of the digits.

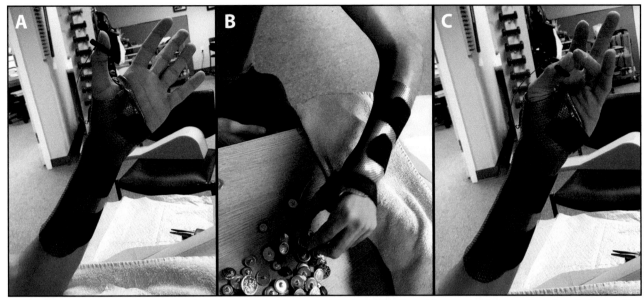

Figure 11-12. (A) Extensor pollicis longus function assisted with a dynamic orthosis. (B) Client able to complete tasks of pinch and release with a dynamic orthosis. (C) Active thumb flexion.

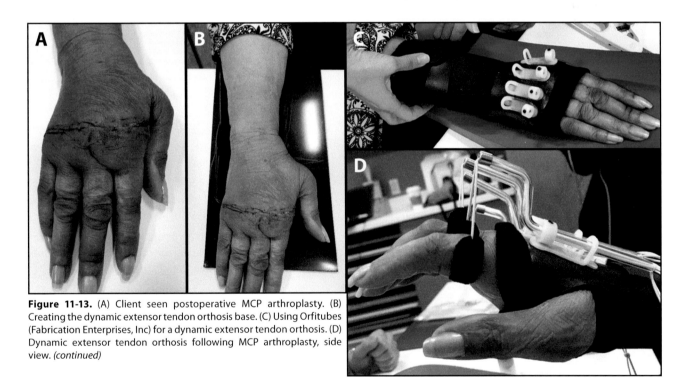

Figure 11-13. (A) Client seen postoperative MCP arthroplasty. (B) Creating the dynamic extensor tendon orthosis base. (C) Using Orfitubes (Fabrication Enterprises, Inc) for a dynamic extensor tendon orthosis. (D) Dynamic extensor tendon orthosis following MCP arthroplasty, side view. *(continued)*

The dynamic MCP joint extension orthosis is typically fabricated 5 days after reconstruction surgery. The tension of the dynamic splint is set to maintain full MCP joint extension at rest and allow maximal active MCP joint flexion. The orthosis is worn at all times for a total of 6 weeks. Then, the orthosis is worn only in the evenings. The client is allowed to begin light-duty hand activities during the day. At 12 weeks, the orthosis is discontinued, and the client resumes unrestricted activity (Figure 11-13).

Radial Nerve Palsy

The classic deformity in radial nerve palsy is the client's inability to extend the wrist and the loss of finger extension at the MCP joints, as well as an inability to extend and abduct the thumb. Orthotic fabrication is designed to preserve motion, enable function, and prevent overstretching of the denervated muscles. Orthoses for clients with radial nerve palsy may provide stability for the wrist while enabling the digits to extend at the MCP joints in order to

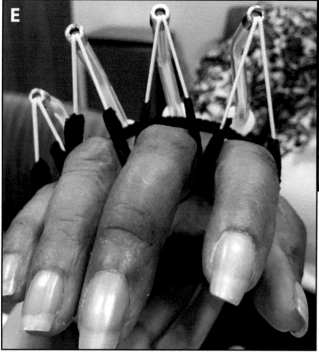

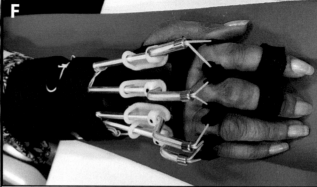

Figure 11-13 (continued). (E) Dynamic extensor tendon orthosis following MCP arthroplasty, front view. (F) Dynamic extensor tendon orthosis following MCP arthroplasty showing addition of buddy strap between index and middle finger to help prevent rotation and overlapping of fingers.

release objects. Alternatively, they may enable the tenodesis motion of wrist extension with finger flexion and wrist flexion with finger extension. There are many different designs and options. The clinician should assess each specific client and fabricate the most appropriate orthosis to assist in the recovery of radial nerve function (Figure 11-14).

Stiffness

Guidelines for the wearing and use of dynamic orthoses for stiffness can be found in multiple studies describing the commercially available Dynasplint (Dynasplint Systems, Inc). According to their standardized protocol, it is recommended to use any dynamic orthosis for up to a maximum of 6 to 8 continuous hours per day or night, allowing for intermittent periods of therapeutic exercise, functional activity, and rest. Individualized wearing schedules should be based on client needs and tolerance (Figure 11-15).

See Box 11-3 for helpful hints for the fabrication of orthoses for mobilization.

Summary

- Knowledge of the benefits, indications, and contraindications of mobilization orthoses will help the practitioner choose the most appropriate orthotic design for each specific client.

- Knowledge of the phases of healing, key anatomical structures of the UE, and how these are affected by the use of mobilization orthoses will help the practitioner determine the most appropriate orthotic mobilization design and wearing schedule.

- Objective and subjective outcome measures should be performed prior to fabrication of a mobilizing orthosis so that its effectiveness can be accurately assessed after a given time period.

- All outriggers and components must be securely bonded to the base orthosis so that parts do not break or cause harm to the client.

- Tension should be applied at a minimum initially and gradually increased while carefully monitoring the effect.

- The goals of a mobilization orthosis and the specifics of each individual wearing schedule will vary depending on each client's needs and clinical condition.

- Mobilization orthoses are fabricated on a base orthosis. The design chosen depends on the client's clinical condition, current functional needs, specific indications requested by the referring physician, and practitioner preference.

- Each orthosis must be molded to the individual anatomy for the best fit. Post-fabrication critique and checkout help identify areas for modification and optimize client comfort.

In Your Client's Shoes

As a practitioner, it is very important to appreciate the impact of the UE injury on the client who requires a mobilization orthosis and its effect, both positive and negative, on your client's daily occupations. The orthosis will most likely interfere with many, if not all, of your client's daily

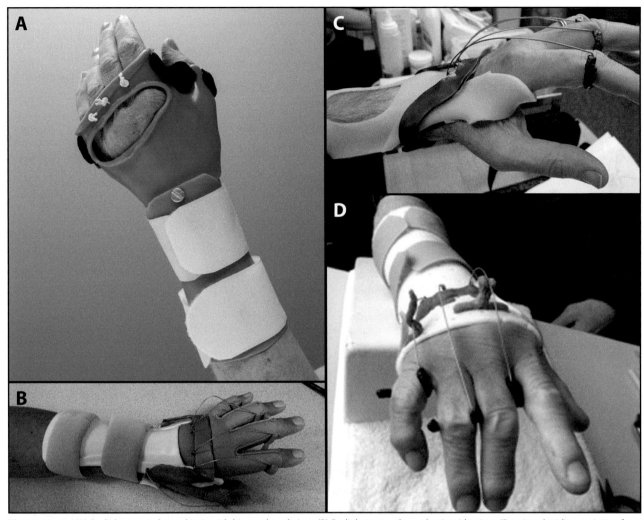

Figures 11-14. (A) Radial nerve palsy orthosis with hinge, dorsal view. (B) Radial nerve palsy orthosis with wires. (Reprinted with permission from Kim Conti.) (C) Radial nerve palsy orthosis with wires. (D) Radial nerve palsy orthosis with wires.

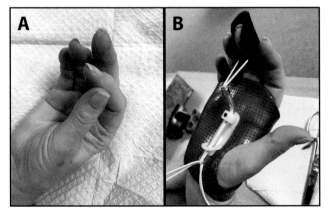

Figure 11-15. (A) Stiff digit after trauma. (B) Dynamic orthosis for the stiff digit.

Box 11-3. Helpful Hints

- Make sure the thermoplastic orthotic base is very well formed to prevent sliding and movement when traction forces are applied.

- Make sure to monitor the client and orthotic fit frequently.

- Start with a minimum amount of force and add more force gradually.

- Create an outrigger system that is easily adjustable.

- Record ROM measures and functional goals prior to beginning the use of mobilization orthoses in order to gauge effectiveness of the intervention.

activities. You should experience how it feels to wear a mobilization orthosis for an extended period of time. This experience will enable you to be client centered when using mobilization orthoses as an intervention strategy in your practice. You must consider how to instruct your client on the importance of the wearing schedule and the benefits of compliance for maximum benefits.

References

Benaglia, P. G., Sartorio, F., & Franchignoni, F. (1999). A new thermoplastic splint for proximal interphalangeal joint flexion contractures. *Journal of Sports Medicine and Physical Fitness, 39*, 249-252.

Lucado, A. M., & Li, Z. (2009). Static progressive splinting to improve wrist stiffness after distal radius fractures: A prospective case series study. *Physiotherapy Theory and Practice, 25*(4), 297-309.

Lucado, A. M., Li, Z., Russell, G. B., Papadonikolakis, A., & Ruch D. S. (2008). Changes in impairment and function after static progressive splinting for stiffness after distal radius fracture. *Journal of Hand Therapy, 21*, 319-325.

McGrath, M. S., Ulrich, S. D., Bonutti, P. M., Marker, D. R., Johanssen, H. R., & Mont, M. A. (2009). Static progressive splinting for restoration of rotational motion of the forearm. *Journal of Hand Therapy, 22*, 3-9.

Parent-Weiss, N., & King, J. (2006). Static progressive forearm rotation contracture management orthosis design: A study of 28 clients. *Journal of Orthotics and Prosthetics, 18*(3), 63-67.

Veltman, E. S., Doornberg, J. N., Eygendaal, D., & van den Bekerom, M. P. (2015). Static progressive versus dynamic orthosis for posttraumatic elbow stiffness: A systematic review of 232 clients. *Archives of Orthopaedic and Trauma Surgery, 135*(5), 613-617.

Wang, J., Erlandsson, G., Rui, Y.-J., & Li-Tsang, C. (2014). Efficacy of static progressive splinting in the management of metacarpophalangeal joint stiffness: A pilot clinical trial. *Hong Kong Journal of Occupational Therapy, 24*(4), 45-50.

Suggested Reading

Alsancak, S., Altinkaynak, H., & Kinik, H. (2006). Elbow orthosis to re-establish elbow extension motion. *Journal of Prosthetics and Orthotics, 18*(4), 106-110.

Bhat, A. K., Bhaskaranand, K., & Nair, S. G. (2010). Static progressive stretching using a turnbuckle orthosis for elbow stiffness: A prospective study. *Journal of Orthopaedic Surgery (Hong Kong), 18*(1), 76-79.

Bonutti, P. M., Windau, J. E., Ables, B. A., & Miller, B. G. (1994). Static progressive stretch to re-establish elbow range of motion. *Clinical Orthopedics and Related Research, 303*, 128-134.

Chung, K. C., Burns, P. B., Wilgis, E. S., Burke, F. D., Regan, M., Kim, H. M., & Fox, D. A. (2009). A multicenter clinical trial in rheumatoid arthritis comparing silicone metacarpophalangeal joint arthroplasty with medical treatment. *Journal of Hand Surgery, 34*(5), 815-823.

Doornberg, J. N., Ring, D., & Jupiter, J. B. (2006). Static progressive splinting for posttraumatic elbow stiffness. *Journal of Orthopedic Trauma, 20*(6), 400-404.

Flowers, K. R. (2002). A proposed decision hierarchy for splinting the stiff joint, with an emphasis on force application parameters. *Journal of Hand Therapy, 15*(2), 158-162.

Gallucci, G. L., Boretto, J. G., Dávalos, M. A., Alfie, V. A., Donndorff, A., & De Carli, P. (2014). The use of dynamic orthoses in the treatment of the stiff elbow. *European Journal of Orthopaedic Surgery & Traumatology, 24*(8), 1395-1400.

Gallucci, G. L., Boretto, J. G., Dávalos, M. A., Donndorff, A., Alfie, V. A., & De Carli, P. (2011). Dynamic splint for the treatment of stiff elbow. *Shoulder & Elbow, 3*(1), 52-55.

Gelinas, J. J., Faber, K. J., Patterson, S. D., & King, G. J. (2000). The effectiveness of turnbuckle splinting for elbow contractures. *Journal of Bone and Joint Surgery (British Volume), 82*(1), 74-78.

Green, D. P., & McCoy, H. (1979). Turnbuckle orthotic correction of elbow flexion contractures after acute injuries. *Journal of Bone and Joint Surgery (American Volume), 61*(7), 1092-1095.

Hannah, S. D., & Hudak, P. L. (2001). Splinting and radial nerve palsy: A single-subject experiment. *Journal of Hand Therapy, 14*(3), 195-201.

Lindenhovius, A. L., Doornberg, J. N., Brouwer, K. M., Jupiter, J. B., Mudgal, C. S., & Ring, D. (2012). A prospective randomized controlled trial of dynamic versus static progressive elbow splinting for posttraumatic elbow stiffness. *Journal of Bone and Joint Surgery (American Volume), 94*(8), 694-700.

Liu, H. H., Wu, K., & Chang, C. H. (2011). Treatment of complex elbow injuries with a postoperative custom-made progressive stretching static elbow splint. *Journal of Trauma, 70*(5), 1268-1272.

McClure, P. W., Blackburn, L. G., & Dusoid, C. (1994). The use of splints in the treatment of joint stiffness: Biologic rationale and an algorithm for making splints. *Physical Therapy, 74*, 1101-1107.

McGrath, M. S., Ulrich, S. D., Bonutti, P. M., Smith, J. M., Seyler, T. M., & Mont, M. A. (2008). Evaluation of static progressive stretch for the treatment of wrist stiffness. *Journal of Hand Surgery, 33*, 1498-1504.

Schwartz, D. A. (2012). Static progressive orthoses for the upper extremity: A comprehensive literature review. *Hand, 7*(1), 10-17.

Schwartz, D. A., & Janssen, R. G. (2007). Static progressive splint for composite flexion. *Journal of Hand Therapy, 18*(4), 447-450.

Sueoka, S. S., & Detemple, K. (2011). Static-progressive splinting in under 25 minutes and 25 dollars. *Journal of Hand Therapy, 24*(3), 280-286.

Ulrich, S. D., Bonutti, P. M., Seyler, T. M., Marker, D. R., Morrey, B. F., & Mont, M. A. (2010). Restoring range of motion via stress relaxation and static progressive stretch in posttraumatic elbow contractures. *Journal of Shoulder and Elbow Surgery, 19*, 196-201.

Wang, J., Erlandsson, G., Rui, Y., & Xu, X. (2011). Composite flexion splint for the stiff hand. *Journal of Hand Therapy, 24*(1), 66-68.

Test Your Knowledge

SHORT ANSWER

1. A dynamic mobilization orthosis is based on what type of tissue loading?

2. A static progressive orthosis uses what type of components as outriggers?

3. A stiff joint can benefit from what type of mobilization orthosis?

4. What type of mobilization orthosis would be helpful for someone with loss of wrist extension due to a nerve laceration?

5. What are some contraindications for fabrication of a mobilization orthosis for an elderly client?

MULTIPLE CHOICE

6. Orthoses that incorporate nonelastic components to apply torque to a joint are called:
   a. Dynamic orthoses
   b. Serial static orthoses
   c. Static progressive orthoses
   d. None of the above

7. Dynamic orthoses are often used to aid in functional activities, as with clients who have:
   a. Peripheral nerve injuries
   b. Traumatic amputations
   c. Fractures
   d. Repetitive strain injuries

8. Serial static orthoses are used to facilitate holding a stiff joint:
   a. In its end-range position to increase PROM
   b. In its most comfortable position to increase PROM
   c. In its most painful position to increase PROM
   d. In a position without stress to increase PROM

9. Static progressive orthoses apply force with the use of:
   a. Elastic components
   b. Nonelastic components
   c. Rubber bands and elastic threads
   d. All of the above

10. The applied force in the orthosis is adjustable by the client or therapist in a:
    a. Dynamic orthosis
    b. Serial static orthosis
    c. Immobilization orthosis
    d. Static progressive orthosis

11. When comparing dynamic orthoses and static progressive orthoses:
    a. Both types of mobilization orthoses start with a base and have an outrigger.
    b. Both types of orthoses need to adhere to basic orthotic fabrication principles.
    c. Only dynamic orthoses need flared edges.
    d. A and B.

12. The indications for static progressive orthoses might be:
    a. Crush injuries
    b. Multiple fractures
    c. Scar tissue, stiffness
    d. All of the above

13. During the initial stage of healing:
    a. Edema lasts less than 1 week.
    b. No orthoses are necessary.
    c. Pain and edema predominate.
    d. Static progressive orthoses are important.

14. Care must be taken to avoid the overly aggressive use of mobilizing forces. This may cause:
    a. A renewal of the inflammatory process
    b. An increase in edema
    c. Reddened tissue
    d. All of the above

15. When there is a bony block to movement, such as heterotrophic ossification or exostosis formation, use of the following type of mobilization orthosis is appropriate to regain motion:
    a. Static progressive orthoses
    b. Serial static orthoses
    c. Dynamic orthoses
    d. No type of orthosis is appropriate.

16. Client appropriateness for static progressive orthoses includes the following factor:
    a. Sensory status of the hand
    b. The ability to follow directions
    c. Understanding of the principles involved
    d. All of the above

CASE STUDIES

Case Study 1

Matthew is a 37-year-old, right-hand–dominant male computer engineer who sustained a fracture of the left distal radius in a snowboarding injury 3 months ago. He wore a cast for 6 weeks and began finger exercises on the doctor's recommendations but did not attend therapy. After cast removal, the doctor did not recommend further treatment but advised Matthew that he would regain his motion gradually. However, at his last follow-up, Matthew raised concerns about lack of wrist motion. The doctor then recommended that he see a specialist for further evaluation and treatment because Matthew was limited in both wrist flexion and extension ROM. Matthew reports that his wrist is very stiff and tight when he wakes up in the morning, but with exercises and heat, he is able to get his hand moving and use it throughout the day.

He presents for therapy with a prescription that reads:
Status post distal radius fracture—left:
1. *Evaluate and treat.*
2. *ROM: active and passive.*
3. *Provide orthoses as needed.*

Your assessment:

Matthew presents to therapy for an evaluation of the left wrist and hand. The left wrist joint displays only mild swelling. Active/passive ROM is measured as follows:

- Wrist extension 15/20 degrees
- Wrist flexion 20/28 degrees

Finger ROM is within normal limits. Grip and pinch strength are also within functional range. Pain was evaluated using the visual analog scale and rated as 3/10 with activity on the left and 1/10 at rest. Matthew is not worried about the pain because he understands that this is telling him he is overdoing his activity level. However, he is quite concerned about the lack of wrist motion because he wants to remain active with sports and outdoor activities.

Using different clinical reasoning approaches, answer the following questions about this client and the prescribed orthosis.

Procedural Reasoning

1. What client factors are important to consider when determining the most suitable orthotic design for this client?

2. Which mobilization orthotic design would be most appropriate for this client? Why?

3. What LTTM properties are important to consider?

4. Describe the instructions you would give this client on:
   - How to care for the orthosis
   - Wearing schedule
   - Precautions
   - Exercises/activities

Pragmatic Reasoning

5. What resources are available to fabricate this orthosis (time, materials, expertise)?

6. Are you able to clearly document the need for this orthosis?

7. Does evidence-based practice support the use of this orthosis for this client's diagnosis?

Interactive Reasoning

8. What are the client's goals and valued occupations?

9. What impact will the client's injury and use of the orthosis have on his activities of daily living (ADL)?

Conditional Reasoning

10. What factors will influence this client's compliance to the wearing schedule of this orthosis?

Narrative Reasoning

11. How does this condition and, more specifically, this orthotic intervention affect this client's valued occupations?

12. What activities is this client most concerned about?

Ethical Reasoning

13. Does the client understand the need for the orthosis?

14. Does the client have the resources to be able to pay for the orthosis (as applicable)?

15. What other options are available to this client if he lacks the resources necessary to pay for the orthosis?

16. Write one short-term goal (1 to 2 weeks) and one long-term goal (6 to 8 weeks) for this client.

Case Study 2

Linda is a 28-year-old, right-hand–dominant, stay-at-home mom who injured her right hand when she fell while walking the family dog. Linda states she fell right on top of her hand as it hit the pavement. She was seen by an orthopedic surgeon, who diagnosed Linda with right fourth and fifth metacarpal fractures. Linda was treated for 6 weeks with an immobilization cast in wrist extension and the ulnar fingers in MCP joint flexion with these digits free to flex somewhat at the PIP and distal interphalangeal (DIP) joints. The injury happened about 8 weeks ago. Linda's main complaints are that her hand now is very stiff and she cannot make a tight fist to hold things. She has trouble "bending the ring and little fingers, like on my other hand." Linda now presents for therapy with a prescription that reads:

Right fourth and fifth metacarpal fractures:

1. *Evaluate and treat.*

2. *Provide orthosis as needed.*

3. *Active and passive ROM exercises.*

Your assessment:

The MCP joints on the right hand are slightly swollen in comparison to the left. Linda's active wrist motion is as follows:

- Wrist extension: 30 degrees
- Wrist flexion 40 degrees

Active MCP joint motion is as follows:

- Extension/flexion:
  - Index: 10/50 degrees
  - Middle: 10/55 degrees
  - Ring: 10/40 degrees
  - Little: 15/35 degrees

PIP and DIP flexion and extension are within normal limits. Pain was evaluated using the visual analog scale and rated as 3/10 with finger movement and 0/10 at rest. Linda denies any numbness, tingling, or other sensory symptoms in her right thumb.

Linda reports that she is having difficulties with many ADL, including self-dressing, doing household chores, and cooking for her family. She is eager to regain full motion and function in her injured right hand.

Using different clinical reasoning approaches, consider the following questions about this client and the prescribed orthosis. Some questions may be directed more toward the client, and some questions may be directed more toward you as the practitioner for reflection.

Procedural Reasoning

1. What client factors are important to consider when determining the most suitable mobilization orthotic design for this client?

2. Which mobilization orthotic design would be most appropriate for this client? Why?

3. What LTTM properties are important to consider?

4. Describe the instructions you would give this client on:
   ○ How to care for the orthosis
   ○ Wearing schedule
   ○ Precautions
   ○ Exercises/activities

Pragmatic Reasoning

5. What resources are available to fabricate this orthosis (time, materials, expertise)?

6. Are you able to clearly document the need for this orthosis?

7. Does evidence-based practice support the use of this orthosis for this client's diagnosis?

Interactive Reasoning

8. What are the client's goals and valued occupations?

9. What impact will the client's injury and use of the orthosis have on her ADL?

Conditional Reasoning

10. What factors will influence this client's compliance to the wearing schedule of this orthosis?

Narrative Reasoning

11. How does this injury and, more specifically, this orthotic intervention affect this client's valued occupations?

12. What activities is this client most concerned about?

Ethical Reasoning

13. Does the client understand the need for the orthosis?

14. Does the client have the resources to be able to pay for the orthosis (as applicable)?

15. What other options are available to this client if she lacks the resources necessary to pay for the orthosis?

16. Write one short-term goal (1 to 2 weeks) and one long-term goal (6 to 8 weeks) for this client.

SPECIAL PROJECTS

1. Create a dynamic or static progressive orthosis based on an article from the Practice Forum in the *Journal of Hand Therapy*. Discuss the diagnosis, its impact on function, and how a client might benefit from the orthosis in terms of ADL.

2. Research a specific hand therapy diagnosis outlined in this textbook leading to lack of active and passive motion. Review the current evidence to support the use of orthotic intervention to help assist a client with lack of motion. Create the orthosis.

Appendix

STUDENT ASSIGNMENTS

1. Define all of the key terms used in this chapter.

2. Explain the differences between dynamic and static progressive orthoses to a fellow student.

3. How would you describe the concept of torque to a fellow student? A client?

4. How would you plan a wearing schedule for a static progressive orthosis for the elbow? On what could you base this plan?

5. Describe the benefits of LLPS to a classmate.

6. Describe the idea of TERT to a classmate.

Multiple Choice Answer Key

6. c
7. a
8. a
9. b
10. d
11. d
12. d
13. c
14. d
15. d
16. d

Glossary

Activation Time: The length of time it takes thermoplastic material to soften in the splint pan to allow the practitioner to mold the orthosis.

Adhesion: Scar tissue at the site of repair, causing loss of gliding and movement of the involved tendon.

Angulation: Refers to the direction in which the fracture "ends" move either volarly or dorsally.

Annular Pulleys: Circular pulleys located on the volar aspect of the digits that function to keep the flexor tendons close to the bone and joint axes during movement.

Antideformity Position: Another term used to describe the position of the digits, thumb, and wrist in an orthosis that minimizes the risk of joint and/or soft tissue contractures.

Ape Hand Deformity: A position of the hand and wrist following injury to the median nerve characterized by extension of the thumb CMC and MCP joints, and inability to abduct and oppose the thumb.

Axis: The center of a joint where rotation or movement occurs.

Ball Design: A type of wrist hand immobilization orthosis that is fashioned over a ball during fabrication where the practitioner can separate each digits into abduction.

Biomechanics: The study of mechanics, or forces, on the musculoskeletal system.

Bony Prominences: Areas where a bone lies immediately below the surface of the skin.

Boutonniere Deformity: A finger deformity where the PIP joint is positioned in flexion and the DIP joint hyperextends.

Bowstringing: Loss of critical pulley function causing movement of the tendon away from the joint axis, and loss of joint movement.

Boxer's Fracture: A fracture involving the fifth metacarpal bone.

Brachial Plexus: A network of nerves found in the axilla that supply innervation to all the muscles in the upper extremity.

Brachial Plexus Palsy: Injury to the brachial plexus at birth.

Buddy Strapping or Taping: The use of strapping or an orthosis to link the injured finger to an adjacent uninjured digit(s) to prevent further injury.

Camper's Chiasm: A split in the flexor digitorum superficialis tendon where the flexor digitorum profundus tendon travels through it.

Camptodactyly: A condition of non-traumatic PIP joint flexion contractures apparent at birth (Type I), later in adolescence (Type II), or associated with other syndromes.

Carpometacarpal (CMC) Joint: The joint formed by the base of the first metacarpal and the trapezium.

Schofield, K., & Schwartz, D. *Orthotic Design and Fabrication for the Upper Extremity: A Practical Guide* (pp 227-233). © 2019 Taylor & Francis Group.

Central Slip: A continuation of the extensor tendon that travels over the PIP joint and attaches to the base of the middle phalanx.

Circumduction: Movement of the thumb in a circular fashion.

Close-Packed Position: The articular surfaces of a joint are in maximum contact with each other, and the joint capsule and collateral ligaments and joint capsule are taut, or tight.

Collagenase Injection: Injection of collagenase into the Dupuytren's diseased cord(s) in order to disrupt the collagen bonds, which weakens the cord.

Complex Forearm Fractures: Those that involve both the radius and ulna, and may also include injury to the proximal radioulnar and/or distal radioulnar joints.

Compressive Force: Creation of force when two forces are applied perpendicular to a structure, causing the two parts to come together.

Cone Design: A type of wrist hand immobilization orthosis that places the digits around a conical form.

Conformability/Drapability: The ability of thermoplastic material to conform or drape and mold around the contours of an individual's anatomy.

Constraint Induced Movement Therapy (CIMT): A therapy protocol to encourage movement in an affected limb by restraining the opposite limb in an orthosis or cast.

Creep: Of soft tissue to prolonged stress.

Cruciate Pulleys: Cross-shaped pulleys located on the volar aspect of the digit that function to keep the flexor tendons close to the joint axis during movement.

Cubital Fossa: The volar aspect of the elbow in anatomical position that contains many important soft tissue structures.

Cubital Tunnel: A tunnel of muscle, ligament, and bone on the inside of the elbow through which the ulnar nerve passes.

Cubital Tunnel Syndrome: Compression of the ulnar nerve at the elbow as it courses through the cubital tunnel.

De Quervain's Tenosynovitis: A condition that involves the two tendons of the first dorsal compartment of the wrist, abductor pollicis longus, and extensor pollicis brevis.

Dislocations: Direction of dislocation is named for the distal bone segment: A dorsal dislocation refers to dorsal displacement of the middle phalanx, while a volar dislocation refers to volar displacement of the middle phalanx.

Distal Humerus: The end of the humerus where it joins with the ulnar and radius to form the elbow joint.

Distal Radioulnar Joint: The distal articulation between the two forearm bones, the radius and the ulna.

Dorsal: An anatomical term used to describe the back part of the body segment in anatomical position.

Dorsal Blocking Orthosis: Extension restriction orthosis with the wrist, MCP, PIP, and DIP joints included for 3 to 4 weeks. The wrist is typically positioned between 10 and 20 degrees of flexion, the MCPs at 40 to 50 degrees flexion, and the PIP/DIP joints in extension.

Dorsal Design: A type of wrist immobilization orthosis that rests on the back of the hand, wrist, and forearm.

Dupuytren's Contracture: Characterized by progressive thickening of the fascia below the skin, which draws the digits in toward the palm.

Duran (Modified): A treatment protocol for flexor tendon repairs using an extension restriction orthosis. The client performs passive digit flexion exercises within the orthosis 10 to 20 times per hour during the day. The modified Duran protocol uses a strap to position the IP joints in extension between exercises and at night.

Dynamic Orthoses: Orthoses with a static base and moveable parts used to help clients regain passive range of motion and/or to stretch tight or contracted soft tissue structures. They incorporate outriggers with variable tension such as springs, coils, or elastic components to assist in function or place force on stiff joints or soft tissue.

Dysesthesias: Reports of pain from normally nonpainful touch.

Early Active Motion: A treatment protocol for tendon repairs that includes initiation of early active contraction of the muscle-tendon unit to achieve more natural gliding and excursion at the repair site.

Effort Force: The segment or component of a lever system that provides the effort or force needed to support the fulcrum.

Elastic Deformation: In response to stress, the tissue reverts back to its original length when the force on it is removed.

Equilibrium: When an object is at rest and does not move.

Erb's Palsy: Injury to the C5-C6 nerve roots of the brachial plexus.

Excursion: The length of movement of tendons with muscle contraction.

Extension Lag: Loss of active PIP and/or DIP joint extension.

Extensor Mechanism: A complex arrangement of tendon structures, fibers, and ligaments that lie on the dorsal and lateral aspects of the digit that contribute to extension of the MCP, PIP, and DIP joints.

Extra-Articular Fractures: The fracture does not involve the articulating surfaces.

Extrinsic Healing: Extrinsic healing occurs as a result of blood supply from the vincula and deposition of collagen cells on the outside of the tendon at the repair site.

Extrinsic Muscles: Muscles in the forearm and hand that originate proximally in the forearm and insert on or distal to the wrist.

Fibroplasia: The second stage of wound healing characterized by a proliferation of fibroblasts, the cells that contribute to the collagen production for wound healing.

First-Class Lever: A lever system where the fulcrum is between the effort force and the resistance force.

Flaccidity: Absence of muscle tone and deep tendon reflexes, and inability to move the extremity actively.

Flexion Contracture: Limited PIP extension.

Flexor and Extensor Retinaculum: Strong fibrous bands that serve to hold the tendons that cross the wrist close to the wrist joint axis during movement.

Fall on an Outstretched Hand (FOOSH): Fall on an outstretched hand.

Force: The amount of stress placed on the tissue or joint to mobilize it.

Fracture: A medical term used when a bone is broken.

Fracture Reduction: Setting of the fractured bone segments together in alignment.

Fulcrum: The component of a lever system where the lever rests or is supported and on which it moves or pivots when force is placed on it.

Functional Hand Position: A resting position of the hand characterized by wrist extension, MCP joint flexion, slight PIP and DIP joint flexion, and thumb abduction.

Gamekeeper's Thumb: Injury to the ulnar collateral ligament of the thumb. The term originated from the repetitive stress placed on this ligament by Scottish gamekeepers as they euthanized rabbits.

Gliding: Movement of the tendons within their connective tissue.

Hard End Feel: Firm pressure is required to mobilize a stiff joint further than the limitation.

Health Care Common Procedural Coding System Codes (HCPCS codes): A five-character alphanumeric code used in the United States where the first letter describes the type of service billed and the other four numeric characters describe the specific type of service provided.

Hypertonicity: An increase in muscle tone with resistance to active and passive movement, and hyperactive stretch reflexes.

Hypotonicity: Low muscle tone characterized by weakness and impaired ability to resist the force of gravity during active movement.

Immediate Controlled Active Motion (ICAM): A protocol for extensor tendon repair in zones V through VII. The yoke orthosis is worn together with a wrist extension immobilization orthosis. The yoke orthosis is designed to hold one or two digits in relative extension compared to the adjacent digits.

Immobilization Orthosis: Orthoses that have no movable parts used to immobilize a body part, prevent movement, encourage rest of injured structures, and provide support.

Inflammatory: The first stage of wound healing after trauma or surgery with a tissue response of edema and inflammatory reaction.

Interosseous Membrane: A fibrous membrane that unites the radius and ulna together.

Interphalangeal (IP) Joint: The joint formed by the thumb proximal phalanx and distal phalanx.

Intra-Articular Fractures: Fractures that involve the articulating surfaces of the bones in a joint.

Intra-Articular Joint Injuries: Refers to complex injuries that involve a fracture of the bone on the joint surface.

Intrinsic Healing: Intrinsic healing occurs as a result of nutrition from the synovial fluid surrounding the tendon within the sheath and formation of new tendon cells at the repair site.

Intrinsic Muscles: Muscles that originate and insert distal to the wrist.

Intrinsic Plus Position: A term used to describe the position of the digits, thumb, and wrist in an orthosis that minimizes the risk of joint and/or soft tissue contractures. The interossei and lumbrical muscles (collectively, the intrinsic muscles) actively contract to flex the MCP and extend the PIP and DIP joints.

Joint Dislocation: When the articulating surfaces of a joint are no longer in contact with each other.

Juncturae Tendinum: Tendinous slips that connect the extensor digitorum tendons.

Kleinert: A treatment protocol for flexor tendon repairs that also includes elastic traction on the involved digit(s) holding the digit(s) in flexion, and the client performs active extension against the resistance of the elastic traction followed by passive flexion.

L-Codes: Codes that are part of the HCPCS codes used to report and bill for fabrication and fitting of specific orthoses for the upper extremity.

Lateral Bands: Two slips of tendon that arise from the sides of the extensor tendon just proximal to the PIP joint, travel on either side of the proximal phalanx and PIP joint, and join together over the dorsal aspect of the middle phalanx to form the terminal extensor tendon that attaches to the distal phalanx.

Lever Arm: Refers to the length of the orthosis on each side of the joint axis of motion.

Lever Systems: A rigid structure or object that can rotate or move around a fixed axis when force is applied to it. There are three different types, or classes, of lever systems: first, second, and third class.

Long Opponens: A type of thumb and wrist immobilization orthosis that immobilizes the wrist, thumb CMC, and/or the MCP and IP joints.

Low-Load Prolonged Stretch (LLPS): The principle of applying a low load of stress to tissue or a stiff joint over a long duration of time.

Low-Temperature Thermoplastic Material (LTTM): Materials that are activated by heat that can be formed around body segments to make an orthosis.

Mallet Finger: A disruption to the extensor tendon at its attachment on the distal phalanx, causing a flexion deformity of the DIP joint.

Memory: The ability of thermoplastic material to return to its original shape and size once it has been stretched out and then reactivated/reheated.

Metacarpophalangeal (MCP) Joint: The joint formed by the thumb metacarpal and proximal phalanx.

Metacarpophalangeal (MCP) Ulnar Drift: Common deformity seen with Rheumatoid arthritis where the MCP joints drift in an ulnar direction.

Mobilization Orthosis: An orthosis that has adjustable parts called *outriggers*, such as turnbuckles, hinges, or others, and is designed to apply low-load stress to contracted, stiff tissues to improve joint and tissue movement, or to facilitate upper extremity function by substituting for weak or paralyzed muscles.

Modified Weeks Test: A measurement helpful in decision making regarding which type of orthosis to use for a stiff joint.

Needle Fasciotomy: Use of a needle to repeatedly pierce the skin of Dupuytren's diseased cords.

Neoprene Orthoses: A type of thumb orthosis that uses neoprene material, either by itself or with the addition of thermoplastic components for rigidity. These orthoses offer less rigidity and comfort for those who need less stability but some support for their thumb joint(s).

No Man's Land: Flexor tendon zone II from the insertion of the flexor digitorum superficialis tendons just distal to the PIP joint to the distal palmar crease near the metacarpal head. The flexor digitorum superficialis and flexor digitorum profundus travel together in the same sheath and are frequently injured together.

Oblique Retinacular Ligament: A ligament that attaches to the sides of the proximal phalanx on the volar surface and connects distally to the lateral bands. It lies volar to the PIP joint's lateral axis and dorsal to the DIP joint's lateral axis. As a result, it contributes to PIP flexion and DIP extension.

Open-Packed Position/Position of Deformity: The articular surfaces of a joint are in minimum contact with each other, and the collateral ligaments and joint capsule are lax, or loose.

Open Reduction With Internal Fixation (ORIF): Treated surgically with open reduction with internal fixation either with a plate, pins, wires, or a combination.

Opposition: Combined movements of thumb adduction, metacarpophalangeal joint flexion, internal rotation, and radial deviation of the proximal phalanx over the MCP joint.

Orthoses: Term used to describe more than one orthosis.

Orthosis: An external rigid or semi-rigid device that is used to support, align, prevent, or correct deformity; improve function; or restrict movement of a body part following injury, disease, or surgical intervention.

Orthotic Fabrication: The process, or science, of creating an orthosis.

Orthotic Intervention: Use of an orthosis as an intervention strategy.

Osteoarthritis (OA): A condition where the cartilage lining the articular joint surfaces degenerates and thins. It occurs in large, weightbearing joints, as well as joints that are subject to repeated stress as a person ages, or because of past injury to the articulating surface(s) of a joint. It can affect only one joint or multiple joints in the body.

Outrigger: Components added to the orthosis base to hold the mechanism through which force or stress is applied to the body part.

Palmar Abduction: Position of the thumb where the thumb is in wide abduction directly under the second digit.

Palmar Aponeurosis: A thin, strong layer of fascia attached to the palmaris longus tendon that helps to form the palmar skin creases and assists with grasp.

Paresthesia: Symptom of numbness and tingling usually due to nerve compression.

Peripheral Nerves: The portion of the nervous system that is outside the brain and spinal cord. There are three main peripheral nerves that supply motor and sensory function in the upper extremity: radial, median, and ulnar.

Plastic Deformation: In response to stress, the tissue will maintain its new length even without the force.

Position of Safe Immobilization (POSI): The position of the digits, thumb, and wrist in an orthosis that minimizes the risk of joint and/or soft tissue contractures.

Prehension: Ability to reach, grasp, and manipulate objects with the thumb and fingers together.

Proximal Radioulnar Joint: The proximal articulation between the two forearm bones, the radius and the ulna.

Pseudo-boutonneire: A finger that presents with a PIP flexion contracture but has no DIP joint involvement, meaning the DIP joint can be passively flexed.

Pulley Ring: A ring formed from thermoplastic material and placed around the proximal phalanx of the finger when the pulley has been repaired along with the flexor tendon to offer protection during healing.

Radial: An anatomical term used to describe the body segment on the side of the radius and thumb.

Radial Collateral Ligament: A ligament on the radial side of the thumb MCP joint.

Radial Deficiency: A congenital anomaly with failure of formation along the radial border of the upper extremity.

Radial Head: Distal portion of the radius that articulates with the humerus.

Radial Neck: Portion of the radius just proximal to the radial head.

Relative Motion Orthosis or Yoke Orthosis: Relative motion orthosis for tendon injuries are to limit full flexion or extension at the MCP joint(s), limit full tendon excursion and thus protect a repair from excessive stress, and facilitate increased motion at the more distal PIP and DIP joints.

Resistance Force: The segment of the lever system that resists the effort force.

Resistance to Stretch: How easy or difficult it is to stretch thermoplastic material around a body part once it is activated.

Rheumatoid Arthritis (RA): An autoimmune disease that typically affects the wrist and small joints in the hand, and usually occurs on both sides of the body. The synovial tissue within joints and surrounding tendon sheaths is targeted by the body's immune system.

Rigidity: An increase in muscle tone, with muscles on both sides of a joint affected, resulting in loss of voluntary movement in all directions that a joint moves. Also refers to how strong and supportive the material is.

Scaphoid Fracture: A break in the scaphoid bone. These can occur in the middle (waist), proximal pole, or tubercle.

Scar Maturation: The final stage of wound healing that is characterized by an increase in scar collagen fibers and their maturation and reorganization.

Second-Class Lever: A lever system where the fulcrum is on one end, the resistance force is in the middle, and the effort force is at the other end.

Serial Cast or Serial Orthosis: A PIP extension orthosis (from thermoplastic material or plaster of Paris) fabricated with the joint held in maximum extension and worn continuously for several days or up to 1 week without removal by the client.

Serial Static: A method of holding a stiff joint in its end range position in order to increase passive range of motion.

Shear Force: Force created when two external forces are applied parallel to a structure.

Short Arc Motion (SAM) Protocol: A rehabilitation treatment protocol for clients following a surgically repaired central slip injury in zones III and IV.

Short Opponens: A type of thumb immobilization orthosis that includes the thumb CMC joint and, most often, the thumb MCP joint as well. The IP joint may also be included depending on the purpose of the orthosis.

Skier's Thumb: An acute injury to the thumb MCP ulnar collateral ligament resulting from a fall that forces a ski pole from the hand, rupturing the ligament.

Skin Creases: Creases that correspond to where the joints of the elbow, wrist, and hand move.

Soft End Feel: Passive movement in a joint that gives way with a small amount of pressure.

Sprain: An injury to ligaments associated with a synovial joint.

Stages of Healing: Describes the different stages of normal wound healing of tissue following surgery or trauma.

Static: An orthosis without an outrigger or movable part that immobilizes a body segment.

Static Progressive: Orthoses that incorporate an outrigger with constant tension designed to progressively reposition a stiff joint in its maximum tolerated end-range position.

Subluxation: Misalignment of joint surfaces, or partial dislocation of a joint.

Supracondylar: A reference point above the condyles.

Surface Impressionability: The surface of the thermoplastic material and whether it easily marks up with fingerprints and etching or has a dense and strong surface that does not mark easily.

Swan Neck Deformity: A finger deformity where the PIP joint rests in hyperextension and the DIP joint in flexion.

Synovial Joint: Joints that permit free motion between the bones they joint together. This is the most common type of joint in the body.

Tendinitis: A common condition where a tendon becomes inflamed or irritated.

Tenodesis Effect: This occurs when the digit and thumb flexor muscles that cross the wrist (flexor digitorum superficialis, flexor digitorum profundus, and flexor pollicis longus) passively flex when the wrist actively extend, creating a passive grasp. The digits and thumb passively extend when the wrist moves into flexion, causing release or extension of the digits and thumb.

Tensile Force: Force created when two forces are applied perpendicular to a structure, causing parts of the structure to pull apart.

Thermoplastic: Material that can be softened in hot water and molded directly onto an individual's body part.

Third-Class Lever: A lever system where the fulcrum is on one side, the effort force in the middle, and the resistance is at the other end.

Three-Point Fixation: One pressure point over the fracture site, and two pressure points on either side of the fracture.

Thumb Boutonniere Deformity: A position of the thumb characterized by thumb MCP joint flexion and IP joint hyperextension.

Thumb-in-Palm Deformity: The thumb is adducted tightly into the palm due to spasticity.

Thumb Spica: A term used to describe a thumb orthosis that immobilizes the wrist, CMC, and/or the MCP and IP joints.

Thumb Swan Neck Deformity: A position of the thumb characterized by thumb MCP hyperextension and IP joint flexion.

Torque: Extent to which a force tends to cause rotation of an object around an axis, such as a bone around a joint.

Torque Angle Curve: A graph depicting the amount of force applied to a stiff joint and the resulting passive range of motion gained.

Total End Range Time (TERT): Amount of time the joint is held in its end range position.

Trigger Finger: Inflammation of the flexor tendon sheath, irritation of the tissues, and subsequent narrowing of the space beneath the A1 pulley, causing a snapping or triggering as the finger flexes or extends.

Tuft Fracture: A crush-type injury to the tip of the distal phalanx resulting in multiple fracture fragments and a very painful fingertip.

Ulnar: An anatomical term used to describe the body segment on the side of the ulna and fifth digit.

Ulnar Claw Hand: Clawing or flexing of the ulnar digits at the PIP and DIP joints with MCP joint hyperextension due to ulnar nerve dysfunction.

Ulnar Collateral Ligament: A ligament on the ulnar side of the thumb MCP joint. This ligament is involved with gamekeeper's or skier's thumb.

Valgus: Lateral deviation of the forearm in relation to the humerus when the upper extremity is in anatomical position.

Varus: Medial deviation of the forearm in relation to the humerus when the upper extremity is in anatomical position.

Velcro Hook: Material that is used to secure or anchor Velcro loop onto the completed orthosis.

Velcro Loop: Strapping material that is used to secure the orthosis onto the body part.

Vincula: Small vessels arising from the digital arteries giving blood supply to the flexor tendons.

Volar: An anatomical term used to describe the front part of the body segment in anatomical position.

Volar Design: A type of wrist immobilization orthosis that rests on the palmar side of the hand, wrist, and forearm.

Wide Awake Local Anesthesia No Tourniquet (WALANT): Surgical procedures performed under local anesthesia without tourniquet, allowing the client to be awake throughout the proceedings.

Working Time: The length of time a low-temperature thermoplastic material stays soft to allow the practitioner time to mold the orthosis.

Wrist Cock-Up: A common term used to describe a wrist immobilization orthosis.

Zig-Zag Deformity: A deformity seen in rheumatoid arthritis characterized by ulnar deviation of the wrist, radial deviation of the metacarpals, and ulnar deviation of the digit MCP joints.

Prefabricated Immobilization Orthoses

Prefabricated immobilization orthoses refer to orthoses that are commercially available for purchase through vendors and/or distributors. These orthoses can be a valuable resource when clinicians do not have the time, experience, or materials available for custom fitting of orthoses on their clients. Prefabricated orthoses are available in many different designs and in different sizes. The challenge facing clinicians is getting the most appropriate orthosis and making sure it fits correctly. The same general rules of determining the best orthotic design still apply. The clinician must consider the client and his or her specific diagnosis, the proper positioning of the limb in the orthosis, the fit, and the wearing schedule. The clinician should be familiar with the various designs on the market in order to determine the best option for each client.

Prefabricated orthoses are available for every specific joint of the upper extremity. Clinicians can often learn about new designs at trade shows and conferences or look for these items in catalogs and online.

Modifications can sometimes be made to prefabricated orthoses. For example, the flexible metal insert can be adjusted in a commercially available wrist support, and additional straps can be added as needed. Prefabricated orthoses made from low-temperature thermoplastic material can be heated, flared, or trimmed to create a more comfortable and well-fitting orthosis. However, prefabricated orthoses made from high-temperature thermoplastic materials cannot be easily modified. Clinicians should measure their clients carefully to order the correct size and eliminate the need for major modifications.

Some clients may present with allergies and/or sensitivities to latex, neoprene, or other materials used in prefabricated orthoses. Clinicians should check the materials used in each prefabricated orthosis and make the client aware of its properties. A suggestion of wearing a liner or cotton socks underneath the orthosis may help to alleviate skin irritability.

Suggested Reading

Coppard, B. M., & Blanchard, S. (2014). Orthotic processes, tools, and techniques. In B. M. Coppard & H. Lohman. *Introduction to orthotics: A clinical reasoning and problem-solving approach* (4th ed., pp. 27-52). St. Louis, MO: Elsevier Mosby.

Harris, R. (2014). Prefabricated orthoses. In M. L. Jacobs & N. M. Austin. *Orthotic intervention for the hand & upper extremity* (2nd ed., pp. 308-325). Baltimore, MA: Lippincott, Williams & Wilkins.

Index

abnormal tone
    wrist and hand immobilization orthoses for, 86-87
    wrist immobilization orthoses for, 64-65
adducted thumb, orthoses for, 109-110
adhesions, with tendon healing, 195
anatomical landmarks
    in making forearm-based orthoses, 49
    of upper extremity, 34
anatomical location terminology, 6
anterior elbow immobilization orthoses, 132
    design of, 133-134
anti-claw orthosis pattern, 151, 158, 160
antideformity position, 82, 83, 84
arm, anterior aspect muscles of, 24
arm-based orthosis, 8
arthritis. *See also* osteoarthritis; rheumatoid arthritis
    digit-based orthoses for, 169-171
    forearm- and hand-based thumb orthoses for, 103-105
    wrist and hand immobilization orthoses for, 85-86, 89-90, 94
    wrist immobilization orthoses for, 62-64

ball-based wrist and hand immobilization orthoses, 90
biceps brachii, 24
biceps injuries, distal, 130
biomechanics
    of digit-based immobilization orthoses, 179-180
    of elbow, wrist, and hand immobilization orthoses, 131-132
    of mobilization orthoses, 214
    principles of, 36-38
    of tendon management orthoses, 203-204
    of wrist and hand immobilization orthoses, 91-92
    of wrist immobilization orthoses, 64-67
blocking orthoses, 160-161
    dorsal, 204-205, 208
        check-out for, 204-205
        check-out form for, 210
        for flexor tendon injuries, 196, 197
bones
    of thumb, 29-30

of upper extremity, 16-17
bony prominences
    padding for, 66-67
    protection of in tendon management, 203-204
    of thumb, 30
    of upper extremity, 19-20
boutonniere deformity
    clinical test for, 177
    digit-based orthoses for, 170, 177-178
    orthotic management of, 175
bowstringing, 33
boxer's fractures, hand-based orthoses for, 144-147, 163-164
brachial plexus, 19, 21
brachial plexus palsy, 82
brachialis, 24
brachioradialis, 24
buddy strapping, 145
    for finger joint injuries, 172-173
burns
    hand-based orthoses for, 152
    wrist and hand immobilization for, 84, 94

Camper's chiasm, 33
camptodactyly, digit-based orthoses for, 182-183
carpal tunnel syndrome, wrist immobilization orthoses for, 58-60
carpometacarpal (CMC) joint, 102, 103
carpus, subluxation of, 85
carrying angle, 24
central slip, 177
cerebral palsy, 82
    spasticity/adducted thumb in, 109-110
circumduction, 27
circumferential orthoses
    digit-based, 169, 180
    forearm-based thumb, 112
    hand-based, 145
    wrist immobilization, 70, 72
claw hand deformity, 150

Printed in the United States
by Baker & Taylor Publisher Services